Brain-Based
Communication Disorders

Brain-Based Communication Disorders

Leonard L. LaPointe, PhD
Bruce E. Murdoch, PhD, DSc
Julie A. G. Stierwalt, PhD

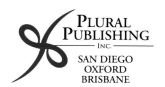

PLURAL
PUBLISHING
INC.

SAN DIEGO
OXFORD
BRISBANE

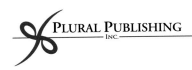

PLURAL PUBLISHING
INC.

5521 Ruffin Road
San Diego, CA 92123

E-mail: info@pluralpublishing.com
Web site: http://www.pluralpublishing.com

49 Bath Street
Abingdon, Oxfordshire OX14 1EA
United Kingdom

Typeset in 11/13 Palatino Book by Flanagan's Publishing Services, Inc.
Printed in Malaysia by Four Colour Print Group

Library of Congress Cataloging-in-Publication Data

LaPointe, Leonard L.
   Brain-based communication disorders / Leonard L. LaPointe, Bruce E. Murdoch, and
Julie A.G. Stierwalt.
         p. ; cm.
   Includes bibliographical references and index.
   ISBN-13: 978-1-59756-194-5 (alk. paper)
   ISBN-10: 1-59756-194-0 (alk. paper)
   1. Communicative disorders. 2. Brain damage. I. Murdoch, B. E., 1950- II. Stierwalt,
Julie A.G. III. Title.
   [DNLM: 1. Communication Disorders. 2. Central Nervous System Diseases—
complications. WL 340.2 L315b 2010]
   RC423.L3397 2010
   616.8—dc22
                                                                  2010006211

Contents

[Note: Throughout the text all terminology introduced will be defined and explained to ensure readability at a first year introductory level.]

Foreword

I first heard about this book when it was only a gleam in the authors' eyes, and I could hardly wait for it to materialize. There were a lot of reasons to be excited about it. Among them were the following: (1) These authors know what they are talking about. (2) They are sublime communicators who write with style, wit, and an enviable ability to make complex matters relatively easy to understand. (3) Another reason is that across the English speaking world, curricula for students are organized, not surprisingly, into starting with the fundamentals before moving on. And, finally, (4) although a plethora of books is available on all of the topics included in *Brain-Based Disorders of Communication and Swallowing*, this is the only one I know of that really does reduce them to "essentials." This solves a problem for beginning students. Confronted with too many facts and too much detail, the result often is to turn them away from this corner of the speech-language pathology universe, and to deny them a glimpse at the stars and galaxies and nebulae that probably would have fascinated a lot of them. There is plenty of time to learn this rich and complex field, and read that weighty literature, but if students are turned off in the beginning, it is not likely to happen.

And now the book is here. Read it with pleasure, safe in the knowledge that it is a wonderful way to begin your understanding of neurogenic communication and swallowing disorders. And do stop to enjoy the elegance of its writing, and learn from it as well.

Audrey L. Holland
University of Arizona

Preface

The world was a different place in 1861. The Civil War raged in the United States and brothers fought a horrific battle at Ball's Bluff in Virginia. The Canellas meteorite struck the earth near Barcelona, Spain. The telegraph left the Pony Express obsolete and horses with mail pouches stopped racing across the American West. Charles Darwin burst on the scene with the publication of *Origin of the Species*. Xian Feng, a Chinese Emperor, died and was succeeded by his 6-year-old son. Explorers Burke and Wills set out with camels and horses and 18 men to cross Australia's outback from South to North. Both died on the return trip of exhaustion and hunger. San Francisco was rocked by a series of small tremors, followed by a major earthquake on July 4.

In France, history was being made as well. Tremors across the intellectual communities were created by Pierre Paul Broca, who opened a dialogue on brain and language by presenting the first of two landmark papers (Broca, 1861a, 1861b). These papers have since served as a clear demarcation and turning point in the history of understanding brain-based disorders of language and speech. Broca is one of our heroes. He encapsulates all that a good clinician, scholar, and neuroscientist should be. He cared for and about his patients. Broca understood the whirlpool of despair into which a shoemaker from rural France could be plunged by an

unseen stroke in his brain. He guided, nurtured, and studied the small victories of recovery from torn brains in his practice. Clearly, 1861 was a big year. So it came to pass that Carl Sagan (1979) rhapsodized in *Broca's Brain* about the exquisite experience of standing in the *Musée de l'Homme* as he contemplated and gazed upon the preserved brain of Pierre Paul Broca (June 28, 1824–July 9, 1880) this scientific giant of the 19th century who contributed so much of what we know about the localization of articulate speech in the brain of humans. Broca was a French physician, anthropologist, and eventually a senator who believed that by studying the brains of cadavers and correlating the known experiences and behaviors of the former possessor of the organs, human behavior could be revealed, associated with brain function, and better understood. For that purpose, he collected hundreds of human brains in jars of the preservative formalin. Upon his death in 1880, with exquisite irony, his own brain was preserved in formalin and added to the collection in the museum, along with hundreds of skulls that Broca had used in his comparative cephalometric studies. When Sagan happened upon Broca's brain in the museum, along with that of Broca's milestone patient "Tan" Leborgne, he was awestruck by the irony of it all. Here was Broca, for whom the region of the frontal lobe of the cortex that he had described was subsequently named, with his own Broca's area discernible. Sagan was mesmerized by the incongruity of all of this. In *Broca's Brain*, he used that visit to the Museum of Man to launch philosophical questions that challenge some core ideas of human existence and consciousness such as *"How much of that man known as Paul Broca can still be found in this jar?"*

These questions were pondered again as we looked upon the brains of Broca's patients in the Dupuytren Museum in Paris in July of 2009. This question and other brain puzzles are pondered in the essay, "Broca's brain: Brother, wherefore art thou?" (LaPointe, 2010). Indeed, we are indeed in the debt of this French scientist and scholar as well as of his patients whose brains rest even today in these jars.

In 2010 the world is different and the world is the same. Twitter, social networking, texting, and 24-hour information access have created digital autism and consume us as we text our way off of the curbs into the traffic of perpetual connectivity. Neural imaging that would have appeared to be magic in 1861 is now commonplace. Diffusion tensor imaging (DTI) and magnetoencephalography (MEG) are guiding us to better visions of broken brains and their consequences. Sophisticated ways of viewing brain activity have led to speculations about the study of different gamma oscillation patterns for true versus false memories and even into the seeming brain science fiction of "mind gaming" or thought controlled activities. What was rudimentary in 1861 and speculative in 2010 may be commonplace in days to come. But people with brain-based communication disorders still will require attention and intervention by clever and

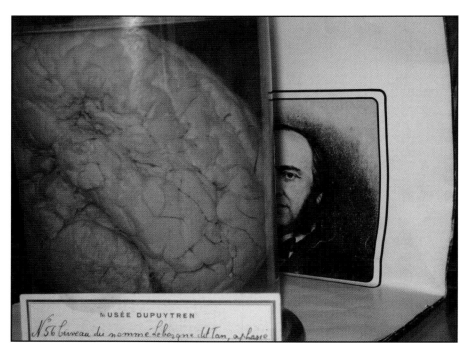

The brain of Broca's patient LeBorgne ("Tan") in formalin at the Dupuytren museum in Paris (LaPointe photo).

educated experts. That is what this book is all about.

Brain-Based Communication Disorders introduces the reader to the major clinically recognized types of acquired speech/language, cognitive, and swallowing disorders encountered by clinicians working with child and adult neurologic cases. The text provides contemporary and state-of-the-art content on these disorders in terms of their neuropathologic bases, clinical symptomatology, and prognosis. Basic anatomy and physiology of human communication and swallowing are introduced, as well as the neural mechanisms controlling speech, language, cognitive, and swallowing functions. In addition to the traditional acquired speech/language disorders of the nervous system (aphasia; neuromotor speech disorders), content including communication impairments caused by traumatic brain injury, multisystem blast injuries, and degenerative disorders of the nervous system also is provided. The reader also is introduced to the principles that govern the assessment and treatment for both pediatric and adult populations. We are indebted to those who passed before, such as Pierre Paul Broca who showed us the path. We are indebted as well to all those who have undergone the slings and arrows of brain damage from whom we have learned. We hope the future generations of brain scientists and clinicians will grow in their ability to understand and to help.

References

Broca, P. (1861a). Perte de la parole, ramollissement chronique et desstruction partielle du lob antérieur gauche de cerveau. *Bulletins de la Société d'Antrhopologie, 62,* 235–238.

Broca, P. (1861b). Remarques sur le siége de la faculté du langage articulé, suivies d'une observation d'aphemie (Perte de la Parole). *Bulletins et memoires de la Société Anatomique de Paris, 36,* 330–357.

LaPointe, L. L. (2010). *Voices: Collected essays on language, laughter, and life.* Albany, NY: Cengage Delmar Publishing.

Sagan, C. (1979). *Broca's brain: Reflections on the romance of science.* New York, NY: Random House.

To our friend and colleague Sadanand Singh
(1934–2010) whose vision we have embraced.
May the dolphins guide you.

1

The Neurologic Basis of Speech and Language

Left Cerebral Hemisphere Infarction

Roland Cappa, a prominent lawyer in a small country town was admitted to hospital having experienced a sudden collapse at his downtown office. At 62 years of age, Roland was highly successful and hard working and had been developing a brief for a large public liability case that was due to be heard at the district court the following day. On admission, although conscious, Roland was unable to speak and exhibited a paralysis down the right side of his body. A neurologic and neuroradiologic examination confirmed that Roland had suffered a stroke. A computerized tomographic (CT) scan and subsequent magnetic resonance imaging (MRI) scan revealed the presence of a large brain lesion (infarction) involving the cerebral cortex of the left frontal lobe with extension into the adjacent subcortical white matter and also extending to include a small section of the parietal lobe. The neuroradiologist considered the lesion to be consistent with blockage of the upper division of the middle cerebral artery. At 3 months post cerebrovascular accident (CVA), Roland's paralysis had resolved to a mild weakness (hemiparesis) primarily affecting his right arm with lesser involvement of his left leg. Although he retained his ability to comprehend speech, Roland's speech was nonfluent and characterized by agrammatism (telegraphic speech). His speech-language pathologist diagnosed his communication disability as nonfluent or Broca's aphasia.

Cerebellar Tumor

Sara Jones is an 8-year-old, right-handed school girl who had been developing normally until the age of 6 years. At that time, Sara progressively developed signs of being listless and uncoordinated. She also experienced nausea and vomiting daily. A CT scan revealed the presence of a large brain tumor involving Sara's cerebellum (the tumor was classified as a cerebellar astrocytoma). Surgery was performed to remove the tumor and involved complete removal of the left cerebellar hemisphere and a portion of the right cerebellar hemisphere. Neither radiotherapy nor chemotherapy were administered as part of the treatment regimen. At the time of her referral to the Centre for Neurogenic Communication Disorders Research at The University of Queensland, Sara presented as a happy, intelligent girl with a moderate motor speech disturbance characterized by articulatory inaccuracy, a slow rate of speech, and an equal and even stress pattern. Her speech disorder was diagnosed as an ataxic dysarthria.

Peripheral Nerve Lesion

Janet Wise, a 25-year-old secretary, was having difficulty carrying out her daily duties. Over the previous 12 months she had become increasingly excitable and nervous, exhibiting a moist skin, rapid pulse, elevated metabolic rate, and protrusion of the eyes. Blood tests confirmed the presence of elevated levels of thyroid hormone and Janet subsequently was recommended for surgery to treat her hyperthyroidism. Unfortunately for Janet, while performing a thyroidectomy (reduction in the size of the thyroid gland), her surgeon accidentally severed her left recurrent laryngeal nerve as it ascended in the neck in proximity to the trachea (windpipe). The left recurrent laryngeal nerve is a branch of the Xth cranial or vagus nerve and regulates the functioning of the majority of the laryngeal muscles. Consequently, Janet's left vocal cord was paralyzed in a position just to the side of the mid-line (paramedian position) leading to a flaccid dysarthria characterized by dysphonia, reduced loudness, and a harsh and breathy quality to her voice.

Brainstem Lesion

Josie Mohr, a 9-year-old, right-handed school girl was referred to the Centre for Neurogenic Communication Disorders Research for treatment for a severe articulatory deficit arising from bilateral paralysis of her tongue. Josie had been developing normally and was enjoying her third year of school when she suffered a brainstem infarction following partial occlusion of her vertebral arteries secondary to arteritis when she was 7 years old. An MRI scan demonstrated infarction in the medial aspect of the medulla oblongata that compromised the nucleus of the XIIth (hypoglossal) nerve bilaterally. A neurologist diagnosed her resulting condition as medial medullary syndrome. An oral examination conducted by Josie's speech-language pathologist revealed that Josie had atrophy (muscle wastage) on both sides of her tongue. Tongue movement was severely restricted and Josie had particular difficulty producing high front vowels and consonants that require elevation of the tongue tip to the alveolar ridge or hard palate (e.g., t, d, n, l, etc.) for their production. Josie's speech disorder was diagnosed as a flaccid dysarthria arising from damage to the origins (nuclei) of the XIIth cranial nerves in the brainstem.

Introduction

Speech and language function is highly dependent on processes that take place in the human nervous system. Consequently, many of the speech and language disorders encountered by speech-language pathologists in their clinics are the outcome of injury and damage to some part of the nervous system. Such injury may involve the brain, the spinal cord, or the peripheral nerves that regulate the functioning of the speech production mechanism and may be caused by a myriad of conditions such as trauma, stroke (cerebrovascular accidents), infectious disorders (e.g., encephalitis), demyelinating conditions (e.g., multiple sclerosis), neoplastic disorders (e.g., brain tumors), degenerative brain disorders (e.g., Parkinson's disease), metabolic disorders (e.g., Wilson's disease), and toxic conditions (e.g., heavy metal poisoning). Importantly, the type and nature of the speech and/or language disorders that result from damage to the nervous system depends largely on the location of the damage within the nervous system. For example, injury to the left cerebral hemisphere usually is associated with a range of language disorders called aphasias. Damage to the cerebellum, on the other hand, usually is associated with a speech disorder called ataxic dysarthria whereas lesions that disrupt the origins of the cranial nerves that regulate the contraction of the muscles of the speech production mechanism in the brainstem are associated with a speech disorder called flaccid dysarthria. The four cases outlined at the start of this chapter were selected to demonstrate the diversity of sites in the nervous system that, if damaged by trauma, stroke, and other neurologic insults, can lead to speech and/or language disorders. The speech and language disorders described in association with these four cases, however, represent only a small sample of the large range of brain-based communication impairments encountered by speech-language pathologists in their clinics. The majority of these communication disorders are described in later chapters of this book. Prior to describing and discussing the signs, symptoms, and neuropathologic processes that underlie the various brain-based speech and language disorders, these disorders need to be defined and the reader provided with at least an introductory knowledge of the anatomy of the human nervous system.

Brain-Based Speech and Language Disorders: Definitions

Communication in the form of speech and language activities is regulated by and therefore dependent on processes that take place in the nervous system. Overall, three major groups of brain-based communication impairments—aphasia, dysarthria and apraxia—result from damage to the nervous system. The neurologic basis for each of these three groups of disorders is best understood by reference to the neurologic processes involved in a spoken conversation between two people:

> *John:* Mary, would you like to go the movies tonight?
>
> *Mary:* Yes, John, they are showing the latest movie starring Brad Pitt.

Prior to producing his question in the form of spoken output, John first had to form a symbolic concept of the intended question in the language centers of his brain. Once formulated, John's question to Mary then had to be transferred to the areas of the brain responsible for determining the sequence of contraction of the muscles of the speech production mechanism (e.g., the muscles of respiration, larynx, soft palate, tongue, lips, jaw) to produce John's question as spoken output. The latter process is often referred to as motor programming. Subsequent to motor programming, John's question then had to be externalized as speech through the coordinated contraction of the muscles of the speech pro-

duction apparatus, a process regulated by the transfer of nerve impulses from the motor areas of the brain to the speech production muscles via pathways collectively referred to as the motor pathways. The words spoken by John in the form of sound waves, in turn, had to be detected by receptors in Mary's inner ear and then conveyed to the auditory and language centers of her brain where they were perceived and interpreted. Subsequently, Mary had to formulate her response in the language centers of her brain and then pass her response to the motor areas of the brain for motor programming and execution.

Disruption to the first process involving the organization and concepts and their symbolic formulation and expression leads to a group of language disorders that collectively are referred to as aphasias. Aphasia has been defined as the loss or impairment of language function caused by brain damage. The various types of aphasia are described more fully in Chapter 4.

Impairment in the second process involving the programming of the sequence of muscle contractions required to produce speech leads to a communication disorder called apraxia of speech. This disorder manifests primarily as errors in the articulation of speech and secondarily by what are considered by many clinicians to be compensatory alterations of prosody (e.g., pauses, slow rate, equalization of stress). Although the muscles of the speech mechanism are neither paralyzed nor weak, individuals with apraxia of speech have difficulty speaking because their brain damage prevents them from carrying out, voluntarily and on command, the sequence of muscle contractions involved in speaking.

Disruption of the third process involving the motor production of speech leads to a group of speech disorders collectively referred to as dysarthrias. Dysarthria can result from any of the basic neural processes involved in the transfer of nerve impulses from the motor areas of the brain to the muscles of the speech production apparatus. The clinical features of the various different forms of dysarthria are described in Chapter 8.

Dysarthria and apraxia of speech involve disruption of the motor control of speech and, therefore, are referred to as motor speech disorders. In contrast, aphasia is considered to be a language disorder. Although each of the three disorders is distinctive, they can occur in combination and consequently many of the clients with neurologic disorders seen by speech-language pathologists may exhibit features of more than one of these disorders. The remainder of this chapter is devoted to providing the reader with an overview of the relevant neuroanatomy necessary to understand the mechanisms that underlie the occurrence of brain-based communication disorders.

Gross Anatomy of the Nervous System

For ease of description, the nervous system often is arbitrarily divided into a number of parts, which may give students of neuroanatomy the false impression that these parts function in isolation of one another. Prior to embarking on a description of the major components of the nervous system; therefore, it is important to stress that the descriptive divisions are artificial and that the nervous system functions as an entity, not as a series of isolated parts. With this important knowledge in the background, the gross anatomy of the nervous system will be outlined.

The nervous system is comprised of two large divisions: the central nervous system and the peripheral nervous system (Figure 1–1). The central nervous system is comprised of the brain and spinal cord; the major components of the peripheral nervous system are

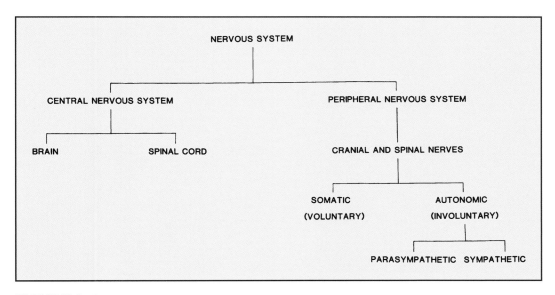

FIGURE 1–1. Basic organization of the nervous system.

the nerves, which arise from the base of the brain (called cranial nerves) and the spinal cord (called spinal nerves). In total, there are 12 pairs of cranial nerves and 31 pairs of spinal nerves. The peripheral nervous system may be further subdivided into the somatic and autonomic nervous systems, the somatic nervous system including those nerves that regulate contraction of skeletal muscles (e.g., the muscles of the limbs, muscles of the speech production mechanism) and the autonomic nervous system including the nerves involved in regulation of involuntary structures such as the heart, smooth muscles of the gastrointestinal system and exocrine glands (e.g., sweat glands).

Cells and Tissues of the Nervous System

Cells

Cells form the basic anatomic and functional units of all of the organ systems of the human body. In the case of the nervous system, the nerve cell or neuron represents the basic functional unit as the neurons that are responsible for the conduction of nerve impulses from one part of the body to another, such as from the brain to the muscles of the speech production mechanism to produce the movement of the lips, tongue, and so on for speech production. The nervous system is made up of millions of neurons that are held together and supported by a variety of specialized nonconducting cells call neuroglia.

Although there are a number of different types of neurons (e.g., motor neurons, which regulate the contraction of muscles; sensory neurons, which convey information from sensory receptors

to the central nervous system), most consist of three basic parts: a cell body (also known as a soma or perikaryon); a variable number of short processes called dendrites (meaning "treelike"); and a single, usually elongated, process called an axon, which in the majority of neurons is surrounded by a segmented fatty insulating sheath called the myelin sheath. A schematic representation of a typical motor neuron is shown in Figure 1–2.

Within the central nervous system, axons are responsible for conveying nerve impulses from one part of the central nervous system to another and often are collected into bundles called tracts or pathways (e.g., some tracts called the corticospinal tracts, connect the motor areas of the cerebral cortex to the spinal cord, see below). Some axons leave the central nervous system and connect the central nervous system to structures such as muscles or sensory receptors in the peripheral parts of the body. The latter axons are collected into bundles that form the various cranial and spinal nerves. The term "nerve" is defined as a group of fibers that travel together in the peripheral nervous system, with any one nerve containing thousands of axons.

The neuroglia (often simply called glial cells), in contrast to neurons, do not conduct nerve impulses and contribute to brain function mainly by supporting neuronal function. The major types of neuroglia found in the central nervous system include astrocytes, oligodendrocytes, ependymal cells, and microglia. A specialized type of neuroglial cell found in the peripheral nervous system is called a Schwann cell. These cells form the myelin sheath of axons found in the peripheral nervous system. Occasionally, neuroglial cells undergo pathologic growth and in doing so form various

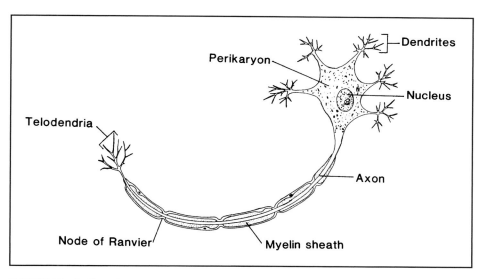

FIGURE 1–2. Structure of a typical motor neuron (from Murdoch, 1990. Reprinted with permission).

types of tumors that may involve the brain or spinal cord (e.g., astrocytoma, ependymomas).

In order to regulate various body activities, such as speech and language functions, neurons do not work in isolation but rather form neural networks. Consequently, the activity of any specific neuron is determined by input from many other neurons that form part of that neural network. The points at which two neurons communicate with each other are referred to as synapses. Each synapse represents a region of functional but not anatomic continuity between the axon terminal of one neuron (the presynaptic neuron) and the dendrites, cell body, or axon of another neuron (the postsynaptic neuron). The synapse is an area where a great degree of control can be exerted over nerve impulses. At the synapse, nerve impulses can be either blocked (inhibited) or facilitated. There may be thousands of synapses on the surface of a single neuron. When one considers that there are billions of neurons, the complexity of the circuitry of the nervous system is staggering.

Transmission of nerve impulses from the pre- to the postsynaptic neuron involves the release of chemical transmitter substance from the terminal portion (bouton terminal or synaptic knob) of the presynaptic neuron. There are many kinds of neurotransmitter substance, some of which facilitate (excitatory transmitters) nerve impulse conduction in the postsynaptic neuron and others that inhibit (inhibitory transmitters) nerve impulse conduction in the postsynaptic neuron. Some of the more common neurotransmitter substances include acetylcholine, norepinephrine, serotonin, dopamine, and gamma-amino-butyric acid (GABA).

When released from the synaptic knob, the chemical transmitter diffuses across a gap called the synaptic cleft between the bouton terminal and the membrane of the postsynaptic neuron to either excite or inhibit the postsynaptic neuron.

As neurotransmitter substance is located only on the presynaptic side, a synapse can transmit in only one direction.

Neuroeffector junctions are functional contacts between axon terminals and effector cells. Structurally, neuroeffector junctions are similar to synapses with the exception that the postsynaptic structure is not a neuron but rather a muscle or gland. The type of neuroeffector junction of most relevance to speech-language pathologists is the junction with skeletal muscles as this type of muscle tissue comprises the muscles of the speech mechanism. Neuroeffector junctions with skeletal muscles are termed motor end plates.

Tissues

Both the brain and spinal cord are comprised of two different types of tissue, gray matter and white matter. The gray matter is made up mainly of neuron cell bodies and their closely related processes, the dendrites. White matter is comprised primarily of bundles of long processes of neurons (mainly axons), the whitish appearance resulting from the lipid insulating material (myelin). Cell bodies lack the white matter. Both the gray and white matter, however, contain large numbers of neuroglial cells and a network of blood capillaries.

In the brain, most of the gray matter forms an outer layer surrounding the cerebral hemispheres. This layer, which varies from around 1/16" to 5/32" (1.5 mm to 4 mm) thick, is referred to as the cerebral cortex (cortex meaning "rind" or "bark"). Within the spinal cord, the distribution of gray and white matter is largely the reverse to that seen in the brain, the gray matter forming the central core of the spinal cord, which is surrounded by white matter.

The Central Nervous System

The Brain

Weighing approximately 3.09 lbs (1400 gm) in the average human, the brain is the largest and most complex mass of nerve tissue in the body. Located in the skull, the brain is surrounded by three fibrous membranes called the meninges and is suspended in a fluid called cerebrospinal fluid. Within the brain are a series of fluid-filled cavities called the ventricles. The brain can be divided into three major parts: the cerebrum, the brainstem and the cerebellum (Figure 1–3).

The Cerebrum. The cerebrum is the largest portion of the brain, representing approximately seven-eighths of its total weight. Centers that govern all sensory and motor activities (including speech production) are located in the cerebrum. In addition, areas that determine reason, memory and intelligence as well as the primary language centers also are located in this region of the brain.

The surface of the cerebrum is highly folded or convoluted. The convolutions are called gyri (gyrus, singular) whereas the shallow depressions or intervals between the gyri are referred to as sulci (sulcus, singular). If the depressions between the gyri are deep, they are then called fissures. A very prominent fissure, called the longitudinal fissure, is located in the midsagittal plane and almost completely divides the cerebrum into two separate halves or hemispheres, called the right and left cerebral hemispheres. The longitudinal fissure can be viewed from a superior view of the brain as shown in Figure 1–4.

The cerebral cortex is the convoluted layer of gray matter covering the cerebral hemispheres. The cerebral cor-

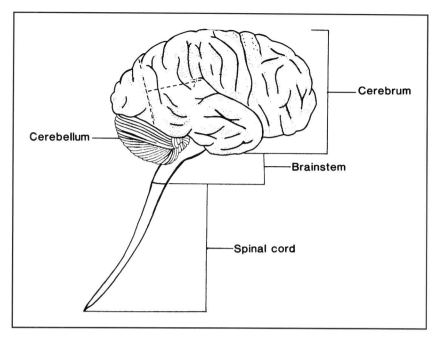

FIGURE 1–3. Major parts of the central nervous system (from Murdoch, 1990. Reprinted with permission).

tex comprises about 40% of the brain by weight and it has been estimated that it contains in the region of 15 billion neurons. Based on observations on animals, especially monkeys and chimpanzees as well as from studies of humans undergoing brain surgery, it appears that different regions of cerebral cortex serve different functional roles. These functional areas of the cortex include motor, sensory, and association areas.

The motor areas control voluntary muscular activities whereas the sensory areas are involved with the perception of sensory impulses (e.g., vision and audition). Three primary sensory areas have been identified in each hemisphere, one for vision, one for hearing, and one for general senses (e.g., touch). The association cortex (also called the "uncommitted cortex" because it obviously is not devoted to some primary sensory function such as vision, hearing, touch, smell and so on, or motor function) occupies approximately 75% of the cerebral cortex. Three main association areas are recognized: prefrontal, anterior temporal, and parietal-temporal-occipital area. Overall, they are involved in a variety of intellectual and cognitive functions.

Beneath the cerebral cortex, each cerebral hemisphere consists of white matter within which there are a number of isolated patches of gray matter. These isolated patches of gray matter are referred to as the basal nuclei. The basal nuclei, or ganglia, serve important motor functions and, when damaged, are associated with a range of neurologic disorders including Parkinson disease, chorea, athetosis, and dyskinesia, all of which may cause dysarthria. Anatomically, the basal ganglia consist of the caudate

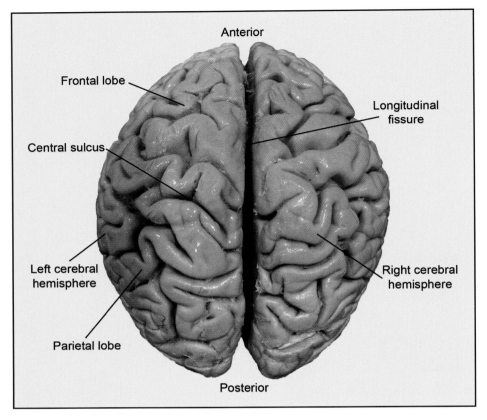

FIGURE 1–4. Superior view of the brain.

nucleus, the putamen, the globus pallidus, and the amygdaloid nucleus. Some neurologists include another nucleus, the claustrum, as part of the basal ganglia. Collectively, the globus pallidus and the putamen are referred to as the lenticular nucleus (lentiform nucleus), so called because its shape is similar to that of a biconvex lens. The lenticular nucleus combined with the caudate nucleus make up what is known as the corpus striatum, so called because of the striated (striped) nature of this region of the brain. The relative positions of the basal ganglia to other structures within the cerebral hemispheres are shown in Figures 1–5A and 1–5B.

The white matter underlying the cerebral cortex consists of myelinated nerve fibers arranged in three principal directions. First, there are association fibers. These transmit nerve impulses from one part of the cerebral cortex to another part in the same cerebral hemisphere. The fibers comprising the second group are known as commissural fibers. These transmit nerve impulses from one cerebral hemisphere to the other. By far the largest commissure is the corpus callosum, a mass of white matter that serves as the major pathway for the transfer of information from one hemisphere to the other. The third group of fibers that make up the subcor-

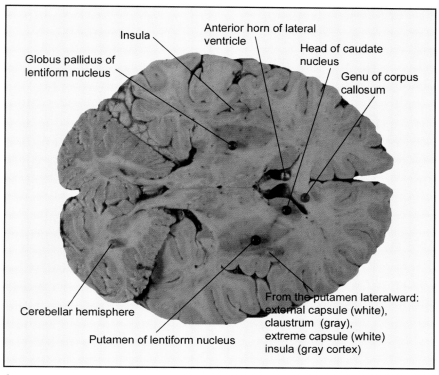

Insula

Anterior horn of lateral
ventricle

Globus pallidus of
lentiform nucleus

Head of caudate
nucleus

Genu of corpus
callosum

Cerebellar hemisphere

From the putamen lateralward:
external capsule (white),
claustrum (gray),
extreme capsule (white)
insula (gray cortex)

Putamen of lentiform nucleus

A

FIGURE 1–5. A. Horizontal section through the brain showing the relative positions of the basal ganglia (from Murdoch, 1983. Reprinted with permission). *continues*

tical white matter are projection fibers. These form the ascending and descending pathways that connect the cerebral cortex to the lower central nervous system structures such as the brainstem and spinal cord.

Each cerebral hemisphere is a "mirror-twin" of the other and each contains a full set of centers for governing the sensory and motor activities of the body. Each hemisphere also is largely associated with activities occurring on the opposite (contralateral) side of the body. For instance, the left cerebral hemisphere is largely concerned with motor and sensory activities occurring in the right side of the body. Although each hemisphere has a complete set of structures for governing the motor and sensory activities of the body, each hemisphere tends to specialize in different functions. For example, in most people, speech and language is largely controlled by the left cerebral hemisphere. The left hemisphere also specializes in hand control and analytical processes. The right hemisphere specializes in such functions as stereognosis, the sense by which the form of objects is perceived (e.g., if a familiar object such as a coin or key is placed in the hand it can be recognized without looking at it), and the perception of space.

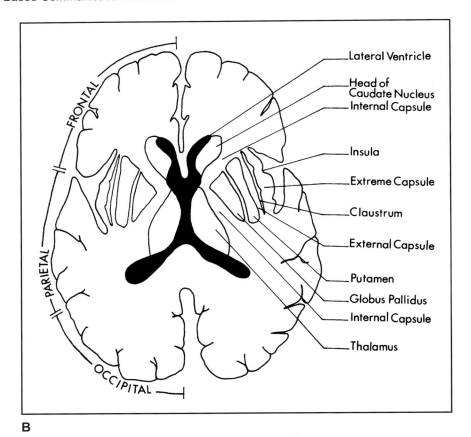

B

FIGURE 1–5. *continued* **B.** Diagrammatic representation of a horizontal section of the cerebral hemisphere showing the anatomy of the basal ganglia (from Murdoch, 1990. Reprinted with permission).

The cerebral hemisphere that controls speech and language is referred to as the dominant hemisphere.

Each cerebral hemisphere can be divided into six lobes. These include the frontal, parietal, occipital, temporal, central (also called the insula or island of Reil), and limbic lobes. The six lobes are delineated from each other by several major sulci and fissures, including the lateral fissure (fissure of Sylvius), central sulcus (fissure of Rolando), cingulate sulcus and the parieto-occipital sulcus. A superior view of the brain reveals two lobes; the frontal and parietal, separated by the central sulcus (see Figure 1–4).

Four lobes, namely the frontal, parietal, temporal, and occipital lobes can be seen from a lateral view of the cerebrum (Figure 1–6). The boundaries of the lobes on the lateral cerebral surface are as follows: the frontal lobe is located anterior to the central sulcus and above the lateral fissure; the parietal lobe is located posterior to the central sulcus, anterior to an imaginary parieto-occipital line (this runs parallel to the parieto-occipital sulcus, which is found on the medial surface of the hemisphere in the longitudinal fissure) (Figure 1–7) and above the lateral fissure and its imaginary posterior continuation toward the occipital pole; the temporal lobe is located below the lateral fissure and anterior to the imaginary parieto-occipital line.

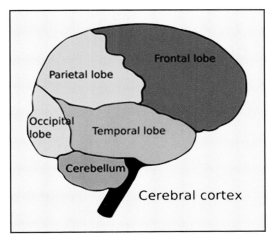

FIGURE 1–6. Lateral view of the right cerebral hemisphere.

The central lobe or insula is not visible from an external view of the brain. It is hidden deep within the lateral fissure. To view the central lobe, the lateral fissure must be held apart or the opercula removed (Figure 1–8). Those parts of the frontal, parietal, and temporal lobes that cover the external surface of the insula are called the frontal operculum, parietal operculum, and temporal operculum, respectively.

The limbic lobe is a ring of gyri located on the medial aspect of each cerebral hemisphere. The largest components of this limbic lobe include the hippocampus, the para-hippocampal gyrus, and the cingulated gyrus, some of which can be examined from a midsagittal view of the brain (see Figure 1–7).

Each of the six lobes appears to be specialized with respect to the function. Located in the frontal lobes are the centers

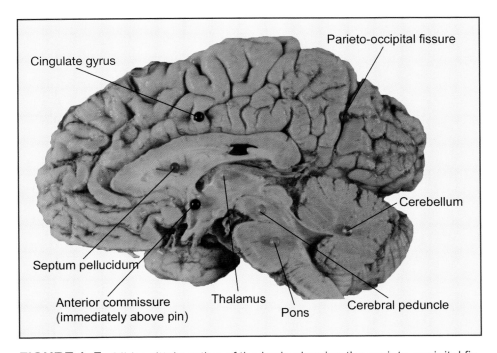

FIGURE 1–7. Midsagittal section of the brain showing the parieto-occipital fissure (from Murdoch, 2009. Reprinted with permission).

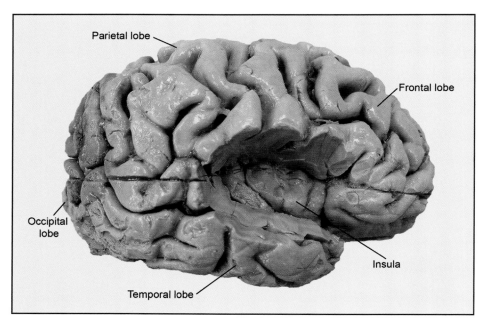

FIGURE 1–8. Lateral dissection of the brain showing the insula (frontal, parietal and temporal operculae removed) (from Murdoch, 2010. Reprinted with permission).

for the control of voluntary movement, the so-called motor areas of the cerebrum. Immediately anterior to the central sulcus is a long gyrus called the precentral gyrus (Figure 1–9). This gyrus, also known as the primary motor area or motor strip, represents the point of origin of the nerve fibers that carry voluntary nerve impulses from the cerebral cortex to the brainstem and spinal cord. In other words, the nerve cells in this area are responsible for the voluntary control of skeletal muscles on the opposite side of the body. Electrical stimulation of the primary motor area causes the contraction of muscles primarily on the opposite or contralateral side of the body. The nerve fibers that leave the primary motor area and pass to either the brainstem or spinal cord form what are known as the direct motor pathways or pyramidal pathways.

All parts of the body responsive to voluntary muscular control are represented along the precentral gyrus in something of a sequential array. A map showing the points in the primary motor cortex that cause muscle contractions in different parts of the body when electrically stimulated is shown in Figure 1–10. These points have been determined by electrical stimulation of the human brain in patients having brain operations under local anesthesia.

The map as shown is referred to as the motor homunculus. It should be noted that the areas of the body are represented in an almost inverted fashion, the motor impulses to the head region originating from that part of the precentral gyrus closest to the lateral sulcus, whereas impulses passing to the feet are initiated from an area located within the longitudinal fissure. The size of the

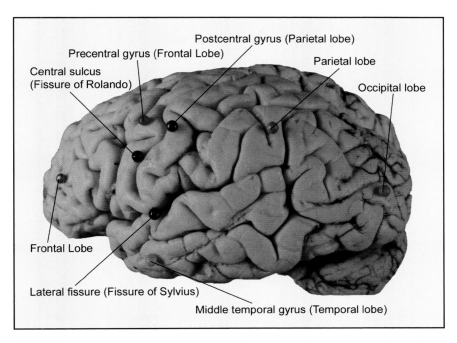

FIGURE 1–9. Lateral view of the left cerebral hemisphere (from Murdoch, 1983. Reprinted with permission).

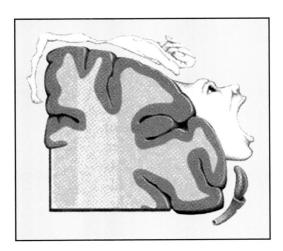

FIGURE 1–10. The motor homunculus.

area of precentral gyrus devoted to a particular part of the body is not strongly related to the size of that body part. Rather larger areas of the motor strip are devoted to the parts of the body which have a capacity for finer and more highly controlled movement. Consequently, the area devoted to the hand is larger than that given to the leg and foot. Likewise, because the muscles of the larynx are capable of very discrete and precise movements, the area of precentral gyrus devoted to their control is as large or larger than the area given to some of the big leg muscles that are capable of only more gross movements.

In addition to the primary motor area, several other motor areas have been located in the frontal lobes by simulation studies. These latter areas include the premotor area, the supplementary motor area, the secondary motor area, and the frontal eye field. Another important area of the frontal lobe is Broca's area. Also known as the motor speech area, Broca's area is one of two major cortical areas that have been identified as having specialized language functions and appears to be necessary for the production of fluent, well-articulated speech. Broca's area is described in more detail later in this chapter.

The parietal lobe is involved in a wide variety of general sensory functions. The sensations of heat, cold, pain, touch, pressure, and position of the body in space and possibly some taste sensation all reach the level of consciousness here. The primary sensory area for general senses (also called the somaesthetic area or sensory strip) occupies the postcentral gyrus. Each sensory strip receives sensory signals almost exclusively from the opposite side of the body (a small amount of sensory (touch) information comes from the same ipsilateral side of the face). As in the case of the motor strip, the various parts of the body can be mapped along the postcentral gyrus to indicate the area devoted to their sensory control. The proportion of the sensory strip allocated to a particular body part is determined by the sensitivity of that part. Consequently, a large area of the postcentral gyrus is assigned to highly sensitive areas such as the lips and hand (particularly the thumb and index finger) and a smaller area assigned to less sensitive areas such as the trunk and legs.

In addition to the postcentral gyrus, two other gyri in the parietal lobe also are of importance to speech-language pathologists. These are the supramarginal gyrus and the angular gyrus. The supramarginal gyrus wraps around the posterior end of the lateral fissure; the angular gyrus lies immediately posterior to the supramarginal gyrus and curves around the end of the superior temporal gyrus. In the dominant hemisphere (usually the left), these two gyri form part of the posterior language cen-

ter, an area involved in the perception and interpretation of spoken and written language. The posterior language center is described more fully later in this chapter.

The temporal lobe is concerned with the special sense of hearing (audition) and at least some of the neurons concerned with speech and language are located here. The primary auditory area is not visible from a lateral view of the brain because it is concealed within the lateral fissure. The floor of the lateral fissure is formed by the upper surface of the superior temporal gyrus. This surface is marked by transverse temporal gyri. The two most anterior of these gyri, called anterior temporal gyri or Heschl's convolutions, represent the primary auditory area. The posterior part of the superior temporal gyrus, which is evident on the lateral surface of the temporal lobe, together with that part of the floor of the lateral fissure that lies immediately behind the primary auditory area (an area called the planum temporal) constitute the auditory association area. In the dominant hemisphere, the auditory association area also is known as Wernicke's area, another important component of the posterior language center.

The occipital lobe is concerned primarily with vision. The primary visual area is located in the posterior part of the occipital lobe. The limbic lobe, also known as the rhinencephalon (smell brain), is associated with olfaction, autonomic functions, and certain aspects of emotion, behavior, and memory. Although the functions of the central lobe are uncertain, it is believed that it also operates in association with autonomic functions.

The Brainstem. If both the cerebral hemispheres and the cerebellum are removed from the brain, a stalklike mass of central nervous system tissue remains, the brainstem. The brainstem is comprised of four major parts. From rostral (head) to caudal (tail), these include the diencephalon, midbrain (mesencephalon), pons (metencephalon), and medulla oblongata (myelencephalon). The relationship of these components to one another can be seen in Figure 1–11.

The Diencephalon. The diencephalon (or "Tweenbrain") lies between the cerebral hemispheres and the midbrain. It consists of two major components, the thalamus and hypothalamus. The thalamus is a large rounded mass of gray matter measuring about 1.25" (3 cm) anteroposteriorly and 5/8" (1.5 cm) in two other directions. Located above the midbrain, it is not visible in surface views of the brain. It can be seen, however, from a midsagittal section of the brain (see Figure 1–11). The thalamus is one of the major sensory integrating centers of the brain and is sometimes referred to as the gateway to the cerebral cortex. All of the major sensory pathways with the exception of the olfactory pathways pass through the thalamus on their way to the cerebral cortex. The thalamus, therefore, receives sensory information via the sensory pathways, integrates that information, and then sends it on to the cerebral cortex for further analysis and interpretation. In addition to its sensory activities, the thalamus is functionally interrelated with the major motor centers of the cerebral cortex and can facilitate or inhibit motor impulses originating from the cerebral cortex.

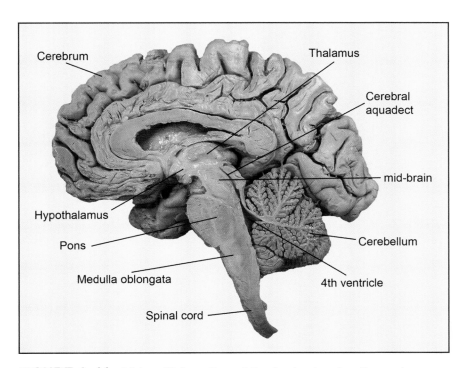

FIGURE 1–11. Midsagittal section of the brain showing the major components of the brainstem.

The hypothalamus lies below the thalamus (see Figure 1–11). When examined from an inferior view of the brain (Figure 1–12), the hypothalamus can be seen to be made up of the tuber cinereum, the optic chiasma, the two mammillary bodies, and the infundibulum. The tuber cinereum is the name given to the region bounded by the mammillary bodies, optic chiasma, and beginning of the optic tracts. The infundibulum, to which is attached the posterior lobe of the pituitary gland is a stalklike structure that arises from a raised portion of the tuber cinereum called the median eminence. The median eminence, the infundibulum, and the posterior lobe of the pituitary gland together form the

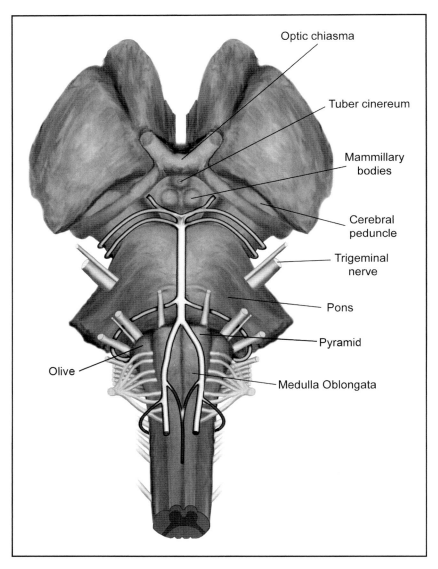

FIGURE 1–12. Inferior view of the brainstem (from Murdoch, 2009. Reprinted with permission).

neurohypophysis (posterior pituitary gland). The mammillary bodies are two small hemispherical projections placed side by side immediately posterior to the tuber cinereum. They contain nuclei important for hypothalamic function. The optic chiasma is a crosslike structure formed by the partial crossing over of the nerve fibers of the optic nerves. Within the optic chiasma, the nerve fibers originating from the nasal half of each retina cross the midline to enter the optic tract on the opposite side.

Although the hypothalamus is only a small part of the brain, it controls a large number of important body functions. The hypothalamus controls and integrates the autonomic nervous system, which stimulates smooth muscle, regulates the rate of contraction of cardiac muscle, and controls the secretions of many of the body's glands. Through the autonomic nervous system, the hypothalamus is the chief regulator of visceral activities (e.g., it controls the heart rate, the movement of food through the digestive system, and contraction of the urinary bladder). The hypothalamus also is an important link between the nervous and endocrine systems. It regulates the secretion of hormones from the anterior pituitary gland and actually produces the hormones released from the posterior pituitary. The hypothalamus also controls aspects of emotional behavior such as rage and aggression. It also controls body temperature and regulates water and food intake and is one of the centers that maintains the waking state. The hypothalamus also has a role in the control of sexual behavior.

The Midbrain. The midbrain is the smallest portion of the brainstem and lies between the pons and diencephalon. The midbrain is traversed internally by

a narrow canal called the cerebral aqueduct (aqueduct of Sylvius), which connects the third and fourth ventricles and divides the midbrain into a dorsal and ventral portion. A prominent elevation lies on either side of the ventral surface of the midbrain (see Figure 1–12). These two elevations are known as the cerebral peduncles and consist of large bundles of descending nerve fibers. The dorsal portion of the midbrain contains four rounded eminences, the paired superior and inferior colliculi (collectively known as the corpora quadrigemina) (Figure 1–13). The four colliculi comprise the roof or tectum of the midbrain. The superior colliculi are larger than the inferior colliculi, and are associated with the visual system. The inferior colliculi, on the other hand, act as relay nuclei on the auditory pathways to the thalamus.

The Pons. The pons lies between the midbrain and medulla oblongata and anterior to the cerebellum, being separated from the latter by the fourth ventricle. The term pons means bridge. The pons takes its name from the appearance of its ventral surface, which essentially is that of a bridge connecting the two cerebellar hemispheres.

Although the pons consists mainly of white matter, it does contain a number of nuclei. These nuclei include the motor and sensory nuclei of the trigeminal nerve (cranial nerve V), the facial nucleus (cranial nerve VII), and the abducens nucleus (cranial nerve VI). A nucleus involved in the control of respiration, the pneumotaxic center, also is located in the pons. Major sensory fibers also ascend through the pons. The pons also acts as a synaptic or relay station for motor fibers conveying impulses from the motor areas of the cerebral cortex to the cerebellum.

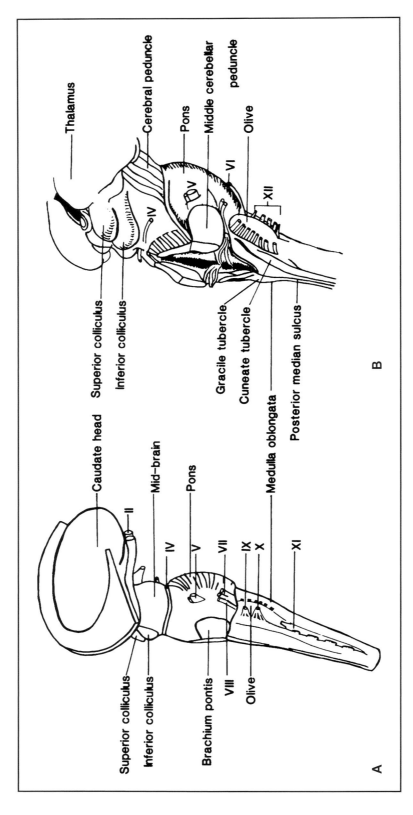

FIGURE 1–13. **A.** Lateral view of the brainstem. **B.** Dorsolateral view of the brainstem (from Murdoch, 1990. Reprinted with permission).

The Medulla Oblongata. The medulla oblongata is continuous with the upper portion of the spinal cord and forms the most caudal portion of the brainstem. It lies above the level of the foramen magnum and extends upward to the lower portion of the pons. The medulla is composed mainly of white fiber tracts. Among these tracts are scattered nuclei that either serve as controlling centers for various activities or contain the cell bodies of some cranial nerve fibers.

On the ventral surface of the medulla in the midline is a fissure that is bordered by two ridges, the pyramids (see Figure 1–12). The pyramids are composed of the largest motor tracts that run from the cerebral cortex to the spinal cord, the so-called corticospinal tract (pyramidal tracts proper). Near the junction of the medulla with the spinal cord, most of the fibers of the left pyramid cross to the right side and most of the fibers in the right pyramid cross to the left side. The crossing is referred to as the decussation of the pyramids and largely accounts for why the left cerebral hemisphere controls the voluntary motor activities of the right side of the body and the right cerebral hemisphere the voluntary motor activities of the left side of the body. On either side of the medulla are oval elevations called the olives, which contain the inferior olivary nucleus (see Figure 1–12).

The medulla contains a number of important cranial nerve nuclei including the nucleus ambiguus (which gives rise to the motor fibers which are distributed to voluntary skeletal muscles via the IXth, Xth, and cranial portion of the XIth nerves) and hypoglossal nucleus (which gives rise to the motor fibers which pass via the XIIth nerve to the muscles of the tongue). In addition to containing the nuclei for various cranial nerves, the medulla also contains a number of nuclei that initiate and regulate a number of vital activities such as breathing, swallowing, regulation of heart rate, and the caliber of smaller blood vessels.

The Cerebellum. The cerebellum (small brain) lies behind the pons and medulla and below the occipital lobes of the cerebrum (see Figures 1–7 and 1–11). Grossly, it may be seen to be composed of two hemispheres, the cerebellar hemispheres, which are connected by a median portion called the vermis (Figure 1–14). The cerebellum is attached to the brainstem on each side by three bundles of nerve fibers called the cerebral peduncles.

In general terms, the cerebellum refines or makes muscle movements smoother and more coordinated. Although it does not in itself initiate any muscle movements, the cerebellum continually monitors and adjusts motor activities that originate from the motor areas of the brain or peripheral receptors. It is particularly important for coordinating rapid and precise movements such as those required for the production of speech. Damage to the cerebellum is often reported to be associated with a motor speech disorder called ataxic dysarthria.

The Spinal Cord

The spinal cord is the part of the central nervous system that lies below the level of the foramen magnum. Protected by the vertebral column, the spinal cord lies in the spinal or vertebral canal and, like the brain, is surrounded by three fibrous membranes, the meninges. It is cushioned by cerebrospinal fluid and held in place by the denticulate liga-

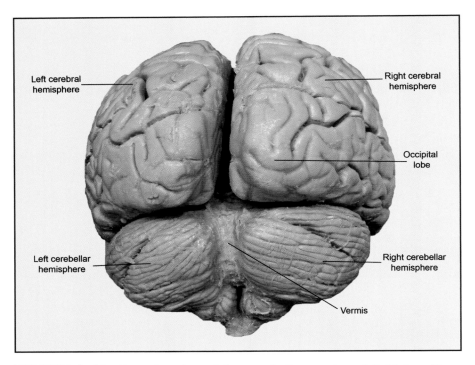

Left cerebral
hemisphere

Right cerebral
hemisphere

Occipital
lobe

Left cerebellar
hemisphere

Right cerebellar
hemisphere

Vermis

FIGURE 1–14. Posterior view of the cerebellum and occipital lobes (from Murdoch, 2010. Reprinted with permission).

ments. It is comprised of well-demarcated columns of motor and sensory cells (the gray matter) surrounded by the ascending and descending tracts that connect the spinal cord with the brain (the white matter). A transverse section of the spinal cord shows that the gray matter is arranged in the shape of the letter "H," with anterior and posterior horns and a connecting bar of gray matter (Figure 1–15). A lateral horn of gray matter is also present in the thoracic part of the cord. A narrow cavity called the central canal is located in the connecting bar of gray matter.

The spinal cord is divided into five regions, each of which takes its name from the corresponding segment of the vertebral column. From top to bottom, these regions include the cervical, thoracic, lumbar, sacral, and coccygeal regions. Thirty-one pairs of spinal nerves arise from the spinal nerves arise from the spinal cord. Eight of these nerves arise from the cervical region, twelve from the thoracic, five each from the lumbar and sacral regions and one from the coccygeal region. Each spinal nerve is formed by the union of a series of dorsal and ventral roots, the dorsal roots carrying only sensory fibers, which convey information from peripheral receptors into the spinal cord, and the ventral roots, which contain only motor fibers that act as a final pathway for all motor impulses leaving the spinal cord.

The Peripheral Nervous System

The three principal components of the peripheral nervous system are the cra-

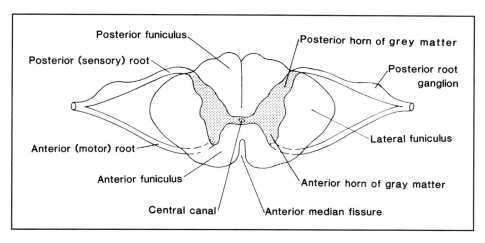

FIGURE 1–15. Transverse section of the spinal cord (from Murdoch, 1990. Reprinted with permission).

nial nerves, the spinal nerves, and the peripheral portions of the autonomic nervous system.

The Cranial Nerves

Twelve pairs of cranial nerves arise from the base of the brain. With only one exception, the olfactory nerves which terminate within the olfactory bulbs, all cranial nerves either originate from or terminate within the brainstem. The cranial nerves are numbered by Roman numerals according to their position on the brain from anterior to posterior. The names given to the cranial nerves indicate either their function or destination. Some cranial nerves are both sensory and motor. Others, however, are either sensory or motor only. Table 1–1 summarizes the principal features of the 12 cranial nerves including their names and peripheral connections.

Cranial nerves are responsible for the control of the majority of muscles comprising the speech mechanism. In particular, cranial nerves V, VII, IX, X, XI, and XII are vital for normal speech production and, for this reason, the anatomy of the latter nerves is described in more detail below.

Trigeminal Nerves (V). The trigeminal nerves emerge from the lateral sides of the pons and are the largest of the cranial nerves (see Figures 1–13 and 1–16). Each trigeminal nerve is composed of three branches: the ophthalmic branch, the maxillary branch, and the mandibular branch. Of the three branches, the ophthalmic and maxillary are both purely sensory, whereas the mandibular is mixed sensory and motor.

The ophthalmic branch exits the skull through the superior orbital fissure and provides sensation from the cornea, ciliary body, iris, lacrimal gland, conjunctiva, nasal mucous membrane, and the skin of the eyelid, eyebrow, forehead, and nose. The maxillary branch leaves the skull through the foramen rotundum and supplies sensory fibers to the skin of the cheek, lower eyelid, side of the nose and upper jaw, teeth of the upper jaw, and mucous membrane of the mouth and maxillary sinus.

Table 1–1. Summary of the Cranial Nerves

Nerve		Function
I	Olfactory	Smell
II	Optic	Vision
III	Oculomotor	Four extrinsic eye muscles (medial, inferior and superior recti, inferior oblique) and levator palpebrae. Parasympathetic to iris diaphragm of eye (constriction) and ciliary muscles of eye (lens accommodation)
IV	Trochlear	One extrinsic eye muscle (superior oblique)
V	Trigeminal	
	Motor root	Muscles of mastication and tensor tympani
	Sensory root	Cranial-facial sensation
VI	Abducens	One extrinsic eye muscle (lateral rectus)
VII	Facial	
	Motor root	Muscles of facial expression and stapedius
	Intermediate root (nervus intermedius)	Parasympathetic innervation of submandibular and sublingual salivary glands. Taste from anterior two-thirds of tongue
VIII	Vestibulocochlear nerve	
	Vestibular nerves	Balance
	Cochlear nerve	Hearing
IX	Glossopharyngeal	Stylopharyngeus muscle. Parasympathetic innervation to parotid salivary gland. Sensation from pharynx and taste from posterior one-third of tongue
X	Vagus	Pharyngeal and laryngeal muscles and levator veli palatini. Parasympathetic innervation of thoracic and upper abdominal viscera
XI	Accessory	
	Cranial portion	Joins the vagus to supply the muscles of the larynx and pharynx
	Spinal portion	Sternocleidomastoid and trapezius muscles
XII	Hypoglossal	All intrinsic and most extrinsic tongue muscles

The mandibular branch unites with the motor root immediately after it exits from the cranial cavity via the foramen ovale. The motor root arises from the motor nucleus of the trigeminal in the pons. Because the trigeminal nerve is

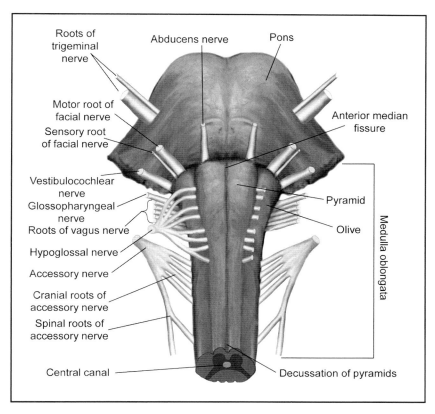

FIGURE 1–16. Inferior view of the pons and medulla oblongata showing the origins of cranial nerves V to XII (from Murdoch, 2010. Reprinted with permission).

mainly sensory, the motor root is much smaller than the sensory portion. Sensory fibers in the mandibular branch provide sensation from the skin of the lower jaw and the temporal region. In the mouth, they supply the lower teeth and gums and the mucous membrane covering the anterior two-thirds of the tongue. The motor fibers of the mandibular branch innervate the muscles of mastication, which include the temporalis, masseter, and medial and lateral pterygoid muscles. In addition, the motor fibers supply the mylohyoid, anterior belly of the digastric, the tensor veli palatine, and the tensor tympani of the middle ear.

The functioning of the motor portion of the trigeminal nerve can be tested clinically by observing the movements of the mandible. Normally, when the mouth is opened widely, the mandible is depressed in the midline. In unilateral trigeminal lesions, however, the mandible deviates toward the paralyzed side due to the unopposed contraction of the pterygoid muscles on the active side (i.e., the side opposite to the lesion) when the mouth is opened. As a further test of trigeminal function, the masseter and temporalis muscles should be palpated while patients clench their teeth. In patients with unilateral lesions, it will be noted that the muscles of mastication on the same side as the lesion will either fail to contract or contract only weakly. When bilateral trigeminal lesions are present, the muscles of mastication on both sides will undergo flaccid paralysis.

Facial Nerve (VII). Each facial nerve emerges from the lateral aspect of the brainstem at the lower border of the pons, in the pontomedullary sulcus, in the form of two distinct bundles of fibers of unequal size (see Figure 1–16). The larger, more medial bundle arises from the facial nucleus of the pons and carries motor fibers to the muscles of facial expression. The smaller, more lateral bundle carries autonomic fibers and is known as the nervus intermedius. The two roots run together for a short distance in the posterior cranial fossa to enter the internal auditory meatus in the petrous temporal bone along with the VIIIth nerve (auditory nerve). Within the temporal bone, the facial nerve passes through the facial canal and eventually emerges from the skull at the stylomastoid foramen. From here, the motor fibers are distributed to the muscles of facial expression including the occipito-frontalis, orbicularis oris, and buccinator. Other muscles supplied by the facial nerve include the stylohyoid and the posterior belly of the digastric. Within the facial canal, a small number of motor fibers are given off to supply the stapedius muscle in the middle ear.

The autonomic fibers of the facial nerve supply the submandibular and sublingual salivary glands as well as the lacrimal gland in the orbit.

The motor portion of the facial nerve is tested by observing the patient's face, both at rest and during the performance of a variety of facial expressions such as pursing the lips, smiling, corrugating the forehead, blowing out the cheeks, showing the teeth, and closing the eyes against resistance. Normally, all facial movements should be equal bilaterally. Unilateral facial nerve lesions cause weakness or paralysis of the half of the face on the same side as the lesion. At rest, the face of patients with unilateral flaccid paralysis of the muscles of facial expression appears to be asymmetrical. The mouth on the affected side droops below that on the unaffected side and saliva may constantly drool from the corner. In addition, due to loss of muscle tone in the orbicularis oris muscle, the lower eyelid may droop causing the palpebral fissure on the affected side to be somewhat wider than on the normal side. When the patient smiles, the mouth is retracted on the active side but not on the affected side. Likewise, when asked to frown, the frontalis muscle on the contralateral side will corrugate the forehead; however, on the side ipsilateral to the lesion, no corrugation will occur.

In bilateral facial nerve paralysis, as might occur in Moebius syndrome, saliva may drool from both corners of the mouth. The seal produced by compression of the lips may be so weak that the patients cannot puff out their cheeks and the lips may be slightly parted at rest.

Glossopharyngeal Nerve (IX). Each glossopharyngeal nerve arises from the medulla oblongata as a series of rootlets at the upper end of the postolivary sulcus (see Figure 1–16). The IXth nerve leaves the cranial cavity via the jugular foramen along with the vagus and accessory nerves.

The glossopharyngeal nerve contains both sensory and motor as well as autonomic fibers. The motor fibers arise from the nucleus ambiguus and innervate the stylopharyngeus muscle. The sensory fibers provide sensation from the pharynx, the posterior one-third of the tongue, the fauces, tonsils, and soft palate. They also carry the sense of taste from the posterior one-third of the tongue.

The autonomic fibers within the IXth nerve regulate secretion from the parotid salivary gland.

Vagus Nerve (X). Each vagus nerve arises from the lateral surface of the medulla oblongata by numerous rootlets, which lie immediately inferior to those which give rise to the glossopharyngeal nerve (see Figure 1–16). It then leaves the cranial cavity via the jugular foramen.

The vagus nerve contains sensory, motor, and autonomic fibers and is the only cranial nerve to venture beyond the confines of the head and neck, supplying structures within the thorax and the upper parts of the abdominal cavity.

After emerging from the jugular foramen, the vagus receives additional motor fibers from the cranial portion of the accessory nerve. The motor fibers of the vagus arise from the nucleus ambiguus and, in combination with those from the accessory nerve, supply the muscles of the pharynx, larynx, and the levator veli palatini and musculus uvulae of the soft palate. The first branch of the vagus nerve important for speech is the pharyngeal nerve, which supplies the levator muscles of the soft palate. As the vagus descends in the neck, it gives off a second branch, the superior laryngeal nerve, which supplies the cricothyroid muscle (the chief tensor muscle of the vocal folds). At a lower level in the neck, a third branch is given off, the recurrent laryngeal nerve, which supplies all of the intrinsic muscles of the larynx except for the cricothyroid and therefore is responsible for regulating adduction of the vocal folds for phona-

tion and abduction of the vocal folds for unvoiced phonemes and inspiration.

The autonomic component of the vagus supplies organs in the thorax and abdomen including the heart, lungs, major airways, and blood vessels and the upper part of the gastrointestinal system.

Functioning of the vagus nerve can be easily checked clinically by noting (1) the quality of the patient's voice; (2) the ability to swallow; and (3) the position and movements of the soft palate at rest and during phonation. Unilateral vagus nerve lesions cause paralysis of the ipsilateral vocal fold leading to dysphonia. The paralyzed fold cannot be abducted or adducted. By asking the patients to open their mouths and say /ah/, movements of the soft palate can be observed. Normally, the uvula and soft palate rise in the midline during phonation. However, unilateral lesions of the vagus nerve cause the palate to deviate to the contralateral side (the side opposite to the lesion) during phonation. In addition, the distance between the soft palate and the posterior pharyngeal wall is less on the paralyzed side and the arch of the palate at rest will droop on the side of the lesion.

In bilateral lesions of the vagus nerves, both sides of the soft palate and both vocal folds may be paralyzed. Both sides of the soft palate rest at a lower level than normal, although their symmetry at rest may appear normal to inexperienced clinicians. However, despite the apparent symmetry, there is less space under the arches of the soft palate and the curvature is flatter. The extent of movement on phonation is reduced. In severe cases, the palate may not rise at all. When observed by either direct or indirect laryngoscopy, abduction and adduction of both vocal folds is severely impaired.

Accessory Nerve. There are two parts to each accessory nerve, a cranial portion that arises from the nucleus ambiguus in the medulla oblongata and a spinal portion that arises from the first five segments of the cervical region of the spinal cord. The cranial accessory emerges from the lateral part of the medulla oblongata in the form of four or five rootlets immediately below those that form the vagus nerve (see Figure 1–16). Prior to leaving the cranial cavity via the jugular foramen, the cranial accessory is joined by the spinal accessory to form the accessory nerve. The spinal accessory fibers arise from the anterior horns of the first five cervical segments of the spinal cord. These fibers emerge from the lateral parts of the spinal cord and unite to form a single nerve trunk that ascends alongside the spinal cord and enters the skull through the foramen magnum to join the cranial accessory.

After exiting through the skull, the cranial accessory leaves the spinal accessory and joins the vagus nerve and is distributed by that nerve to provide motor supply to the muscles of the pharynx, larynx, musculus uvulae, and levator veli palatini muscles. The spinal accessory, on the other hand, provides the motor supply to the trapezius muscle and the upper portion of the sternocleidomastoid muscle.

Disorders of the cranial accessory are recognized clinically as disorders of the vagus nerve whereas disorders of the spinal accessory are evident in atrophy and paralysis of the trapezius and sternocleidomastoid muscle.

Hypoglossal Nerve. Each hypoglossal nerve arises from motor cells in the hypoglossal nucleus and emerges from the medulla oblongata as a series of rootlets in the groove that separates the pyramid and olive (see Figure 1–16).

The nerves leave the cranial cavity via the hypoglossal canal, which lies in the margin of the foramen magnum.

The hypoglossal nerves provide the motor supply to the muscles of the tongue. Tongue muscles can be divided into two groups, the intrinsic muscles, which lie entirely within the substance of the tongue and are responsible for changes in its shape, and the extrinsic muscles. The latter muscles are attached at one end to structures outside the tongue and are responsible for moving the tongue within the mouth. The hypoglossal nerves innervate all of the tongue muscles with the exception of the palatoglossus.

Functioning of the hypoglossal nerves can be tested by observing the tongue at rest and during movement. Unilateral hypoglossal nerve damage is associated with atrophy and fasciculations in the ipsilateral side of the tongue. When observed in the mouth, the tongue on the side of the lesion may appear smaller and the surface corrugated, indicative of atrophy. In some cases, fasciculation of the tongue may be the earliest sign of lower motor neuron disease. When patients are asked to protrude their tongue, it will deviate to the paralyzed side. Another test for weakness of the tongue is to have patients press their tongue against their cheek while the examiner presses against the bulging cheek with their hand.

Spinal Nerves

Each of the 31 pairs of spinal nerves is formed by the union of the dorsal and ventral nerve roots that emerge from each segment of the spinal cord. Once formed in this manner, each spinal nerve leaves the vertebral canal through its intravertebral foramen and ends soon after by dividing into a dorsal ramus (branch) and ventral ramus. The dorsal rami of the spinal nerves segmentally supply the deep back muscles and the skin of the posterior aspect of the head, neck, and trunk. The ventral rami are larger than the dorsal rami and behave quite differently. Whereas the dorsal rami show a segmental arrangement, the ventral rami in the cervical, lumbar and sacral regions form four extensive, intermingled networks of nerves called plexuses. One important plexus of interest to speech-language pathologists is the cervical plexus (so called because it originates from the cervical region of the spinal cord), which gives rise to the phrenic nerve that supplies the respiratory diaphragm. The ventral rami in the thoracic region course in the intercostal spaces to supply primarily the intercostal muscles, which also are important contributors to respiration.

The Autonomic Nervous System

The autonomic nervous system regulates the activity of cardiac muscle, smooth muscle, and the glands of the body (particularly the exocrine glands). In this way, the autonomic nervous system controls the activity of the visceral organs and, among other things, helps to regulate arterial pressure, gastrointestinal motility and secretion, urinary output, sweating, body temperature, and various other functions. As the autonomic nervous system is not implicated in the causation of brain-based communication disorders, it is not covered further here.

The Ventricular System

The ventricular system is a series of cavities within the brain that contain a fluid known as cerebrospinal fluid. The system includes two lateral ventricles, the third ventricle, the cerebral aqueduct (aqueduct of Sylvius), and the fourth ventricle. The shapes and locations of the various brain ventricles are shown in Figure 1–17.

One lateral ventricle extends into each of the cerebral hemispheres. They lie below the corpus callosum, each extending in a large "C" shape from the frontal lobe to the temporal lobe, though with a small spur (posterior horn) extending into the occipital lobe. The lateral ventricles communicate with one another and with the third ventricle through a pair of foramina (holes) known as the foramina of Munro (interventricular foramina). The lateral ventricles are separated medially by a membranous partition know as the septum pellucidum.

The third ventricle is a small slitlike cavity in the center of the diencephalon. The lateral walls of this cavity are formed mainly by the thalamus and to a lesser extent by the hypothalamus. It is connected posteriorly to the fourth ventricle by the cerebral aqueduct. The cerebral aqueduct is a narrow channel running within the midbrain between the corpora quadrigemina and the cerebral peduncles. The fourth ventricle is a cavity that lies between the pons and medulla on one side, and the cerebellum on the other. It continues below into a narrow channel, the central canal, which is present in the lower medulla oblongata and throughout the length of the spinal cord. Cerebrospinal fluid escapes from the ventricular system through three foramina that are present in the roof and walls of the fourth ventricle.

The ventricles are lined by ependymal cells. In each of the four ventricles, there are complex tufts of small blood vessels and modified ependymal cells that form what are known as choroid plexuses. These plexuses are concerned with the formation of cerebrospinal fluid.

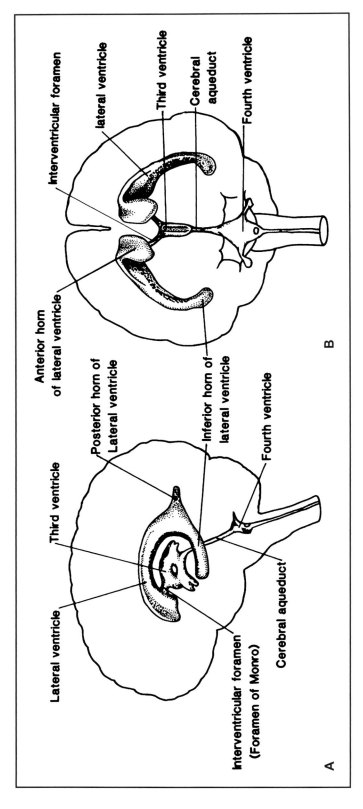

FIGURE 1–17. A. Lateral view of the ventricles. **B.** Frontal view of the ventricles (from Murdoch, 1990. Reprinted with permission).

The Meninges

Three membranes, collectively known as the meninges, surround and protect the brain and spinal cord. From the outside, these are the dura mater, arachnoid, and pia mater. All three envelop the brain and spinal cord (Figure 1–18).

The dura mater is a tough, inelastic outer membrane, made of strong white fibrous connective tissue. In the head, it is comprised of two layers. The outer layer lines and adheres to the skull and is actually the periosteum of the cranial bones. The inner layer of the dura mater covers the brain and in certain locations extends down into the major fissures of the brain, where, it forms three major folds, which divide the skull cavity into adjoining compartments. First, it extends down into the longitudinal fissure forming a membranous partition between the two cerebral hemispheres known as the falx cerebri. A similar, but smaller fold of the inner dura, called the tentorium cerebelli, extends between the occipital lobes of the cerebral hemispheres and the cerebellum in such a way as to form a roof or tent over the cerebellum. Finally, another fold of the inner dura extends between and separates the two cerebellar hemispheres. This latter fold is known as the falx cerebelli.

In certain areas within the skull, the two layers of the dura mater are separated from one another, forming spaces called cranial venous sinuses. These sinuses are filled with blood that flows from the brain to the heart. As we will see later, these sinuses are important in the absorption of cerebrospinal fluid into the bloodstream.

Immediately deep to the dura mater is the second or middle meninge called the arachnoid. The arachnoid is a thin, avascular, delicate, transparent, cobwebby layer. It does not follow each

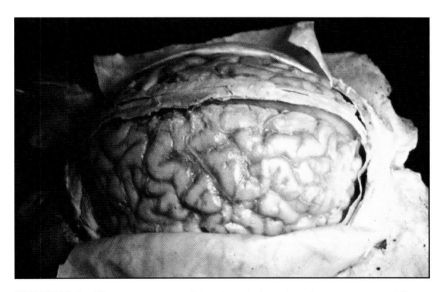

FIGURE 1–18. Dissection of the head showing the meninges (Photo by John A. Beal, PhD, Professor, Louisiana State University Health Sciences Center, 2005. Image available at Wikimedia Commons under the Creative Commons Attribution 2.5 Generic license.).

indentation of the brain but rather skips from gyrus to gyrus. The small space between the arachnoid and the dura mater is known as the subdural space. This space ordinarily is filled with small amounts of lymphlike material. The arachnoid is loosely attached to the inner meninge (the pia mater) by a fine network of connective-tissue fibers (trabeculae), so that a space is created between the arachnoid and the pia mater. This space is called the subarachnoid space. Cerebrospinal fluid circulates through the subarachnoid space.

The pia mater is the innermost meninge and is intimately attached to the brain and spinal cord. It is composed of delicate connective tissue and contains the blood vessels that nourish the neural tissue of the brain and spinal cord. The cerebral blood vessels are adherent to the external surface of the pia mater. Unlike the other two membranes, it dips down into the invaginations of all the sulci of the brain and closely follows the convolutions of the gyri. The pia mater together with the arachnoid are known as the leptomeninges. Inflammation of the meninges is called meningitis, which most often involves the leptomeninges.

The Cerebrospinal Fluid

Cerebrospinal fluid is a clear, colorless fluid that is found in the ventricular system and the subarachnoid space. The brain and spinal cord actually float in the medium. Most of the cerebrospinal fluid is produced by the choroid plexuses of the ventricles of the brain. The volume of cerebrospinal fluid in the ventricles and subarachnoid space is about 120 to 140 ml, with approximately 23 ml in the ventricular system and 117 ml in the subarachnoid space. It has been estimated that cerebrospinal fluid is replaced about once every 6 hours. To maintain a constant volume, therefore, cerebrospinal fluid constantly has to move into the venous sinuses, and hence into the bloodstream.

Cerebrospinal fluid produced in each of the lateral ventricles flows through the interventricular foramen (foramen of Munro) into the third ventricle. More fluid is produced in the third ventricle and all of it flows through the cerebral aqueduct (aqueduct of Sylvius) to the fourth ventricle where more fluid is added. From the fourth ventricle, the fluid escapes into the sub-arachnoid space through one of the three foramina mentioned above. It then circulates around the brain and spinal cord and eventually is reabsorbed into the bloodstream via the venous sinuses in the dura mater.

An obstruction to the passage of cerebrospinal fluid results in a backup of cerebrospinal fluid and an increase in intracranial pressure. This condition, in which there is an accumulation of cerebrospinal fluid in either the ventricular system or subarachnoid space, is called hydrocephalus ("water on the brain").

Hydrocephalus can occur in either adults or children but is most commonly associated with infants who have a congenital abnormality that blocks the flow of cerebrospinal fluid. Hydrocephalus also can occur in adults as a result of tumors, meningitis, and traumatic hemorrhage.

The normal functions of the cerebrospinal fluid are still uncertain. The fluid undoubtedly cushions the brain and spinal cord and minimizes damage that might otherwise result from sudden movements or from blows to the head and spine. The fluid plays a role in the diffusion of materials into and away from the brain, and it might well transport specific substances such as neurohormones from one part of the central nervous system to another.

Cerebrospinal fluid can be sampled by a procedure known as lumbar puncture and a variety of tests carried out to aid the medical diagnosis of a number of neurologic disorders. The same procedure can be used to inject drugs to combat infections.

The Blood Supply to the Brain

Disruption to the blood supply to the brain is a major cause of brain-based communication disorders with the features of the associated speech and/or language disorder being largely determined by the specific cerebral blood vessel(s) involved. Consequently, an understanding of the blood supply to the brain is of fundamental importance to understanding the origins of many of the clinically recognized forms of motor speech and language disorders associated with cerebrovascular pathologies.

Arterial Blood Supply

The arterial blood supply of the contents of the cranial cavity is derived from the paired internal carotid and vertebral arteries. The internal carotid arteries supply blood to the greater part of the cerebral hemispheres. However, the occipital lobes get their chief supply via the vertebral arteries, which also feed the brainstem, and cerebellum. The common carotid arteries ascend in the neck. At the level of the larynx, each divides into an external and an internal carotid artery. Each internal carotid artery enters the cranial cavity through a canal (the carotid canal) in the base of the skull, emerges alongside the optic chiasma and divides into an anterior and middle cerebral artery. The two anterior cerebral arteries are united by a small communicating branch called the anterior communicating artery. Prior to dividing into the anterior and middle cerebral arteries, the internal carotid gives rise to the posterior communicating artery as well as two other small arteries. The posterior communicating artery connects the internal carotid with the posterior cerebral artery and has branches that help supply parts of the hypothalamus, subthalamus, internal capsule, and midbrain.

The vertebral arteries ascend in foramina (openings) in the transverse processes of the cervical vertebrae and enter the cranial cavity through the foramen magnum. On the ventral surface of the brainstem, they join to form a single arterial stem, the basilar artery. This artery ascends in front of the brainstem and ends by dividing into two posterior cerebral arteries. Each of these is joined to the corresponding internal carotid artery by a communicating branch (posterior communicating arteries). This forms what is known as the circle of Willis (i.e., a circle of arteries consisting of the two posterior cerebral arteries, the two anterior cerebral, the two internal carotid arteries and the posterior and anterior communicating arteries) (Figure 1–19). Although the circle of Willis provides a link between the major arteries that supply the brain, under normal conditions there is little exchange of blood between the main arteries through the slender anterior and posterior communicating arteries, as the arterial pressure in the internal carotid arteries is

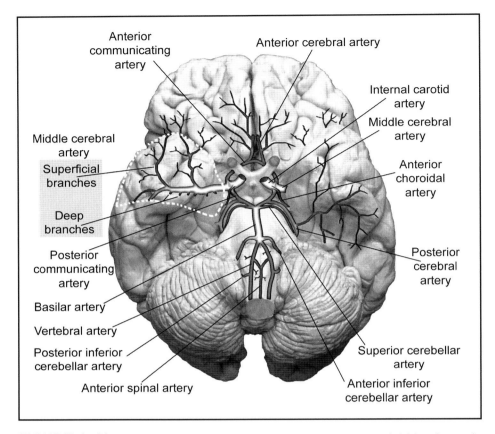

FIGURE 1–19. Ventral surface of the brain showing the arterial blood supply and circle of Willis (from Murdoch, 2010. Reprinted with permission).

similar to that in the basilar artery. The circle of Willis, however, provides alternative but often inadequate routes for blood when one of the major arteries leading into it is occluded. Unfortunately, the circle of Willis and its immediate branches also are common sites for aneurysms (sacs in blood vessel walls caused by weakness in the vessel wall).

The regions of the cerebral hemisphere supplied by the various cerebral arteries are shown in Figure 1–20.

The middle cerebral artery, the largest branch of the internal carotid, travels laterally in the lateral fissure. Eventually, it emerges from the lateral fissure onto the lateral surface of the

cerebral hemisphere, as can been seen from Figure 1–20. Branches of the middle cerebral artery supply almost the entire lateral surface of the hemisphere, including the motor and sensory areas for the face, hand, arm, shoulder, trunk, and pelvis. In the dominant hemisphere, the region supplied by the middle cerebral artery also includes the major speech and language centers, making it the most important artery involved in pathologies associated with the occurrence of aphasia.

The anterior cerebral artery branches off the internal carotid artery near the olfactory tract. It travels along the corpus callosum in the longitudinal fissure and supplies all the medial surface of

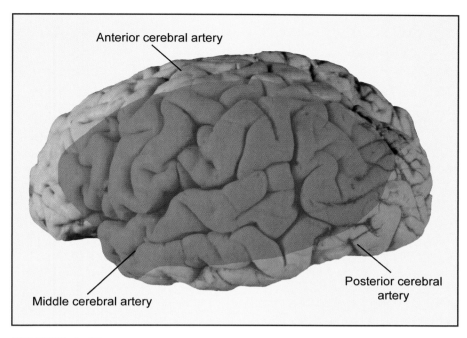

Anterior cerebral artery

Middle cerebral artery

Posterior cerebral artery

FIGURE 1–20. Lateral view of the left cerebral hemisphere showing the distribution of the major cerebral arteries (from Murdoch, 2010. Reprinted with permission).

the cerebral cortex as far back as the parieto-occipital sulcus including the foot and leg areas of the motor strip. The anterior cerebral artery also supplies the undersurface of the frontal lobe.

The posterior cerebral artery branches off the basilar artery at its terminal bifurcation and curves laterally around the midbrain and then dorsally to the temporal and occipital lobes. It supplies the medial and inferior surface of the temporal lobe and the medial surface and pole of the occipital lobe. Branches of the posterior cerebral artery also supply parts of the midbrain and the majority of the thalamus. Whereas the cerebrum is supplied primarily by branches of the internal carotid artery, the brainstem and cerebellum receive their arterial supply via branches of the basilar and vertebral arteries.

Venous Blood Supply

The brain is drained by two sets of veins, both of which empty into the dural venous sinuses which, in turn, empty into the internal jugular veins. These two sets of veins are known as the deep or great cerebral veins and the superficial cerebral veins.

The Blood-Brain Barrier

There is a free and rapid passage of substances between the brain tissue and the cerebrospinal fluid, but there is a barrier between the blood and brain tissue, the blood-brain barrier. This maintains a constant milieu for brain metabolism and is a protection against noxious substances present in the circulation (e.g., waste products such as urea). The barrier is equally effective against antibiotics except when inflammation changes its characteristics.

The capillary network of the central nervous system is extensive, especially in the gray matter. The capillaries in the central nervous system have permeability characteristics that are fundamentally different, however, from those capillaries elsewhere in the body. In fact, the diffusion of most substances is definitely limited, except for fat-soluble compounds and water. The importance of the barrier is that it may prevent potentially therapeutic drugs from reaching the brain. In such cases, these drugs may be administered directly into the cerebrospinal fluid via lumbar puncture.

Speech and Language Centers of the Brain

The French neurologist Paul Broca generally is recognized as being the first to introduce the concept of cerebral dominance when he ascribed speech-language dominance to the cerebral hemisphere contralateral to the preferred hand. Briefly, based on his studies reported in 1861 and 1865, he believed that the speech-language dominant hemisphere in right-handed persons was the left hemisphere, whereas in left-handers the dominant hemisphere was the right hemisphere. Although Broca's correlation of aphasia with focal brain damage in the left hemisphere became widely accepted, we now know that the presumed one-to-one correlation between handedness and dominance for speech-language is over simplistic. Currently, it is believed that approximately 96% of people are left hemispheric dominant for

language, which is related to handedness in the following way: approximately 93% of the population is right-handed and it is estimated that 90 to 99% of all right-handers have their language functions predominantly subserved by the left hemisphere; the remaining 7% of the population are left-handed, with approximately 50 to 70% of the left-handers also having their language functions subserved primarily in the left hemisphere. Within the dominant hemisphere, two major cortical areas have been identified as having specialized language functions. These two areas are located in the perisylvian region (region surrounding the fissure of Sylvius) and include the anterior or motor speech-language area (usually referred to as Broca's area) and the posterior or sensory speech-language area (usually called Wernicke's area) (Figure 1–21).

The two major speech-language areas have been identified largely by the study of patients in whom these areas were damaged by either occlusion of blood vessels or by war injuries. Until relatively recently, the most reliable information concerning the areas of the brain important for language has come from the results of long-term studies of language-disordered patients whose lesions were identified at postmortem examination. Since the mid-1970s, computer tomography has been used to localize lesions associated with various types of language disorders. Using this technique, for the first time, investigators were able to study the relationship between regions of brain damage and disturbances in language function in living subjects, particularly in cases where the lesions involved deep cerebral structures below the level of the cortex. More recently, introduced brain imaging techniques such as positron

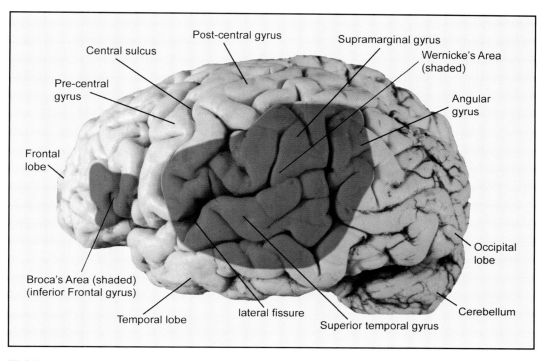

FIGURE 1–21. Lateral view of the left hemisphere showing the major speech-language areas (from Murdoch, 2010. Reprinted with permission).

emission tomography (PET) scanning and magnetic resonance imaging (MRI) scanning have further expanded the ability of researchers to localize lesions associated with specific language disorders in living subjects.

The anterior speech-language area was first identified by Paul Broca in the mid-19th century and, therefore, is commonly referred to as Broca's area. Broca's area occupies the pars opercularis and pars triangularis of the inferior frontal gyrus (also called the third frontal convolution) and lies immediately in front of the part of the cortical motor strip devoted to the peripheral organs of speech.

The posterior speech-language area lies posterior to the fissure of Rolando. The existence of this area was first indicated by Carl Wernicke in the 1870s. Reports in the literature on the location and

extent of the posterior speech-language area vary widely. Wernicke originally indicated that the auditory association cortex of the dominant hemisphere (Wernicke's area) acts as a language center. Subsequent authors have modified and extended this area to include a greater part of the temporal lobe and parts of the parietal lobe. Currently, most descriptions of the posterior speech-language area include within its boundaries the lower half of the postcentral gyrus, the supramarginal and angular gyri, the inferior parietal gyrus, and the upper part of the temporal lobe, including parts of the superior and second temporal gyri and Wernicke's area.

The anterior and posterior speech-language areas communicate with one another via the arcuate fasciculus, a bundle of association fibers that travel as part of a long association tract called the superior longitudinal fasciculus. The arcuate fasciculus sweeps around the insular region and its fan-shaped ends connect parts of the temporal and frontal lobes.

From observations of the speech and language deficits of patients with known lesions sites, it appears that the posterior language area is devoted to tasks having to do mainly with recognition, comprehension, and formulation of language. As this region of the cerebral hemisphere also deals with the reception of sensory stimuli through the auditory, visual, and somatosensory (body sensations) systems, it is believed that language data, which are transmitted through the same modalities, are processed in this area of the left hemisphere. In contrast to the posterior area, the anterior language area is involved with programming and execution of overt acts, such as those that result in speaking, writing, or gesturing.

In addition to the above two areas, a third cortical area that may be involved in speech and language functions has been identified. This third area is small and lies mainly in the medial surface of the frontal lobe (i.e., within the longitudinal fissure) immediately anterior to the foot region of the primary motor strip. It is known as the secondary speech area or the supplementary motor area. Lesions in this area often lead to temporary aphasias and difficulty in producing rapidly alternating movements such as required in the oral region during speech. The entire secondary speech area can be excised, however, without causing a permanent language disorder.

Although the centers described above, including the anterior and posterior language areas and the secondary speech area, comprise the primary speech-language centers of the brain, it is evident that other brain structures also play a role in language function. In particular, these other areas include the parietal, temporal and occipital association areas and various subcortical structures such as the basal ganglia.

References

Beal, J. A. (2005). *Arachnoid*. Retrieved March 19, 2009, from http://commons.wikimedia.org/wiki/File:Human_brain_arachnoid.JPG

Murdoch, B. E. (1983). *An introductory colour atlas of the human brain*. Adelaide, Australia: South Australian College of Advanced Education Press.

Murdoch, B. E. (1990). *Acquired speech and language disorders: A neuroanatomical and functional neurological approach*. London, UK: Chapman and Hall.

Murdoch, B. E. (2010). *Acquired speech and language disorders: A neuroanatomical and functional neurological approach* (2nd ed.). London, UK: Wiley Blackwell.

2

Basic Anatomy and Physiology of the Speech Mechanism

Introduction

In Chapter 1, components of communication were introduced. When you stop to think about it, successful communication is much more complicated than it appears! Consider the following scenario.

Chad and Susan meet up in the student union after class to discuss the concert they had attended the previous night (Figure 2–1).

Susan: "Hey Chad, did you get any sleep last night? I saw you at the concert."

Chad: "Not much, I was so pumped! Dude, that concert really rocked. The crowd was great and the music was phenomenal! What did you think?"

Susan: "I loved it. They are my favorite group. The guitar solos were the best."

Chad: "They are one of my favorite groups too. Did you stick around for autographs after the show?"

Susan: "No, too much of a mob scene for me."

Chad: "Yeah, it was pretty crazy, but totally worth it. I got a poster signed by the entire band, it was awesome."

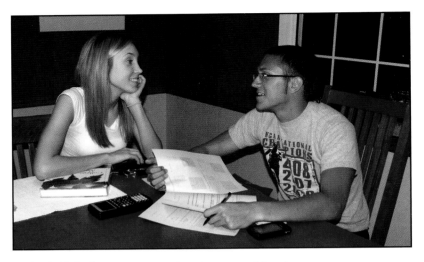

FIGURE 2–1. A conversation between friends.

This exchange contains all the elements of communication introduced in Chapter 1. In order for the conversation to be successful, Susan had to formulate her message using a common *language*. Once formulated, Susan used a variety of structures to convey her message using *speech*. On the other side of the communication partnership, Chad had to hear and understand that message, relying on *speech perception* to do so. An understanding of the message is clear through his appropriate response. The series of events continues to the end of the conversation, illustrating the intricacies of communication.

In Chapter 1, the brain bases of communication were introduced. After reviewing that material, it becomes clear that, for the process of communication, the message begins in the brain. From the brain, signals are passed from the central nervous system (CNS) to the peripheral nervous system (PNS), which innervates the structures and muscles in the periphery that exist away from the brain and spinal cord. Specifically for talking, when the signals reach the muscles at the end of the line, they will act on a variety of systems to produce speech. This whole process appears to be an easy task—after all, we have been doing it since we were children. The ease and automaticity of speech production, however, is deceptive. Most individuals think of speech as being generated by the mouth. However, talking is actually quite complex and involves the careful orchestration of a number of body "systems," all of which contribute to the successful production of speech.

In this chapter, we move away from considering the contributions of the brain and expand our view of communication, focusing on the systems that contribute to the execution or production of speech: respiration, phonation, resonance, and articulation. Each of these systems relies on the others for the successful production of speech. Simply put, they work in a hierarchy to drive, create, and shape sound into the meaningful units we execute as speech. The respiratory system works at the foundation, providing the driving force (air) that is necessary to create sound or the speech signal. At the next level, the air acts on the phonatory system and sound is created. The sound moves through the upper airways and is directed by the resonance system either through the oral cavity or the nasal passages where the sound is shaped into the meaningful units we recognize as speech. The articulatory system is at the top of the hierarchy, further manipulating the air and sound into vowels and consonants. In order to understand how these systems work together, it is important to have a basic knowledge of their anatomy and physiology. Anatomy is the study of the structure of living things. In the case of the speech mechanism, anatomy is composed primarily of respiratory passageways, structures, and muscles. Physiology complements anatomy in that it examines how anatomic structures work together to carry out function. In this chapter, the anatomy of each of the systems of the speech mechanism is reviewed. At the end of the chapter, the physiology of the structures in speech production is explained.

Anatomy of the Speech Mechanism

The Respiratory System

Respiration is a bodily function with the primary purpose of sustaining life by drawing air into the lungs. Once in the lungs, we use that air to oxygenate our blood and tissues, thus maintaining general health. Through the process of evolution, however, we have imposed a secondary purpose on the respiratory

system (grunts and pointing can only get a person so far). That secondary purpose has been to use the respiratory system as a contributor to assist with speech production. There are several components of the respiratory system, all of which must function properly to support speech. Aspects of the respiratory system include the respiratory tract, the framework that protects and supports the system, and the muscles that act on the system to generate breathing.

The Respiratory Tract

The respiratory tract is displayed in Figure 2–2. In total, the respiratory tract begins at the nose and mouth, travels down through the pharynx (throat) and into the larynx (voice box). From that point, the tract continues down into the lungs where the passage divides multiple times (as much as 24 times in an adult), with each passageway growing smaller until it terminates in the miniature air sacs that make up our lungs. This respiratory tract often is divided into an upper and lower respiratory system with the vocal folds serving as the dividing line that separates the two.

The respiratory tract certainly covers a lot of ground. When we inhale, we pull in air from the atmosphere that surrounds us and it travels all the way down through the respiratory tract. The upper respiratory tract functions to warm, filter, and moisten the air that enters the body before it reaches the lungs. The respiratory tract is lined with a mucous membrane, which assists with those functions by keeping the environment warm and moist and filtering the air as it passes through. Have you ever blown your nose on a windy dusty day? If so, you have personal knowledge of

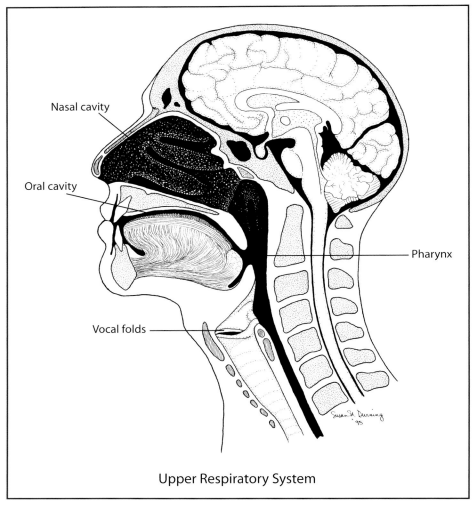

Nasal cavity

Oral cavity

Pharynx

Vocal folds

Upper Respiratory System

A

FIGURE 2–2. A. Diagrammatic representation of the upper respiratory system. From *Anatomy and Physiology Study Guide for Speech and Hearing* by William R. Culbertson, Stephanie S. Cotton, and Dennis C. Tanner. Copyright © 2006 Plural Publishing, Inc. Adapted with permission. *continues*

the filtering properties that are present just in your nose! The lower respiratory system is involved primarily in the air exchange that occurs to keep our blood and tissues oxygenated. The integrity of this entire tract is important for breathing (and, of course, speech). Problems could occur at any point in the respira-tory tract that might cause difficulty. For example, in people with asthma, the tubes leading into the lungs might become inflamed, swelling to the point where it is difficult to breathe. Another example is an individual with sleep apnea (cessation of breathing during sleep). For this individual, the respira-

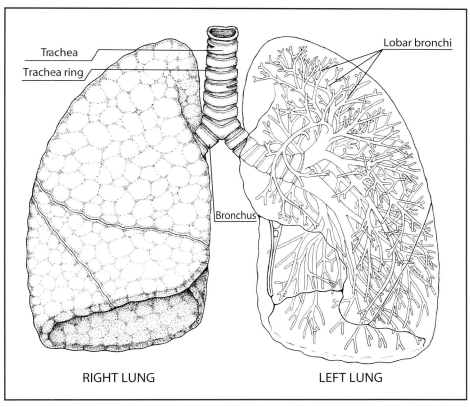

Trachea

Trachea ring

Lobar bronchi

Bronchus

RIGHT LUNG

LEFT LUNG

B

FIGURE 2–2. *continued* **B.** Diagrammatic representation of the lower respiratory system. From *Anatomy and Physiology Study Guide for Speech and Hearing* by William R. Culbertson, Stephanie S. Cotton, and Dennis C. Tanner. Copyright © 2006 Plural Publishing, Inc. Reprinted with permission.

tory tract is open and clear all day; however, during sleep, the muscles relax and can close off the passage so there is no airflow. These illustrations demonstrate the importance of an open, unobstructed respiratory passage.

The Framework for Respiration

The lungs are delicate organs that require protection so they can function properly. Therefore, they are located in the thorax (chest cavity), which provides the necessary support and protection. The thorax is lined by a tough membrane called the pleura, which protects the lungs from puncture or injury and also creates a smooth surface so the lungs can expand and contract continuously (24/7) almost without effort. Surrounding the thorax are bony structures that also lend support and protection (Figure 2–3).

An examination of Figure 2–3 reveals the bony framework that supports the respiratory system. From the posterior (back view), notice the column of vertebrae that includes cervical vertebrae (supporting the neck), thoracic vertebrae

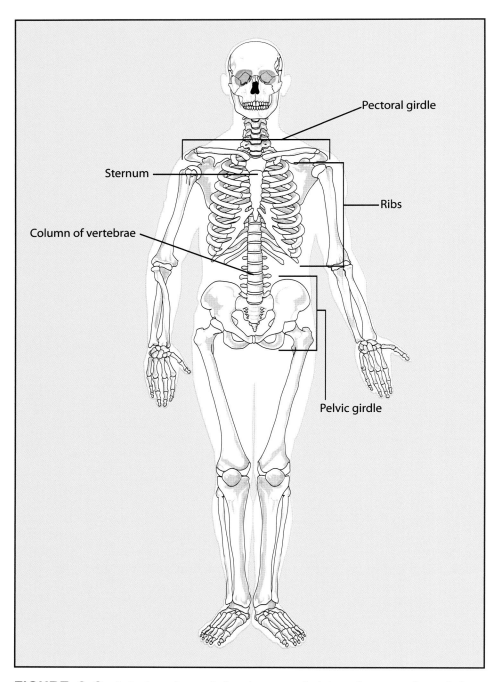

FIGURE 2–3. Anterior view of the human skeleton. Image adapted from Wikimedia Commons. Original image released into public domain by artist.

(supporting the thorax), lumbar vertebrae (supporting the lower back), and the fused sacral and coccygeal vertebrae that form the posterior pelvic girdle and tailbone.

The thoracic vertebrae are unique from the others in that they are the posterior attachment for ribs in the rib cage. There are 12 pairs of ribs and a corresponding 12 thoracic vertebrae that make up the rib cage. Looking at the anterior or front view of Figure 2–3, you can see that the 12 ribs are of varying sizes. Ribs 1 through 7 get progressively larger and are considered "true ribs" because of their direct attachment between the vertebrae in back to the sternum or bony plate in the front. Ribs 8 through 10 are called "false ribs" because they attach to vertebrae in the back, but are indirectly attached to the sternum (through cartilage) in the front. The false ribs begin to get progressively smaller and lead to ribs 11 and 12 which are called "floating ribs" because they are attached to the last two thoracic vertebrae in the back, but the other borders are free floating. If you sit in a very soft chair or couch and you are slumped over, you might feel one of free borders of those "floating ribs" poking you. Considering the rib cage as a whole, notice how its dimensions follow the shape of the lungs. The rib cage with the vertebrae in the back and the sternum in the front offers strong protection for the lungs as well as other vital organs that are located right behind the sternum . . . like the heart!

In addition to the rib cage, there are other bony structures that provide support for respiration. Those structures include the pectoral girdle at the top of the rib cage, and the pelvic girdle located well below the rib cage (see Figure 2–3). The pectoral girdle is made up of the scapulae (shoulder blades) in the back and clavicles in the front. Inferiorly, the pelvic girdle is composed of the coxal (hip) bones, and sacral and coccygeal vertebrae. You might question the relevance of these bony structures when it comes to respiration. In fact, each of these girdles (pectoral and pelvic) serves as a point of attachment for many of the muscles of respiration.

Muscles of Respiration

Up to this point, we have discussed aspects of the respiratory system structure, namely, the passageways where air exchange takes place and the supportive framework that surrounds and protects the lungs. Equally important are the muscles that act on the system, which come into play with breathing. The muscles of respiration attach to bony structures of the thorax and work to expand for the inspiratory (inhale) cycle of breathing and then relax for the expiratory (exhalation) cycle of breathing.

Prior to a discussion of specific respiratory muscles, it is important to review the concepts that relate to muscle physiology. Every muscle has a starting point (origin) and a terminating point (insertion). When muscle contraction occurs, the result is a shortening of the muscle fibers. When the muscle contraction results in movement, that movement typically is in the direction of the point of origin of the muscle. Let's review using the bicep muscle as an example (Figures 2–4A and 2–4B). At rest, the muscle is distributed over the length of the humerus (upper arm) with the point of origin arising from the scapula on the back to the point of insertion on the radius (one of the two bones in the lower arm). When the bicep is contracted, the lower arm is moved up and

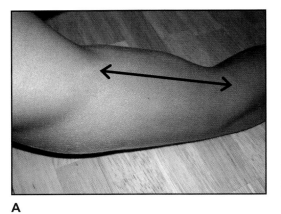 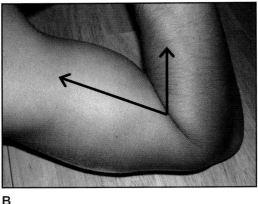

A   B

FIGURE 2–4. **A.** Distribution of muscle fibers in the bicep at rest. **B.** Distribution of muscle fibers at rest, and movement of structures toward the point of insertion with bicep contraction.

toward the point of origin. Such is the case for muscles all over the body. Knowing the origin and insertion of muscles helps us to understand the function of the individual muscles and muscle groups.

Inspiratory Muscles. Perhaps the most important respiratory muscle (certainly the most important for inspiration), is the diaphragm. The diaphragm is located at the base of the rib cage (Figure 2–5) with muscle fibers originating from the ribs, the sternum, and the spinal column. Those fibers course up and insert into a sheet of tendon (aponeurosis) that is located in the center, which makes the structure look a bit like an inverted bowl at the base of the rib cage. We know from the muscle physiology reviewed above that contraction of the diaphragm will result in pulling that aponeurosis down, which expands the thorax. There is a physical principle called Boyle's law that is at work during this process. Simply put, Boyle's law states that if the size or volume of a container increases, the pressure in that container will de-

crease. For breathing, this means that when the diaphragm contracts, expanding the lungs/thorax, the air pressure within the cavity goes down. At that time, the pressure within the lungs is negative, relative to the atmospheric pressure that surrounds us. The result is what is called a pressure gradient (areas of unequal pressure). Because there is an opening (nose) between the two areas of high and low pressure, the air will rush into the lungs in an attempt to equalize (inhalation).

The diaphragm is the inspiratory muscle that works the most; it is most active during quiet breathing, which is the type of breathing we adopt the majority of the time. Looking at Table 2–1, however, you can see that there are additional muscles used for inspiration/inhalation. The listing of muscles is not complete as there are even more muscles that support respiration, but these are the ones that act with the diaphragm for the primary function of breathing. Notice that for the most part (there *are* a few exceptions) the muscles of inhalation are primarily thoracic muscles whose points

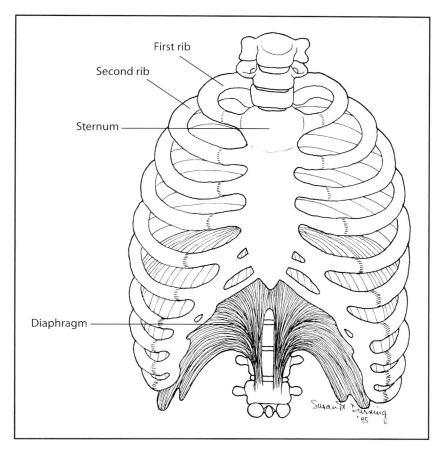

FIGURE 2–5. Inferior view of the diaphragm. From *Anatomy and Physiology Study Guide for Speech and Hearing* by William R. Culbertson, Stephanie S. Cotton, and Dennis C. Tanner. Copyright © 2006 Plural Publishing, Inc. Adapted with permission.

of insertion are below their origin, which will pull the rib cage up, making it bigger and expanding the thorax cavity.

Expiratory Muscles. Now consider the exhalation cycle of breathing. When air rushes in to the thorax during inhalation, the negative pressure within the lungs will equalize with atmospheric pressure. However, the stability is fleeting. Because lungs are somewhat elastic structures, when expanded or stretched, they will want to return to their resting state, much

as a rubber band will quickly return if it is released after being stretched.

If we revisit Boyle's law, we see it take place once again. However, for the exhalation cycle of breathing, the pressure gradient occurs in the opposite direction. As the lungs/thorax returns to resting state, the volume of the cavity decreases. The result is higher pressure now within the lungs when compared to atmospheric pressure. Once again, in an attempt to equalize the pressure, air flows out of the system (exhalation).

Table 2–1. Primary Muscles of Respiration

Cycle of Breathing	Muscle	Location (origin to insertion)	Action
Inhalation	Diaphragm	Base of the rib cage, sternum, and spinal column to the central tendon	The innermost portion (central tendon) of the diaphragm is pulled down
	External Intercostal	Runs from ribs 1–11 to the rib below	Elevates the rib cage
	Internal Intercostal (cartilage portion)	Runs from ribs 1–11 to the rib (medial cartilage portion)	Assists with elevating the rib below at the borders closest to the sternum
	Levatores Costarum (brevis and longis)	Thoracic vertebrae (7–11) to rib below—*brevis*, or two ribs below—*longis*	Elevates those ribs on the posterior rib cage
	Serratus Posterior Superior	Vertebrae (C7–T3) down and laterally to ribs 2–5	Elevates those ribs on the posterior rib cage
	Sternocleido-mastoid	Temporal bone of the skull down to the sternum and clavicle	Assists with the elevation of the rib cage from above
	Scalenus (anterior, middle, & posterior)	Vertebrae (C3–C7) down to the first and second ribs	Elevates ribs 1 and 2
Exhalation	Internal Intercostal (bone portion)	Runs from ribs 1–11 to the rib below (bone portion)	Depresses the rib cage
	Transversus Thoracis	Inner portion of the sternum (lateral borders) to the cartilage portion of ribs 2–6	Depress the rib cage
	Transverse Abdominis	Posterior abdominal wall at the spinal column, runs around the sides of the abdomen to the front of the abdomen from the inner surface of ribs 6–12 down to the pelvic girdle	Compresses the abdomen
	Internal Oblique Abdominis	Pelvic girdle up to the cartilage portion of the lower ribs and the abdominal aponeurosis next to the Rectus Abdominis	Rotates and flexes the trunk, compresses the abdomen

Table 2–1. *continued*

Cycle of Breathing	Muscle	Location (origin to insertion)	Action
Exhalation *continued*	External Oblique Abdominis	The bone portion of ribs 5–12 to the pelvic girdle	Rotates and flexes the trunk, compresses the abdomen
	Rectus Abdominis	Pelvic girdle up to the sternum and cartilage portion of ribs 5–7	Flexes the abdomen
	Serratus Posterior Inferior	Vertebrae T-11 &12 and L1–3 up to ribs 7–12	Depresses the rib cage
	Quadratus Lumborum	Posterior pelvic girdle up to the lower border of rib 12 and lumbar vertebrae 1–5	Fixes the posterior abdominal wall to support abdominal compression

When an individual is just quietly breathing, the exhalation cycle of breathing is just the system returning to rest, there is no active muscle involvement. When active exhalation is required (such as that used for speech), more muscles will be involved. Table 2–1 lists those primary muscles that are used for active exhalation.

The Phonatory System

As described above, the respiratory system functions to provide the air we need for survival. As an intelligent species, however, we have imposed another function in addition to the process of air exchange. In order to talk and use speech for communication, we must have air that drives the system, which is provided by the respiratory system. At the next level, the phonatory system is engaged to create a sound source. The primary structures involved in the phonatory system include a group of cartilages and muscles that form the larynx.

The larynx is a valvelike structure located on top of the trachea. The primary function of the larynx is to protect the airway from anything other than air entering the lungs. When you view the respiratory tract as depicted in Figure 2–2, you see the location of the larynx in the lower pharynx (throat). Also notice that at the level of the larynx, the pharynx divides into two separate pathways. One pathway is for respiration and air exchange as we just discussed in the review of the respiratory system. The other pathway is a component of the digestive system, leading to the stomach. The fact that the respiratory tract and the digestive tract have a common pathway in the pharynx is a bit problematic. It is imperative to the health of the respiratory system that nothing but air enters the lungs, which is where the primary function of the larynx occurs. Because the larynx is a valvelike structure, it can close during the process of eating. In fact, the larynx is sealed off from the pharynx at three levels to ensure that no food or liquid enters the airway. You will read more about that function when you study swallowing in Chapter 10. The larynx is the guardian of the lower airways with its series of valve closures.

Like the respiratory system, we have learned to use the larynx for the overlaid function of communication. Specifically, we use one of the "valves" within the larynx as a vibratory sound source to create a voice. The respiratory tract runs through the larynx but is interrupted at the lateral borders by two folds of tissue (Figure 2–6). The most superior fold is called the ventricular fold (also called the false vocal fold) and the inferior fold is the true vocal fold. When we want to produce speech, we use the air that is coming up from the respiratory system for exhalation and we manipulate the true vocal folds so that they will begin to vibrate. The manipulation that occurs requires an intact framework, careful timing, and coordinated muscle movements within and surrounding the larynx.

Laryngeal Framework

The larynx does not come in contact with the bones of the skeleton. Instead, it is suspended in the neck by muscle and ligaments with the hyoid bone above, and the trachea below. The framework functions as a guardian but also as a supportive structure for the airway that runs through the larynx, which must remain open for breathing at all times

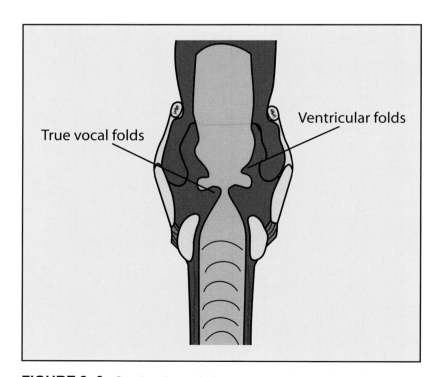

FIGURE 2–6. Section through the larynx and vocal fold. From *Head and Neck Cancer: Treatment, Rehabilitation, and Outcomes* by Elizabeth C. Ward and Corina J. van As Brooks. Copyright © 2007 Plural Publishing, Inc. Adapted with permission.

(with the exception of closing during the swallow). The laryngeal support system is made up of nine cartilages, three of which are paired and three unpaired (Figure 2–7).

The nine structures include an epiglottis, the thyroid cartilage, the cricoid cartilage, arytenoid cartilages (2), corniculate cartilages (2), and two cuneiform cartilages (which are not pictured in Figure 2–7). The thyroid cartilage is the largest of the structures in the larynx and looks somewhat like a shield. The appearance of a shield is interesting as the function of the thyroid is primarily one of protection. The thyroid cartilage supports the airway within to maintain an open glottis (the space between the vocal folds) for breathing and further protects the vocal folds that adduct (join together) for swallowing and voice production. The cricoid cartilage is "class ring" shaped and sits immediately below the thyroid cartilage and on top of the trachea. The ring shape of the cricoid with its narrow band toward the front and larger portion toward the back assists the thyroid in maintaining an open airway. Additionally, the larger back portion of the cricoid serves as a foundation for the

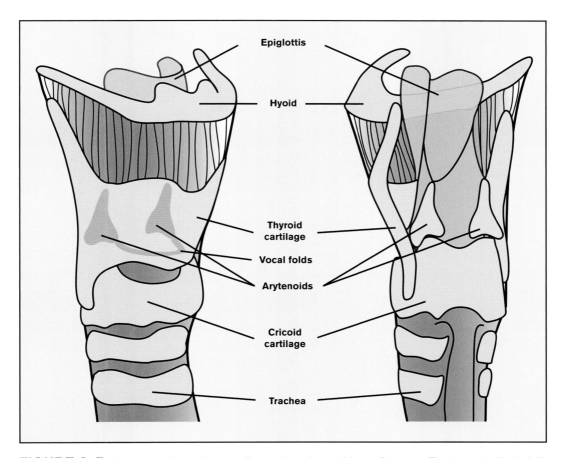

Epiglottis

Hyoid

Thyroid cartilage

Vocal folds

Arytenoids

Cricoid cartilage

Trachea

FIGURE 2–7. Laryngeal cartilages. From *Head and Neck Cancer: Treatment, Rehabilitation, and Outcomes* by Elizabeth C. Ward and Corina J. van As Brooks. Copyright © 2007 Plural Publishing, Inc. Adapted with permission.

arytenoid cartilages. The two arytenoid cartilages are shaped like a pyramid with a convex (curved inward) base below and three projections at each point. The vocal folds are attached to the projection that is directed toward the front of the thyroid (the vocal process), and the convex base of the arytenoid allows them to slide across the back of the cricoid. When the arytenoids slide toward each other, the movement results in bringing the vocal folds together (adduction), a position that is needed for voice production. When the arytenoids slide in the opposite direction, moving the vocal folds apart (abduction), the airway is in an open position, which is necessary for breathing. The very small corniculate cartilages sit atop each arytenoid. The function of these cartilages is unclear (as it is with the cuneiforms); it is thought that they may be vestigial structures that may have had a purpose at one time, but through evolution have become nonfunctional. The epiglottis is a leaf-shaped cartilage that is positioned behind the thyroid cartilage and hyoid bone. The superior boundary of the epiglottis is behind the base of the tongue. The function of the epiglottis is not to support voice production, but instead, the attachments of the epiglottis to the laryngeal framework help it to dip down during swallowing, serving a protective function for the airway.

Laryngeal Muscles

Two groups of muscles (extrinsic and intrinsic) are necessary for laryngeal movements. The term *extrinsic* means that one of the muscle attachments is external or outside the larynx. For example, the sternothyroid is an extrinsic muscle that originates on the head of the sternum and inserts into the side of the thyroid cartilage. As a group, the extrinsic muscles' primary responsibili-ties include stabilizing the location of the larynx and changing its position in the neck (primarily moving up and down). *Intrinsic* muscles are so named because both their attachments (origin and insertion) are within the confines of the laryngeal structure.

Unlike the extrinsic muscles that move the entire larynx, the intrinsic muscles adjust the cartilages within the larynx, changing the shape and configuration of the internal larynx. These finely tuned movements are responsible for voice production. In fact, the muscles of the internal larynx are categorized according to their action on the vocal folds (Table 2–2), classified either as an adductor, abductor, tensor, or a relaxer.

Adduction is an anatomical term meaning "movement toward midline." Applying this concept to the vocal folds would mean bringing the two vocal folds from their lateral position in the larynx to meet at midline, in effect closing the glottis (Figure 2–8A). The lateral cricoarytenoid, the transverse, and oblique arytenoid muscles all function as adductor muscles approximating the folds at midline for glottal closure and voice production. Abduction, on the other hand, is a term for "moving away from midline." Abducted folds open the glottis, a position that is necessary for good air exchange during breathing (Figure 2–8B). The posterior cricoary-tenoid is the only muscle that abducts the folds (Figure 2–9). As an open glottis is needed for breathing, you certainly want this muscle to be working. If through injury or accident, the posterior cricoarytenoid became paralyzed you would need an alternative method of breathing such as a tracheostomy tube (tube placed through the neck to the trachea) or an endotracheal tube (tube placed through the mouth into the trachea).

Table 2–2. Paired Intrinsic Laryngeal Muscles

Muscle	Location (origin to insertion)	Action
Lateral cricoarytenoid	Lateral cricoid cartilage up and back to the lateral (muscular) process of the arytenoid	Adductor
Transverse arytenoid	Lateral margin of the posterior arytenoid to the same location on the opposite arytenoid	Adductor
Oblique arytenoid	Base of the muscular process of one arytenoid up and back to the top (apex) of the opposite arytenoid	Adductor
Posterior cricoarytenoid	Posterior plates of the cricoid cartilage up to the muscular process of the arytenoid above.	Abductor
Cricothyroid	Anterior surface of the cricoid cartilage up to the lateral plates of the thyroid cartilage	Tensor
Thyrovocalis	Inner surface of the thyroid cartilage near the notch back to the vocal process of the arytenoid cartilage.	Tensor
Thyromuscularis	Inner surface of the thyroid cartilage near the notch back to the muscular process and base of the arytenoid	Relaxer

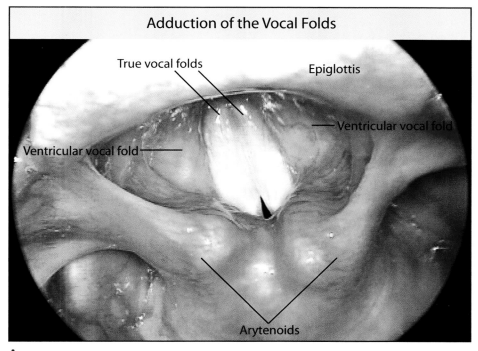

A

FIGURE 2–8. A. Adduction of the vocal folds. *continues*

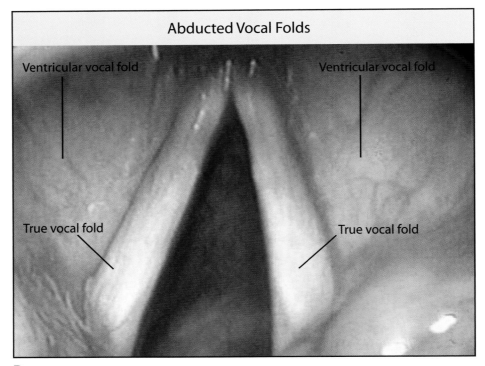

B

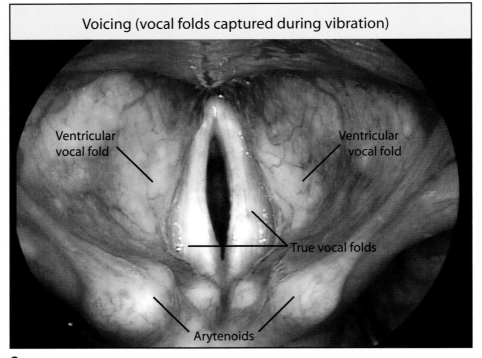

C

FIGURE 2–8. *continued* **B.** Abduction of the vocal folds. **C.** Vocal folds during vibration. From *Textbook of Voice Disorders* by Albert L. Merati and Steven A. Bielamowicz. Copyright © 2007 Plural Publishing, Inc. Adapted with permission.

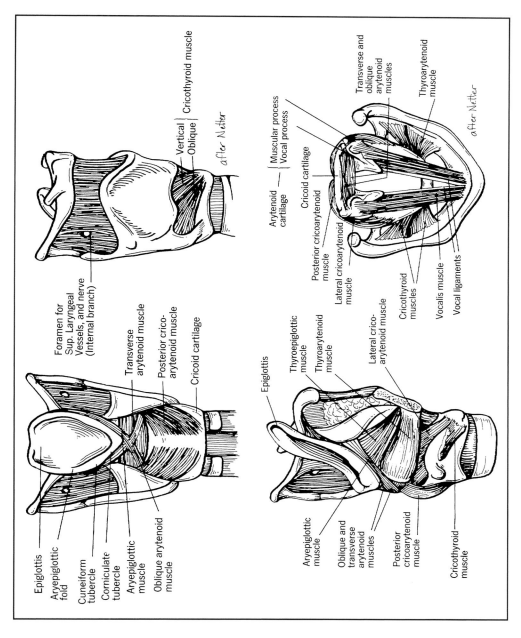

FIGURE 2–9. Intrinsic muscles of the larynx. From *Voice Science* (p. 66), by R. T. Sataloff, 2005, San Diego: Plural Publishing. Copyright © by Plural Publishing, Inc. Reprinted with permission.

Epiglottis
Aryepiglottic fold
Cuneiform tubercle
Corniculate tubercle
Aryepiglottic muscle
Oblique arytenoid muscle

Foramen for Sup. Laryngeal Vessels, and nerve (Internal branch)
Transverse arytenoid muscle
Posterior crico-arytenoid muscle
Cricoid cartilage

Vertical — Oblique } Cricothyroid muscle

after Netter

Epiglottis
Thyroepiglottic muscle
Thyroarytenoid muscle
Lateral crico-arytenoid muscle

Aryepiglottic muscle
Oblique and transverse arytenoid muscles
Posterior cricoarytenoid muscle
Cricothyroid muscle

Arytenoid cartilage — { Muscular process / Vocal process
Cricoid cartilage
Posterior cricoarytenoid muscle
Lateral cricoarytenoid muscle

Transverse and oblique arytenoid muscles
Thyroarytenoid muscle

Cricothyroid muscles
Vocalis muscle
Vocal ligaments

after Netter

The remaining intrinsic muscles describe the nature of the vocal folds rather than their position (Figure 2–8C. Manipulating the vocal folds and changing their tension affects the pitch of the voice. The cricothyroid and the thyrovocalis muscles are considered tensors because contraction of these muscles thins out the folds, increasing the internal tension of the vocal folds. The effect of increased tension in the folds is a faster vibration that will drive pitch higher. The thyromuscularis muscle has the opposite effect. When contracted, the muscles surrounding the thyromuscularis lose tension, becoming more relaxed, almost floppy. A floppy muscle is thicker and heavier causing a slower rate of vibration, lowering the pitch.

Physiology of Phonation. Phonation or voice is created by interrupting the flow of air passing through the larynx on exhalation. Sounds simple, doesn't it? Actually, to generate the voice a careful balance of air pressure and muscle movement is required. To begin, the vocal folds move to an adducted position. Because they are closed against airflow, the air pressure beneath them builds. The increase in air pressure causes the vocal folds to thin at the inferior borders. As the air pressure continues to build, the folds are blown open. When the glottis appears, the *Bernoulli effect* takes place. The Bernoulli effect is another principle of physics, which states that, when matter reaches a point of constriction (in this case airflow through the vocal folds), the speed of airflow increases and the pressure decreases. So when the folds are blown open, the airflow moves faster and negative pressure occurs at the glottis. That negative pressure along with the

elasticity of the tissue in the vocal folds causes the folds to move back together. This process describes just one cycle of vocal fold vibration as illustrated in Figure 2–10, yet the vibratory rate of the average female is 220 Hz, or *220 cycles per second*. In other words, using your voice provides quite a workout! The intrinsic muscles act on the system, further manipulating the nature and position of the vocal folds to change pitch and voicing characteristics for speech.

The Resonance System

Moving from the foundation of the respiratory system and up the vocal tract, the step in the speech mechanism beyond phonation is the resonance system. Similar to the laryngeal system, the resonance system also functions like a valve. The structure that acts like a valve is the soft palate. You can easily distinguish the soft palate yourself by running your tongue back toward the center of the hard palate. Eventually, you will notice a transition of hard palate to soft tissue. That soft tissue is the soft palate, also known as the velum. When air travels from the respiratory system and phonation is initiated, the sound is propagated through the upper airways where the air flows and the sound resonates in the upper chambers (oral cavity, nasal passages). Depending on the position of the velum, the airflow and sound can travel a number of different directions (Figure 2–11).

When the velum is lowered and the lips are open, the air and sound will travel through both the oral and nasal cavities. If the velum remains lowered but the lips are closed, the air and sound will travel through the nasal passage.

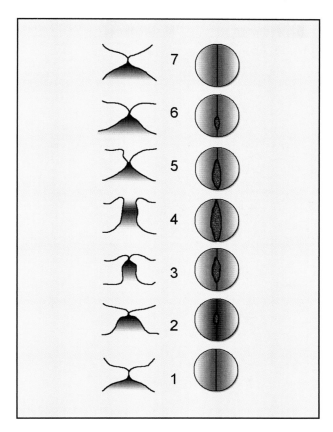

FIGURE 2–10. Airflow through the pharyngeal larynx. From *Voice Disorders* (p. 75), by C. Sapienza and B. Hoffman-Ruddy, 2009, San Diego: Plural Publishing. Copyright © 2009 by Plural Publishing, Inc. Reprinted with permission.

Finally, when the velum is elevated and comes in contact with the posterior pharyngeal wall (the velopharyngeal port), the air and sound will travel through the oral cavity only (Figure 2–11). So the velum functions like a valve in a relay station, directing the airflow and sound according to the speech requirements. So exactly what are speech requirements with regard to nasal resonance and airflow? Only three sounds are considered "nasal" but they are common sounds that are liberally sprinkled through the words we use (there are 8 in this sentence alone!). The nasal sounds are /m/, /n/, and /ng/, like the sound at the end of the word ri<u>ng</u>. In addition to resonant properties, the actual flow of air through the oral cavity also is important for speech production. In fact, 16 of the 25 consonants in the English language require air pressure through the oral cavity in order to be properly articulated (Table 2–3).

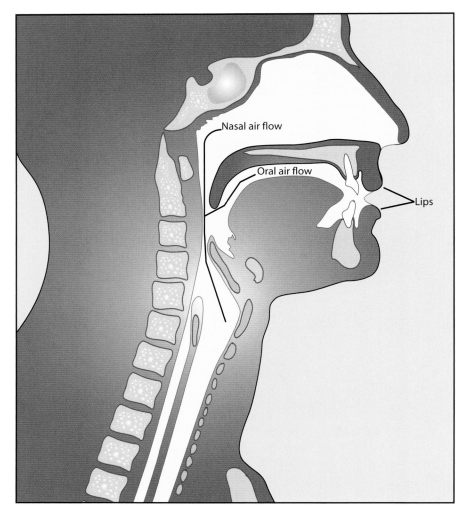

FIGURE 2–11. Airflow directions through the velopharyngeal port and through the oral cavity. Adapted with permission from *Head and Neck Cancer: Treatment, Rehabilitation, and Outcomes* (p. 315), by E. C. Ward and C. J. van As-Brooks, 2007, San Diego: Plural Publishing. Copyright © 2007 by Plural Publishing, Inc.

Muscles of the Resonance System

The velum as a structure is a muscular hydrostat (composed of muscle without an internal skeleton) which makes it exceedingly flexible and easy to move. It must be easy given that it is flopping up and down constantly with every nasal sound that occurs. However, the valve example provided above is perhaps a bit more simplistic than what really exists. Although it is true that the velopharyngeal port is closed by the elevation of the velum, assistance is provided from the sides of the structure as well. That assistance comes from the walls of the

Table 2–3. Speech Sounds That Require Closure at the Velopharyngeal Port

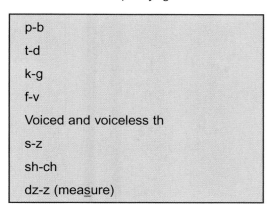

p-b
t-d
k-g
f-v
Voiced and voiceless th
s-z
sh-ch
dz-z (measure)

pharynx, which move toward the velopharyngeal port from the sides. So, rather than a simple lever, velopharyngeal closure occurs with elevation of the velum and lateral movement of the pharyngeal walls almost like a sphincter. The primary muscles of the pharynx that contribute to that closure are the superior constrictor muscles (Figure 2–12).

The muscles of the soft palate, or velum (Figure 2–13) also are categorized according to their action on the velum; elevator, tensor, or depressor. The levator veli palatini is a paired muscle that

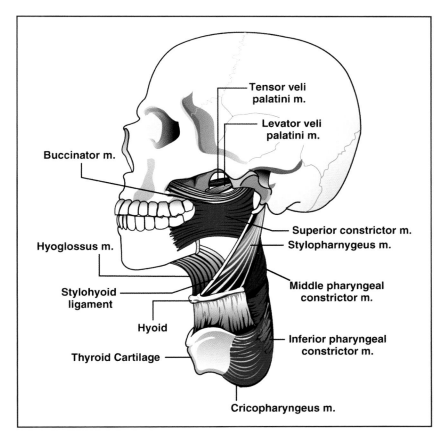

FIGURE 2–12. Superior pharyngeal constrictors. Adapted with permission from *Speech and Voice Science* (p. 286), by A. Behrman, 2007, San Diego: Plural Publishing. Copyright © 2007 by Plural Publishing, Inc.

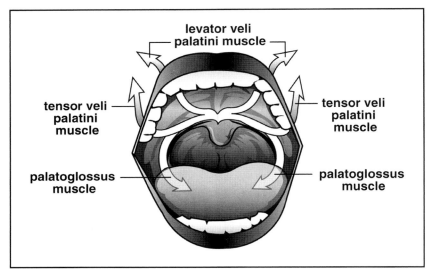

FIGURE 2–13. Muscles of the velum. Adapted with permission from *Speech and Voice Science* (p. 287), by A. Behrman, 2007, San Diego: Plural Publishing. Copyright © 2007 by Plural Publishing, Inc.

makes up the bulk of the soft palate. The muscle originates from the temporal bone of the skull and courses down to insert into an aponeurosis (sheet of tendon) in the velum lateral to the uvula. When contracted, the levator veli palatini elevates the soft palate to close the velopharyngeal port. There are two muscles that are categorized as velum "tensors." Those muscles are the musculus uvula and the tensor veli palatini. The thought is that tensor muscles provide extra tension to the velum when a tight seal is required (sounds requiring high intraoral pressure). In reality, it is unclear how much these two muscles actually assist with closure by providing extra tension. The final two muscles are considered velar depressors. The velum is depressed (put away your antidepressants, I mean *lowered*) during many of the speech sounds, and most of the time for breathing. The muscles that assist with

that function are the paired palatoglossus and the palatopharyngeus muscles.

The Articulatory System

If the speech mechanism is viewed as a hierarchy of component systems, then the articulators would be at the top. With the air provided by the respiratory system, the sound source by the phonatory system, and the resonant characteristics and airflow by the resonance system, the articulators function to shape the sound in the oral cavity into meaningful units that we recognize as speech/language for the process of communication. There are a number of structures, called articulators, that we utilize to help shape and configure the airflow and sound that travels through the oral cavity. These structures include the teeth, hard palate, lips, tongue, and mandible (jaw). Several of these structures are immobile (e.g., teeth, hard palate), providing more of a foundation than actually contributing to the production of sound. The remaining articulators, the lips, tongue, and mandible move freely and their mobility contributes to the production of many sounds (Table 2–4).

Lips

The lips are comprised of muscles, many of which are active during the process of speech. A variety of labial (lip) movements are utilized in producing speech sounds, compression, retraction, rounding, and placement behind the teeth, to provide a few examples. The orbicularis oris is the primary muscle of the lips and surrounds the entire mouth. Additional muscles of facial expression, which function to move the lips in different directions and provide a variety functions that contribute to communication, insert into the orbicularis oris. For example, the Elvis sneer, a wide smile, even a sad frown (Figure 2–14) are all accomplished by muscles that insert into the orbicularis oris.

Mandible

The mandible or lower jaw is another of the dynamic articulators. The jaw functions to provide support for the tongue, and to change the shape of the vocal tract. As the only movable joint of the mandible is at the temporomandibular joint, the movements of the mandible are limited to up, forward, lateral, and down. Therefore, the muscles that move the mandible act to elevate, protrude, or depress the jaw (Figure 2–15). The mandibular elevators consist of the masseter, the medial pterygoid, and the temporalis muscles. The masseter and the medial pterygoid meet and wrap around the angle of the mandible (the bend in the lower jaw located under the ears). The temporalis

Table 2–4. Articulatory Placements for Speech Sounds

Articulators	Speech Sounds			
Lips	p – pull	b – bee	m – my	w – we
Lips + Teeth	f – four	v – vine		
Teeth + Tongue	*th – thick	*th – there		
Tongue + Hard Palate	t – two	d – dime	s – see	z – zoo
	n – new	l – low	sh – show	z – measure
	y – yes	r – ray		
Tongue + Velum	k – key	g – get	ng – ring	
Vocal Folds	h – hay			
Nasal sounds (velum elevated/closed)	m – my	n – new	ng – ring	

*Note that speech sounds may sound different even though they are represented by the same letter. You will understand this phenomenon when you learn about phonetics.

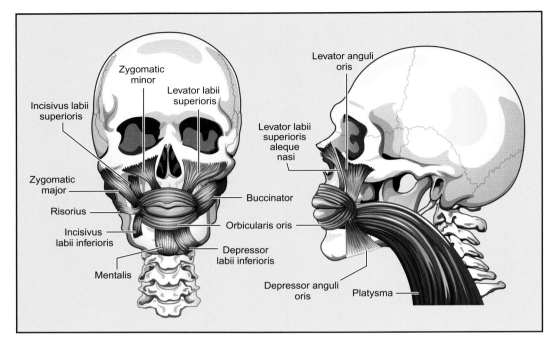

FIGURE 2–14. Facial muscles. From *Preclinical Speech Science* (p. 256), by T. J. Hixon, G. Weismer, and J. D. Hoit, 2008, Plural Publishing. Copyright © 2008 by Plural Publishing, Inc. Reprinted with permission.

can be felt externally by clenching the teeth and feeling the action over the temples. When these muscles contract, they snap or pull the mandible shut. The internal or medial pterygoid protrudes (and actually allows for some lateral movement as well) the mandible, which actually is more applicable to chewing than for speech. The protrusion action contributes to the grinding of food during chewing/swallowing. The mandibular depressors, the digastricus, mylohyoid, geniohyoid, and platysma act to lower the jaw when necessary for chewing as well as speech production.

Tongue

The tongue has been called the most important and active of the articulators. Changing the shape and position of the tongue in the vocal tract results in the production of vowels, and the tongue interacts with other articulators in producing a good number of the consonants. The tongue also is a muscular hydrostat, like the velum. Therefore, it is highly flexible, which is likely why it is so active during speech. Made up of muscle, there are extrinsic and intrinsic muscles responsible for movement (Figure 2–16). As with the extrinsic muscles of the larynx, extrinsic tongue muscles primarily act to move the bulk of the tongue around and the intrinsic primarily change the shape of the tongue. As the tongue is active for such a large selection of speech sounds, it has to be capable of a wide variety of movements (i.e., elevating the tip, protruding through the teeth, creating a groove down midline for airflow to travel

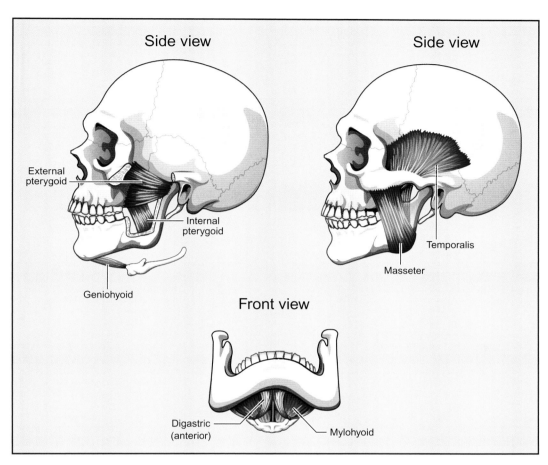

FIGURE 2–15. Muscles of the mandible. From *Preclinical Speech Science* (p. 250), by T. J. Hixon, G. Weismer, and J. D. Hoit, 2008, Plural Publishing. Copyright © 2008 by Plural Publishing, Inc. Reprinted with permission.

FIGURE 2–16. Muscles of the tongue. Public domain at Wikimedia Commons. This faithful reproduction of a lithograph plate from *Gray's Anatomy*, a two-dimensional work of art, is not copyrightable in the United States as per Bridgeman Art Library v. Corel Corp.

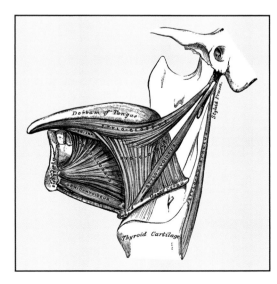

through). What is even more remarkable is the speed and precision with which these actions (and so many more) are carried out. A review of Table 2–4 indicates the sounds that are produced using the tongue.

References

Andreassen, M., Smith, B., & Guyette, T. (1992). Pressure-flow measurements for selected oral and nasal sound segments produced by normal adults. *Cleft Palate-Craniofacial Journal, 12*, 1–9.

Arkebauer, H., Hixon, T., & Hardy, J. (1967). Peak intra-oral air pressures during speech. *Journal of Speech and Hearing Research, 10*, 196–208.

Boone, D., & McFarland, S. (1994). *The voice and voice therapy.* Englewood Cliffs, NJ: Prentice-Hall.

Cassell, M., & Ekaldi, H. (1995). Anatomy and physiology of the palate and velopharyngeal apertures. In R. Shprintzen & J. Bardach (Eds.), *Cleft palate speech management: A multidisciplinary approach* (pp. 45–61). St. Louis, MO: Mosby.

Green, J., Moore, C., Higashikawa, M., & Steeve, R. (2000). The physiological development of speech motor control: Lip and jaw coordination. *Journal of Speech, Language, and Hearing Research, 43*, 239–255.

Green J., & Wang, Y. (2003). Tongue-surface movement patterns during speech and swallowing. *Journal of the Acoustical Society of America, 113*, 2820–2833.

Hirano, M. (1981). *Clincal examination of the voice.* New York, NY: Springer-Verlag Wien.

Hirano, M., Ohala, J., & Vennard, W. (1969). The function of the laryngeal muscles in regulating fundamental frequency and intensity of phonation. *Journal of Speech and Hearing Research, 12*, 616–628.

Hixon, T. J., & Hoit, J. D. (1997). Physical examination of the diaphragm by the speech-language pathologist. *American Journal of Speech-Language Pathology, 7*, 37–42.

Hixon, T. J., & Hoit, J. D. (1999). Physical examination of the abdominal wall by the speech-language pathologist. *American Journal of Speech-Language Pathology, 8*, 335–346.

Hixon, T. J., & Hoit, J. D. (2000). Physical examination of the rib cage by the speech-language pathologist. *American Journal of Speech-Language Pathology, 9*, 179–196.

Hixon, T. J., & Hoit, J. D. (2005). *Evaluation and management of speech breathing disorders: Principles and methods.* Tucson, AZ: Reddington Brown.

Hixon, T. J., Weismer, G., & Hoit, J. D. (2008). *Preclinical speech science: Anatomy, physiology, acoustics, perception.* San Diego, CA: Plural Publishing.

Hollien, H., & Moore, P. (1960). Measurements of the vocal folds during changes in pitch. *Journal of Speech and Hearing Research, 3*, 157–163.

Johnson, A., & Jacobson, B. (1998). *Medical speech-language pathology: A practitioner's guide.* New York, NY: Thieme Medical Publishers.

Kent, R. (1976). Anatomical and neuromuscular maturation of the speech mechanism: Evidence from acoustic studies. *Journal of Speech and Hearing Research, 19*, 421–447.

Kent, R. (1997). *The speech sciences.* San Diego, CA: Singular.

Kent, R., & Vorperian, H. (1995). Development of the craniofacial-oral-laryngeal anatomy: A review. *Journal of Medical Speech-Language Pathology, 3*, 145–190.

Liss, J., Kuehn, D., & Hinkle, K. (1994). Direct training of velopharyngeal musculature. *Journal of Medical Speech-Language Pathology, 2*, 243–249.

Moon, J., Kuehn, D., & Huisman, J. (1994a). Measurement of velopharyngeal closure force during vowel production. *Cleft Palate-Craniofacial Journal, 31*, 356–363.

Moon J., Smith, A., Folkins, J., Lemke, J., & Gartlan, M. (1994b). Coordination of velopharyngeal muscle activity during positioning of the soft palate. *Cleft Palate-Craniofacial Journal, 31,* 45–55.

Netsell, R. (1973). Speech physiology. In F. Minifie, T. Hixon, & F. Williams (Eds.), *Normal aspects of speech, hearing, and language* (pp. 211–234). Englewood-Cliffs, NJ: Prentice-Hall.

Plant, R., & Younger, R. (2000). The interrelationship of subglottic air pressure, fundamental frequency, and vocal intensity during speech. *Journal of Voice, 14,* 170–177.

Seikel, J. A., King, D. W., & Drumwright, D. G. (2005). *Anatomy and physiology for speech, language, and hearing* (3rd ed.). Clifton Park, NY: Thompson Delmar Learning.

Titze, I. (1994). *Principles of voice production.* Englewood-Cliffs, NJ: Prentice Hall.

Ward, E. C., & van As-Brooks, C. J. (2006). *Head and neck cancer: Treatment, rehabilitation, and outcomes.* San Diego, CA: Plural Publishing.

Webster, D. B. (1995). *Neuroscience of communication.* San Diego, CA: Singular Publishing Group.

Zemlin, W. R. (1998). *Speech and hearing science: Anatomy and physiology.* Boston, MA: Allyn and Bacon.

3

Neurological Causes of Communication Disorders

What causes this? One minute she was fine. The love of my life. The one who canoes like a trooper and loves to pick berries by the side of the lake. Next minute it's like a bolt out of the blue and she's babbling, half-paralyzed, and not herself at all. Sure, she had a little high blood pressure. Her whole family does. But she's fit. She does Pilates and runs marathons. What is the little devil inside her head that caused this? How did this happen? I had an argument with her. Is this my fault? Did I bring all this on? Help me. Please explain. This is my soul mate. She is the most flawless person in the world, an angel (Figure 3–1). She loves trees and homeless people and puppies. She adopted an orphan from a Catholic school in India. Why can't she talk or think or remember? Will she continue to get worse? Help me. I feel I'm lost and I sure as hell don't have a GPS to get me out.

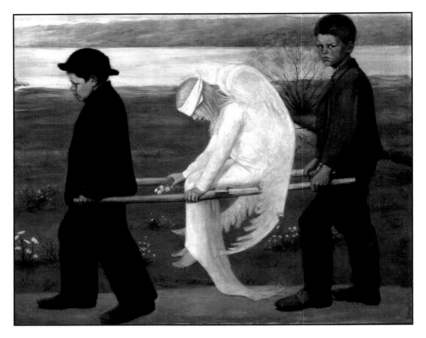

FIGURE 3–1. "The Wounded Angel" by Hugo Simberg. Public domain at Wikimedia Commons.

Introduction

The American Speech-Language-Hearing Association (ASHA) estimates that 49 million Americans have some type of communication disorder. Persons of all ages can be affected by a communication disorder that may result from a variety of causes (e.g., stroke, trauma, or other injury to the brain, injury to facial structure or muscles, neurodegenerative diseases, pediatric cancer, occult differences in neural development as in autism spectrum disorders). These communication disorders can occur in isolation (specific language impairment) or they may coexist with other developmental disorders such as mental retardation or cerebral palsy. In young children, communication disorders represent the most common developmental problem. As broadly defined by ASHA, it is estimated that between 15 and 25% of young children have some form of communication disorder (ASHA, 2009; http://www.asha.org/default.htm).

What Do We Know About the Causes of Communication Disorders?

Frequently, the specific cause of a communication disorder is unknown. Some common problems that coexist with communication disorders include cerebral palsy and other nerve/muscle disorders, traumatic brain injury, stroke, viral diseases, mental retardation, effects of certain drugs, structural impairments such as cleft lip or palate, vocal abuse or misuse, or inadequate speech and language models (ASHA, 2009).

Etiology

The brain is a marvelous thing. It has been rhapsodized in poem and song and called everything from an enchanted loom that weaves a never-ending stream of dissolving patterns to a computer on steroids (Figure 3–2). Listen to Diane Ackerman (2004) talk about the brain:

> Shaped a little like a loaf of French country bread, our brain is a crowded chemistry lab, bustling with nonstop neural conversations. Imagine the brain, that shiny mound of being, that mouse-gray parliament of cells, that dream factory, that petite tyrant inside a ball of bone, that huddle of neurons calling all the plays, that little everywhere, that fickle pleasuredome, that wrinkled wardrobe of selves stuffed into the skull like too many clothes into a gym bag. (p. 1)

Sometimes that mouse-gray parliament of cells; that dream factory creates a nightmare. When the brain goes bad there is misery to pay. Although many diseases or conditions that affect the brain do not result in communication disorders, there is a vast array of disturbances of speech, voice, and language that are a direct consequence of brain damage. Thus, a communication disorder can be the consequence and is many times one of the very first signs of brain dysfunction.

Aphasia is always caused by injury to the brain, most commonly from a stroke, particularly in older individuals. Even though stroke is the most common cause of brain injury resulting in aphasia, it also may occur from head trauma, brain tumors, or brain infections. Not every stroke or brain injury results in aphasia, but the condition of aphasia is never present without some sort of brain

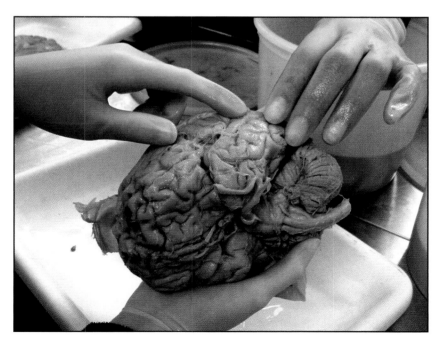

FIGURE 3–2. Brain (LaPointe photo).

damage. Likewise with motor speech disorders. By definition, these disruptions of speech are the result of underlying movement changes in range, direction, velocity, or coordination of movement.

Cerebrovascular Accident

Cerebrovascular accident (CVA) or stroke is by far the leading cause of brain-based communication disorders (Figure 3–3). A stroke takes place when a blood clot blocks a blood vessel or artery, or when a cerebral artery breaks, interrupting blood flow to a portion of the brain. The stroke kills or weakens brain cells in the immediate area. Those neurons or brain cells that are affected by a direct hit usually die within minutes to a few hours after the stroke begins. When brain cells (neurons) die, the abilities they controlled are lost or impaired. This includes functions such as speech, language, movement, sensation, and memory. The specific abilities lost or affected depend on where in the brain the stroke occurs and on the size of the stroke (i.e., the extent of brain cell death). As the left cerebral hemisphere is the area that controls language in upward of 90% of people who are right-handed (the ratio of language dominance is less, but still favors the left hemisphere in left-handed people), nearly all cases of aphasia can be traced to damage in the left cerebral cortex. That does not mean that the right cerebral hemisphere is not involved in any language or language related activities, but certainly the mighty left controls most of language. Three areas of the left cerebral cortex are critical language zones (Figure 3–4). The area around the Sylvian fissure (the peri-Sylvian zone) is an important neighborhood for human language. In that zone of language resides Broca's area (important for the production of speech), Wernicke's area (important for the processing and comprehension of speech), and the PTO cortex (the area of juncture of the parietal, temporal, and occipital lobes of the cerebral cortex; important for reading and word retrieval) (Aphasia.Net, 2010).

These critical areas in the left cerebral hemisphere are those that are vulnerable to damage or lack of oxygen and glucose carried tirelessly by the network of plumbing known as the cerebral vascular system. These vessels of nourishment are ever important to the health of neurons or brain cells. If neurons are deprived of their life-giving nutrients for more than 4 minutes, serious damage can result. First, they weaken and do not fire or transmit neural impulses efficiently, and then after four minutes they die. Brain cells (neurons) are extremely fragile. The constant bath of blood that contains glucose, oxygen, and other nutrients perfuses the brain, and if this perfusion is compromised, the damage begins. That is one of the principal reasons that cardiopulmonary resuscitation (CPR) (Figure 3–5) must be

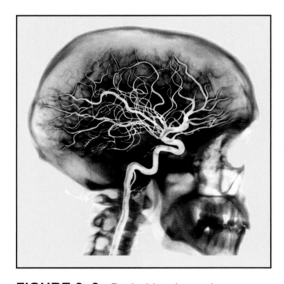

FIGURE 3–3. Brain blood supply.

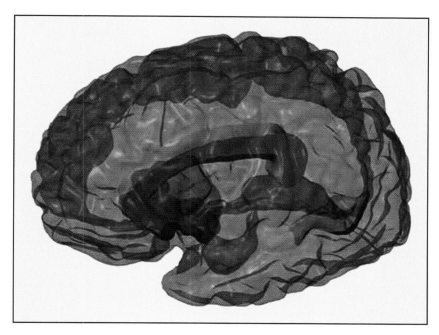

FIGURE 3–4. Speech areas.

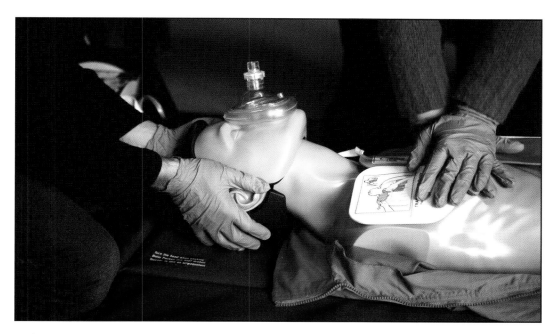

FIGURE 3–5. CPR.

initiated as soon as the heart stops. The heart and cardiac system is responsible for pumping the blood supply into the brain's vascular system and keeping the neurons healthy. By the process of regular chest compressions, the blood can be mechanically forced into the cerebral blood vessels and thus prevent the neurons from losing their vital perfusion of nutrients. In an emergency, when breathing and the pumping of the heart resumes, the CPR that was initiated may have prevented brain damage during the critical interim.

Strokes come in two major types, ischemic and hemorrhagic. Ischemic is a term derived from the word ischemia which means a reduction or loss of blood supply. Hemorrhagic is derived from the term hemorrhage or breaking and leaking of blood (Figure 3–6).

Hemorrhagic Stroke

Hemorrhagic stroke accounts for approximately one out of five strokes and is caused by a blood vessel breaking and leaking blood into or around the brain. The red branchlike structure represents blood vessels and the region of the brain outlined by the gray and red area is the site of the hemorrhage. The gray region represents the brain areas damaged by the stroke. This type of stroke generally is more serious than an ischemic stroke (one caused by a blocked blood vessel). The brain cells normally nourished by the hemorrhaging blood vessel, deprived of oxygen and other nutrients, can perish very quickly. The death of these cells leads to varying states of disability. In the United States, and most likely worldwide, stroke affects women slightly more than it affects men, but the distribution is relatively equal (Aphasia.Net, 2010).

Ischemic Stroke

Ischemic stroke accounts for the vast majority of cerebrovascular accidents. Ischemic stroke occurs when an artery that carries vital nutrients in blood to the brain is blocked. The brain depends on its arteries to bring refreshing blood from the heart and lungs. The blood car-

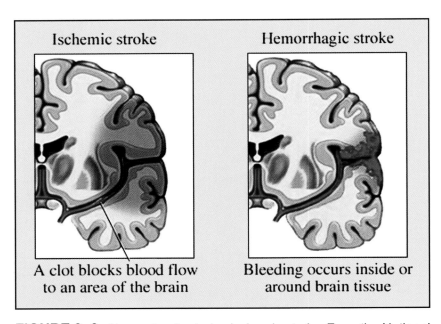

Ischemic stroke

Hemorrhagic stroke

A clot blocks blood flow to an area of the brain

Bleeding occurs inside or around brain tissue

FIGURE 3–6. Hemorrhagic stroke; ischemic stroke. From the National Library of Medicine. Reprinted with permission.

ries oxygen, glucose, and other nutrients to keep the brain alive and functioning, and through the system of veins takes away carbon dioxide and cellular waste. If an artery becomes blocked, the brain cells (*neurons*) cannot generate enough energy to function properly and eventually may die. Ischemic stroke can be caused by many different kinds of diseases. The most common problem is narrowing of the arteries in the neck or head. Most often, this is caused by *atherosclerosis*, or gradual cholesterol or plaque deposits that stick to the insides of the artery. If the arteries become too narrow, blood cells may collect and begin to coagulate or form clots. These blood clots can block the artery where they are formed (*thrombosis*), or can break loose and become trapped to form little dams that restrict blood flow upstream in the brain (*embolism*). Blood clots also can form in other parts of the body (legs, heart, lungs) and travel through the maroon stream to the brain. In the heart, for example, clots can occur as a result of irregular heartbeat (for example, *atrial fibrillation*), heart attack, or abnormalities of the heart valves. Although these are the most common causes of ischemic stroke, there are many other possible causes. Examples include use of recreational street drugs, knife wounds, or other traumatic injuries to the blood vessels of the neck, or abnormal blood clotting. Thromboembolic strokes are responsible for over 50% of all strokes (Stroke Center, 2010).

Mad Cows and Other Prion Diseases

"Within the last few years, unconventional slow CNS infections, the Prion disorders, have been described and defined. In 1997 the second Noble Prize

was awarded in this field to Dr. Stanley Prusiner who has championed the concept of the prion. Our understanding of this group of diseases began with veterinarian virologists and neuropathologists who earlier in this century described spongiform pathology in the disease Scrapie, proved it transmissible, and developed rodent models that have vastly contributed to our understanding." (http://www.path.sunysb.edu/faculty/woz/NPERESS/webclass2p2.htm). Other scientists described spongiform pathology in Creutzfeldt-Jacob disease (C-J disease), which also encouraged the successful transmission experiments. The list of transmissible diseases from animals to humans is large and growing. It includes sporadic, transmissible diseases like Kuru and C-J in humans and Scrapie, Mad Cow disease, and mink encephalopathy in animals. All of these diseases can affect the ability to use language and cognition (State University of New York, Stony Brook, 2010).

Causes and Scope of Brain-Based Disorders

The following table estimates the incidence of the major causes of brain impairment in adulthood in the United States. The estimates are conservative, excluding rare disorders for which reliable data are not available. These statistics are extracted from a very useful Web site designed for caregivers of persons with brain-based disorders (Family Caregiver Alliance, 2009) (http://www.caregiver.org/caregiver/jsp/home.jsp) Worldwide figures on brain-based disorders in general or neurogenic communication disorders more specifically are not available, but educated extrapolation can be conducted to get an idea of the scope of the problem. It is not insignificant. If the data presented for the approximate 294,000,000 population of the United States holds, then one can find the population of any given country and determine the incidence or prevalence of a condition. In the United States, for example, one case of aphasia is expected for every 272 residents. Based on the current population this yields a prevalence of 1,079,600 persons with aphasia. Based on population, therefore we would expect 16,000 Croatians to have aphasia; 10,000 Mongolians; nearly 4 million Indians; 84,000 Taiwanese; 253,000 Turks; and 178,000 South Koreans. Certainly, there are risks to accuracy in extrapolated estimates, but if these data are based on acceptable premises, they can be more useful than having no information; especially for realizing the scope of the problem and planning for the future (World Health Organization, 2007).

For clarification, the term incidence refers to the ratio or expected percentage of a condition or disorder relative to a predetermined number of people (e.g., the incidence of pediatric brain tumors in the United States is 2.1 per 100,000 children). Prevalence, on the other hand is the actual number of people with a disease or condition in a defined community (e.g., 14,683 people in New Zealand have aphasia). Table 3–1 shows an estimated 1.2 million people aged 18 years and older who are diagnosed annually with adult onset brain disease/disorders in the United States. This table also presents an overview of the major etiologies or causes of brain-based disorders. Well over 200 diseases or conditions have associated neurogenic pathologies. These tables present some of the more frequently observed conditions, syndromes, or causes. Many

Table 3–1. Incidence of Adult Onset Brain Disorders in the United States

Diagnosis/Cause	People Diagnosed Annually
Alzheimer's disease	250,000
Amyotrophic lateral sclerosis	5,000
Brain tumor	33,039
Epilepsy	135,500
HIV (AIDS) dementia	1,196
Huntington disease	N/A
Multiple sclerosis	10,400
Parkinson disease	54,927
Stroke	600,000
Traumatic brain injury	80,000
TOTAL ESTIMATED INCIDENCE	1,170,062

more rare or relatively obscure brain-based disorders have been documented in the medical literature, but these are the most likely to be encountered.

More than one million adults in the United States are diagnosed annually with a chronic brain disease or disorder. The need for both long-term care and support for family caregivers is dramatic. Many of these conditions, for example Alzheimer disease, stroke, and Parkinson disease, are associated with increasing age. Given the aging of the United States population, and extrapolated to similar industrialized countries, global figures will increase drastically in the coming decades. This table illustrates the long-term nature of caregiving for many of these conditions. Although it is estimated that one quarter of a million people are diagnosed with Alzheimer's disease annually in the United States, an estimated four million people are living with the disease, many of whom require 24-hour care. Furthermore, the number of households affected by brain impairment only begins to elucidate the impact of brain-based disorders upon family caregivers and the long-term care system. With many individuals requiring 24-hour care, there often are several family members from different households involved in the caregiving process including spouses, adult children, siblings, and friends. Often, these caregivers are juggling the responsibilities of caregiving, child rearing, and employment simultaneously (World Health Organization, 2007).

The brain can be damaged in many ways. Strokes (CVAs) are the most frequent causes of aphasia, but the zones of language can be compromised by traumatic brain injury, infections, diseases, toxicity, or poisons, or any of the other evil influences that can result in malfunction of neurons or brain cells. More about these nonfocal causes of communication disorders in Chapter 5.

Pediatric Conditions

Most of the nasty brain pathologies that can affect adults can also affect children, though in different proportions and with altered consequence since they occur against the backdrop of physical, mental, communicative, cognitive, and social development (Figure 3–7).

Cerebral Palsy

Cerebral palsy (CP) is an umbrella term encompassing a group of nonprogressive, noncontagious conditions that cause

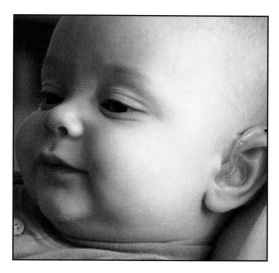

FIGURE 3–7. Baby head.

physical disability in human development. *Cerebral* refers to the affected area of the brain, or the cerebrum (however, the areas of damage have not been localized precisely and the condition most likely involves connections between the cortex and many other parts of the brain such as the cerebellum and basal ganglia). *Palsy* is the rather antiquated term that refers to a disorder of movement. CP is caused by damage to the motor control centers of the developing brain and can occur during pregnancy (about 75%), during childbirth (about 5%) or after birth (about 15%) up to about age three. It is a nonprogressive disorder, meaning the brain damage does not worsen, but secondary orthopedic difficulties are common. There is no known cure for CP. Medical intervention is limited to the treatment and prevention of complications possible from CP's consequences. It, along with the other congenital or postnatal neuromuscular conditions such as all the variants of muscular dystrophy, can play havoc with the developing communication, swallowing, and sometimes cognitive-linguistic systems and create barriers to everyday existence (National Center on Birth Defects, 2010).

Autism Spectrum Disorders

Presumably the disorder has always existed, but not until the middle of the twentieth century was there a label for a disorder that now appears to affect an estimated 3.4 of every 1,000 children ages 3–10, a disorder that causes disruption in families and discontented lives for many children (Figure 3–8). In 1943, Dr. Leo Kanner of the Johns Hopkins Hospital studied a group of 11 children and introduced the label *early infantile autism* into the English language. At the same time a German scientist, Dr. Hans Asperger, described a milder form of the disorder that became known as Asperger syndrome (National Institutes of Mental Health: NIH, 2010). These two disorders were described and are today listed in the *Diagnostic and Statistical Manual of Mental Disorders* DSM-IV (American Psychiatric Association, 2007) as two of the five pervasive developmental disorders (PDD), more often referred to today as autism spectrum disorders (ASD). All these disorders are characterized by varying degrees of impairment in communication skills, social interactions, and

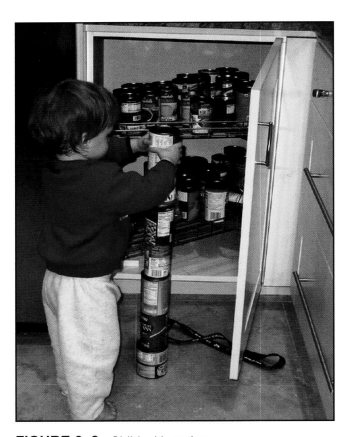

FIGURE 3–8. Child with autism.

restricted, repetitive, and stereotyped patterns of behavior (Jepson, Wright, & Johnson, 2007).

The autism spectrum disorders often can be reliably detected by the age of 3 years, and in some cases as early as 18 months. Florida State University has an active Center for Autism and Related Disorders under the direction of Amy Wetherby and has been a leader in the recognition and development of "red flags" for even earlier identification and intervention. Studies suggest that many children eventually may be accurately identified by the age of 1 year or even younger. The appearance of any of the warning signs of ASD is reason to have a child evaluated by a professional specializing in these disorders. Parents usually are the first to notice unusual behaviors in their child. In some cases, the baby seemed "different" from birth, unresponsive to people or focusing intently on one item for long periods of time. The first signs of an ASD also can be noticed in children who appear to have been developing within normal expectations. Early warning signs are triggered when an engaging, babbling toddler becomes mute, withdrawn, self-abusive, or indifferent to social overtures. Parents notice these changes although sometimes it is a health care professional who first tunes in to them. The pervasive developmental disorders, or autism spectrum disorders, range from a severe form, called autistic disorder, to a milder form, Asperger syndrome. If a child has signs or symptoms of either of these disorders, but does not meet the specific criteria for either, the diagnosis waffles a bit and is called pervasive developmental disorder not otherwise specified (PDD-NOS). Other rare, very severe disorders that are included in

the autism spectrum disorders are Rett syndrome and childhood disintegrative disorder (Jepson et al., 2007).

As is apparent in nearly all subdisciplines or areas of neuroscience, brain-imaging strategies have advanced our knowledge. These new magical tools—computerized tomography (CT), positron emission tomography (PET), single photon emission computed tomography (SPECT), and magnetic resonance imaging (MRI) (Figure 3–9), and functional magnetic resonance imaging (fMRI), have kick-started study of the structure and the function of the brain. This new technology and increasing availability of both normal and autism tissue samples for postmortem brain analysis studies has heartened researchers and facilitated the road to clearer understanding of these brain-based disorders. Postmortem and MRI studies have shown that many major brain structures are implicated in autism. These include the cerebellum, cerebral cortex, limbic system, corpus callosum, basal ganglia, and brainstem. Other research is focusing on the role of neurotransmitters such as serotonin, dopamine, and epinephrine, particularly in their possible role in the repetitive behaviors so characteristic of autism. Research into the myriad network of causes of autism spectrum disorders is being assisted by other recent developments. Evidence points to genetic factors playing a prominent role in the causes for ASD. Twin and family studies point to an underlying genetic vulnerability for the development of ASD. Autism spectrum disorder is a web within an enigma and recent research on this brain-based disorder is beginning to illuminate grains of optimism at the far end of the tunnel (National Institutes of Mental Health: NIH, 2010).

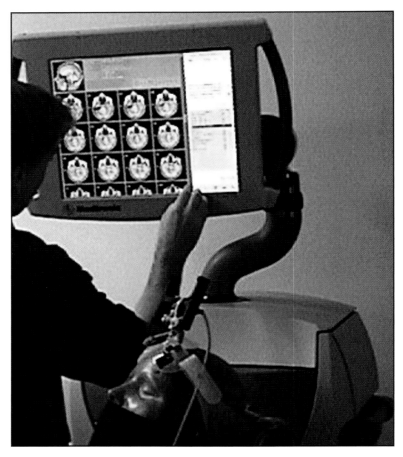

FIGURE 3–9. MRI (LaPointe photo).

Risk Factors

Risk factors for brain-based disorders of communication and swallowing are strongly related to the risk factors for the many types of brain damage. Stroke is the leading cause of aphasia and other disorders of communication. The risk factors for this condition are the most salient and sometimes the least understood. Some stroke risk factors are hereditary. Others are a function of natural aging processes (American Heart Association, 2010). Still others result from a person's lifestyle. You cannot choose your gene pool or alter factors related to

heredity or natural processes, but those resulting from lifestyle or environment can be changed. As nutrition and the nature of a person's activities are within the wonderful world of options, people can reduce the lifestyle aspects of risk for stroke and aphasia. Moderate ingestion of gravy and chili-laden French fries, and laying off the triple bacon cheeseburgers (Figure 3–10) can go a long way to altering the nutrition time bombs that lurk in our arteries waiting to turn into aphasia-causing strokes.

A better balance of fruits, vegetables, grains, and healthy food choices (Figure 3–11) rather than double rich

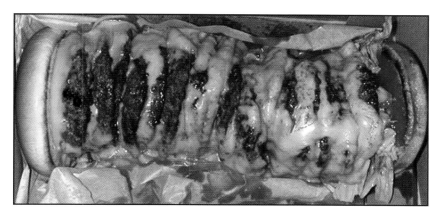

FIGURE 3–10. Cheeseburger.

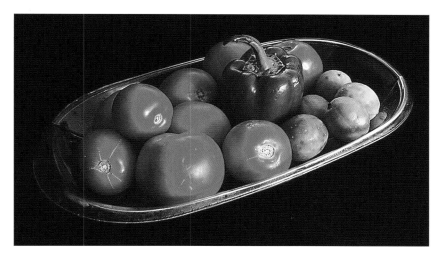

FIGURE 3–11. Fruits (LaPointe photo).

"chunky monkey" ice cream slathered on "death by chocolate" cake can help. Similarly, a lifestyle that incorporates heavy smoking, pouring down double Jager shots chased with less filling brew and an exercise program that consists mostly of chasing little demons around a video game screen is a stroke waiting to happen. In some people later; in many sooner. Lifestyle counts. We can't do much about choosing our relatives, but we can influence how we live our life, and these decisions can affect our likelihood for stroke and disordered communication.

Similarly, as brain trauma is a frequent cause of aphasia as well, our lifestyle choices can alter our probability of ending up with scrambled sentences. Motor vehicular risk takers who practice the Tokyo drift in high-powered cars or drive in a drunken stupor or while texting or chattering away on a cell phone significantly increase their risk for ending up with a bunch of dead brain cells. Not to mention the damage they can cause to people they run into or run over. Brain damage and aphasia arise from many unfortunate sources. We should attempt to control the factors that in fact are under our control. High blood pressure (hypertension), diabetes, smoking, overexuberant alcohol consumption, and buckets of deep fried chicken for breakfast are serious risk factors associated with stroke.

References

Ackerman, D. (2004). *An alchemy of mind.* New York, NY: Simon and Schuster.

American Heart Association. (2010). *Risk factors.* Retrieved February 9, 2010, from http://www.americanheart.org/presenter.jhtml?identifier=9217

American Psychiatric Association. (2007). *Diagnostic and statistical manual of mental disorders. TR* (4th ed.). New York, NY: American Psychiatric Publishing.

American Speech-Language-Hearing Association. (2009). Retrieved April 13, 2009, from http://www.asha.org/default.htm.

Aphasia Net. (2010). *Stroke.* Retrieved February 9, 2010, from http://www.aphasia.net/info/stroke/default.asp

Family Caregiver Alliance. (2009). Retrieved April 13, 2009, from http://www.caregiver.org/caregiver/jsp/home.jsp

Jepson, B., Wright, K., & Johnson, J. (2007). *Changing the course of autism: A scientific approach for parents and physicians.* Boulder, CO: Sentient Press.

National Center on Birth Defects. (2010). *Cerebral palsy.* Retrieved February 9, 2010, from http://www.cdc.gov/cerebral palsy.htm

National Institutes of Mental Health: NIH. (2010). *Autism.* Retrieved February 9, 2010, from http://www.nimh.nih.gov/health/publications/autism/introduction.shtml

State University of New York: Stony Brook. (2010). *Prion disease.* Retrieved February 9, 2010, from http://www.path.sunysb.edu/faculty/woz/NPERESS/webclass2p2.htm

Stroke Center. (2010). *Patients.* Retrieved February 9, 2010, from http://www.strokecenter.org/patients/ais.htm

World Health Organization. (2007). *Neurological disorders: Public health challenges.* New York, NY: World Health Organization Press.

4

Aphasia

A Strange Jumble of Words . . .

Frank Dietz is a 56-year-old married man with two children who lives in Sopchoppy, a small Florida river town close to the state capital and college town of Tallahassee. He is a Vietnam War veteran who served in the Marines during the Tet offensive, a casualty-laden conflict between American armed forces and the Viet Cong. Though several of his platoon mates were killed or critically wounded during this conflict, Frank escaped with a flesh wound to his right buttock. After his evacuation to Japan and recuperation in a Florida Veterans Medical Center, he was discharged from the service and took job as a beer truck driver and distributor for the Budweiser brewing company. He often quipped about his lone medal and wound that he had received a "Purple Heart for my purple ass." Frank is a fisherman and outdoors person with a hearty, rollicking sense of humor and a boisterous laugh. He drove his beer truck through the back roads of rural Florida and delivered Budweiser and other brands of liquid refreshment for 31 years. On his days off he enjoyed driving to the Florida fishing hotspots around Apalachicola and, after a day of scalloping or fishing for red-fish along the tidal rivers or the St. Joe Bay, would swap stories with Gator, Randy, Little Willie, and the regulars at the Indian Pass Raw Bar. Over the years, Frank developed diabetes and high blood pressure and tried to control both with diet and lifestyle change, but was not very successful. His old war wound bothered him slightly after a full day's drive, but he had no other major health complaints, except for two episodes of memory loss, weakness in his right arm, and jumbled speech. Both of these episodes completely cleared within 24 hours and Frank vowed to start watching his weight. On the morning of October 30, Frank was found in the kitchen of his home staring in bewildered fashion and unable to respond to questions. His attempts to speak resulted in what was described as "nonsense words" and "calling his family members the wrong name." He was taken by medical emergency vehicle to the Tallahassee Memorial Hospital and treated for an "acute left hemisphere thromboembolic cerebrovascular accident." In lay terms, Frank had suffered a stroke, a serious medical condition that left him with loss of feeling and loss of movement on the right side of his body, including his lower face. After he was neurologically and medically stable, he was evaluated by the rehabilitation stroke team. The speech-language pathologist administered the Revised Token Test, the Western Aphasia Battery, the Reading Comprehension Battery for Aphasia, and completed a medical, social, and lifestyle history to determine his prestroke and current facility and use of language and speech. Frank was reported to have aphasia. His aphasia was labeled "Nonfluent or Broca's Aphasia characterized by telegraphic speech (agrammatism), reduced sentence and utterance length, and relatively intact comprehension of speech." He also was reported to produce "verbal paraphasias primarily of the semantic-type," and "laborious and imprecise production of speech sounds." His reading was impaired and his writing was more intact than his speech, but mirrored much of his verbal output with frequent misspellings, omission of grammatical function words ("of, an, over, the, to, etc.") and frequent use of unintended but related words, such as "bus . . . no truck . . . I mean bus . . ." for the word "car." During struggling attempts to generate sentences, Frank would frequently revert to saying the phrase, "I see it. I can't see it. Can't see it." Frank would swear a lot during unsuccessful speech attempts and his rehabilitation clinicians were puzzled by his occasional outcry of "Purple ass. Purple ass." Frank was treated successfully for his medical conditions of diabetes and hypertension and made adequate recovery after several weeks of rehabilitation in walking and activities of daily living such as dressing himself and personal grooming. His speech, however, remained densely impaired and affected both the type and amount of social activities in which he participated. Frank was profoundly aphasic and becoming increasingly depressed about his condition. As Frank put it, "No good. Talk. Can't talk. Friends. Gone away. Too hard. I'm too happy. Not happy. When? Talk more? Words. Words mean everywhere."

Introduction

Imagine getting off a train in a completely foreign country, say Azerbaijan or Bulgaria, and having no knowledge of the language being spoken (Figure 4–1). You need to find your way to a backpacker's youth hostel and you haven't the foggiest idea how to get there. You approach a kindly looking elderly gentleman and say, "Pardenk me, Womer, gundoot fry me fall location is Plahnkderper for schtuppy?"

The elderly gentleman gets a puzzled look on his face and says, "Lipsvash mi. Obeecham te kato lud."

He smiles, takes you by the arm, and starts walking toward a ramshackle brick building of small businesses and flats.

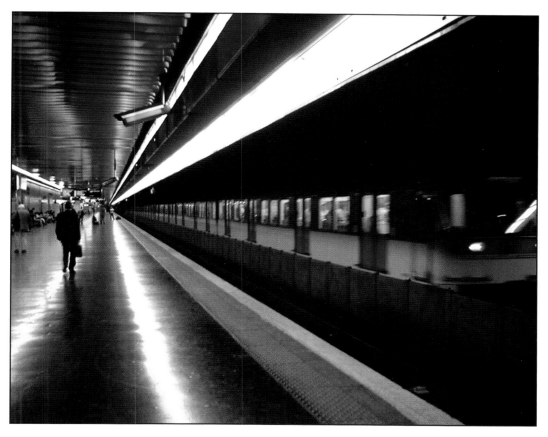

FIGURE 4–1. Railroad station.

You have no idea what he said but you notice a sign above the entrance that reads "Oikokatu Gengatan" (Figure 4–2).

The chill of disorientation and panic begins to set in and you start to realize that you are at the mercy of someone whom you can't understand and who doesn't understand your words. The written or printed word is undecipherable and doesn't look very promising. You are a stranger in a strange land. Your primary means of connecting with everyone else is bizarrely inoperable.

These are the feelings that people with aphasia have described. Betty Penter told me she thought her tongue had been cut out when she awoke from dental oral surgery and was unable to form a meaningful sentence. It was not her tongue at all. She suffered a stroke while under anesthesia and could not talk, understand, read, or write. Arthur Kopit's aviatrix, an airplane stunt woman who suffered aphasia (and whom he memorialized in a remarkable play about aphasia entitled "Wings"), commented on her failure to understand what people were saying to her. She said, "It seemed as though the radio was out; or could pick up only Bucharest!"

We, who have not lost the power of language and speech, can only imagine

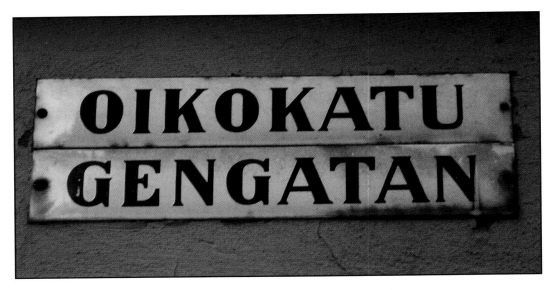

FIGURE 4–2. Entrance sign in foreign language.

or simulate what it must be like. Being transported to a culture, country, or a twilight zone where we cannot make ourselves understood or cannot comprehend what is said is only a small sample of the linguistic and social penalty that must accompany genuine aphasia.

Scope of the Problem

Unlike bubonic plague, aphasia is not an esoteric rare affliction (Figure 4–3). The scope of aphasia is daunting. In the United States, over one million people who have survived the initial insult of brain damage will survive with **aphasia**, the devastating condition of failure to understand or produce the language. This destruction affects a facile language that they mastered long ago, took for granted, and used without as much as a second thought hundreds of times a day. Statistics regarding stroke (also known as cerebrovascular accident or CVA) and aphasia are just as discouraging in other parts of the world.

- Data from 22 European countries indicate that nearly 1 million strokes occur per year in a population of over 500 million.
- In the United Kingdom, more than 100,000 people suffer a stroke every year, 10,000 of whom are still a working age.
- Australia tallies more than 12,000 people per year and stroke is the leading cause of disability Down Under.
- In indigenous Australians, African Americans, and citizens of developing countries and ethnic minorities, the rate of stroke is *double* the number recorded per year compared to Caucasian residents of industrialized nations. (LaPointe, 2005; Data derived from Brain Statistics Table at http://www.braininjurylawtexas.com/brain_statistics.htm)

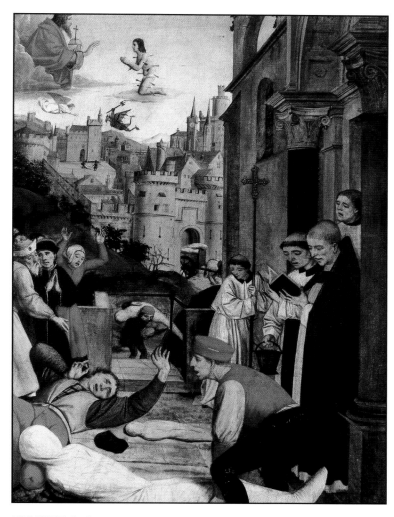

FIGURE 4–3. Diseases. (From "St. Sebastian Interceding for the Plague Stricken," Josse Lieferinxe, 1497–1499. Public domain at Wikimedia Commons).

Definition: What Is Aphasia?

Aphasia is an impairment of language that sabotages the production and the understanding of speech. In some writings, the more accurate term *dysphasia* is used because it refers to a degree of impairment whereas *aphasia* more strictly refers to complete loss of language as a result of brain damage. As in much of our language, usage dictates the preferred term, and at this time the term *aphasia* appears to enjoy the most widespread usage. Everyone who uses the term seems to understand that aphasia refers not only to total loss of language after brain insult, but also all of the gradations and degrees of language impairment as well.

Aphasia affects input as well as output of language use and therefore can degrade the ability to produce or understand the printed or written word as well. People with aphasia can have difficulty reading or writing. As the more basic disorder of aphasia is that of a disturbed or impaired symbol system, aphasia can go beyond just the spoken or written aspects of language. Think for a moment how dependent we are on arbitrary symbol systems that have been incorporated without a second thought into our daily living. Not being able to speak, understand, read, or write is dreadful enough, but the person with aphasia also may have trouble with numbers and mathematics, music notation, telling time, currency or money, or even the more rudimentary symbols such as traffic signals or the warning siren of a fire truck. People who are profoundly hearing impaired since childhood and communicate by sign language can have strokes and find that both the spelling, selection of signs, and order of sign use demonstrate all of the characteristics of aphasia found in hearing, nonsigning persons. Bilingual or polyglot speakers who suffer brain damage in the areas of the brain responsible for linguistic processing frequently discover that there is disparate impairment across native and later learned languages. Sometimes very different patterns emerge across languages as recovery evolves. The characteristics of aphasia are covered in greater detail below.

Aphasia Risk Factors

Risk factors for aphasia are strongly related to the risk factors for the many types of brain damage. As stroke is the leading cause of aphasia, the risk factors for this condition are the most salient (see Chapter 3 section on Risk Factors).

Characteristics of Aphasia

Aphasia is a puzzling and fascinating array of jumbled language. The primary and most obvious observable signs and symptoms include changes in the lexical-semantic sphere of linguistic use. Vocabulary and word selection miscues are the most frequent culprits. The predominant feature of aphasia is in lexical-semantic skill and a person will have inordinate trouble trying to retrieve correct words especially when attempting to name things.

"I know what it is. I rode here to the clinic in it. I rode in our bus . . . no, not bus. Our tray . . . Not train. Our car. Our car. I rode in our car."

Another common problem is the ability to put words together into sentences, and the language difficulty seems more focused on elements of syntax or grammar.

"She never said coming for home for summer. Summer won't be able to home for them."

"Show. Movie. Wife goes movie. Fine show. Too long. Home late."

More commonly multiple aspects of language are impaired in aphasia. Some channels or modalities can be spared or relatively unimpaired while other features or channels are not functional at all. Reading and writing might not be as severely impaired as speaking and understanding. Auditory comprehension can be spared more than reading comprehension. Speaking and producing correctly formulated sentences frequently is more damaged than understanding what others say. Writing is sometimes the only spared modality of expression, but it can be jumbled as well, and a typical attempt to write a note by a person with aphasia could read:

> *Gone past Doctor. So fly supper to gent. Don't worry for Jane, too. Bye.*

The Salad of Aphasic Characteristics

Above we outlined the primary language and related features that result in the mix of ingredients that can be observed in aphasia. It may truly resemble a multicomponent linguistic hodgepodge. Listed below are many of the characteristics that one observes in aphasia, but certainly not all of them.

Speech Production Problems

- Speaks only in single words
- Speaks in short, fragmented phrases
- Anomia (can't name words)
- Paraphasia (use of nonintended words; *chocolate for soup; hanger for airplane*)
- Agrammatism or telegraphic speech (omits small function words such as *of, the, like, but,* etc. so sentences appear like words in a telegram)
- Organizes and speaks words in wrong order
- Switches sounds and/or words (*tephaclone for telephone; wash disher for dish washer*)
- Neologisms, jargon, or new words (*falderbil for Buckingham; cuffolt for silverware; Ferbis for Wertz*)
- Jargon sentences (*I've got some goop in my fingus and my radiator is running funny by the twitcher.*)
- Can't write name or copy words
- Verbal stereotypic or recurrent utterances (*My, my, my. Oh no. No, no no. Anything else but. Anything else but. Jesus, Mary, and Keepsemfromfloppin.*)

Speech Comprehension or Receptive Problems

- Slow to understand messages or sentences
- Can't comprehend normal or fast speech
- Can't follow directions, especially those that exceed one-step commands
- Can't read newspapers or magazines
- Impaired recognition of letters or numbers
- Unreliable yes-no responses
- Can't understand telephone conversations or television newscasts

Severity of Aphasia

Aphasia can be so severe as to make communication almost impossible, or it can be very mild. The mix of what is weakened and what remains strong or intact is highly variable across people with aphasia and is mostly dependent on location, depth, and extent of the underlying brain damage. The severity of aphasia is also a complex issue. Some people are nearly speechless and yet get along very well with alternative or augmentative means of communication and appear to live a full and active life. Others may not even appear to be aphasic but their alteration of language use can create havoc in their lives and radically alter employment or occupational aspects of living. I (L.L.L.) worked with an English professor who was a poet and creative writer. His life was language. He manipulated language in evocative ways that made people laugh, cry, and marvel at his use of words to create images and stories. His aphasia was classified as "mild" when compared to most other stroke survivors who could not talk, but to him his aphasia was a devastating thief that had robbed him of his livelihood and nuanced ability to use language. Similarly, a criminal trial lawyer with whom I worked recovered much of his language after a stroke, but still could not return to the courtroom to create and execute a masterful closing summary to a jury. He said to me, "This was my strong suit. I could organize my thoughts and my language in such a way that I had juries eating out of my hand; I could see them changing their minds as I weaved my summation. I won a lot of cases. Now, I am just an average trial lawyer. I'm no longer on top of the heap. Help me regain my mastery."

The degree of handicap and disability of aphasia is very personal and not very related to the norm-referenced score on a standardized aphasia test. It is much more related to the premorbid or prestroke personal language facility of each individual and the value he or she places on the degree of language loss that they perceive. A frustration of those of us who attempt to remediate these struggling survivors is that we have a difficult time convincing insurers and third-party reimbursers to pay for these services, although they may be equally as devastating as those of the aphasia survivor who is speechless. This is not true in all countries, but surely is a problem in the United States where health care reimbursement for chronic conditions is political, economically driven, and relatively medieval.

Competence Versus Performance

A longtime debate in aphasiology is whether or not the disrupted language of aphasia is a function of a loss of language competence or of performance. That is, are the representations of language and the rules of language lost or erased (linguistic competence loss) or are the representations and rules of language still there and just the result of performance deficits that do not allow a person with aphasia to access language. The jury is still out on the degree to which aphasia is a loss of implicit linguistic competence or a problem in retrieving the use of language that is still there, although the words and thoughts may be buried, veiled, or inaccessible. Some aspects of aphasia, especially in those who are most profoundly impaired, indeed may be the result of the loss of linguistic competence (and this is the predominant view of many neurolinguists who study aphasia). But just as many other aphasiologists feel that aphasia is the result of impaired access (performance) to the linguistic representations and rules of language that indeed are still there and can be revealed under certain circumstances. Many specialists in speech-language pathology who deal with people with aphasia on a nearly daily basis are convinced that the transience and variability of aphasia, and the observation that under certain conditions, language can be stimulated and emitted that previously was not apparent are convinced that impaired access or performance is a potent explanatory model of the nature of aphasia. This is an important argument as it affects the theoretic underpinnings and the very model of aphasia that is embraced. Those who prefer an access or performance model of aphasia (access deficit model) are more likely to recognize the influence and effects of cognitive elements of the interplay of memory, attention, categorization, and organization as important components of the disorder. Cognitive resource allocation skills are viewed by some to be a part of this model of aphasia. Those who view language use as primarily within the domain of linguistic representations and rules are more likely to attribute aphasia solely to their linguistically oriented view of the disorder. Probably both camps are partially correct and it may well not be an either/or supposition. It is fairly certain that implicit linguistic competence cannot be directly measured without confounding the result with performance variables. In the meantime, the energy expended on theoretic and sophistic arm-wrestling in the view of

some might better be spent on developing innovative strategies of intervention and remediation. Theoretic treadmills are great and necessary, but if carried too far, and at the expense of attention to remediation, may appear ever too close to being self-stimulation. The research as well as the debate continues.

Concomitant or Accompanying Problems

The problems that accompany aphasia can be few or many. Generally, the concomitant conditions include those that are physical or medical, emotional, or social. The degree to which any survivor has these difficulties, as with the severity of the aphasia, is related to the location and extent of the brain damage that created the aphasia. Common medical conditions that frequently coincide with the aphasia include hypertension (high blood pressure); diabetes; cardiac or heart disease; obstructive sleep apnea (temporary cessation of breathing during sleep); and problems that may or may not come along with the disorder such as paralysis or weakness of parts of the face or tongue. Commonly, hemiparesis (weakness on one side of the body) or hemiplegia (paralysis of one side of the body) and loss of the sensations of touch, feeling, pain, or temperature along with feelings of numbness or tingling in the extremities (arms and legs) are part of the condition as well. The conditions of apraxia, apraxia of speech, and the dysarthrias may coexist with the aphasic language disorder as may problems in nutrition and swallowing. Those conditions are considered in some detail in Chapters 8 and 9.

Seizures

Sometimes convulsions or seizures accompany aphasia. Epilepsy is a recurrent seizure disorder caused by abnormal electrical discharges from brain cells, often in the cerebral cortex (Figure 4–4). It is not a distinct disease; it is a group of disorders for which recurrent seizures are the main symptom (Neurology channel, 2010). Different forms of epilepsy are either secondary to a particular brain abnormality or neurologic disorder, or are said to be "idiopathic," without any clear cause. The term "seizure disorder" is preferred to "epilepsy" because epilepsy is often incorrectly thought to include some degree of brain damage or the tendency to be violent. **Tonic-clonic (grand mal)** seizures usually begin with an abnormal electrical discharge in a small area of the brain, resulting in a partial seizure. However, the discharge

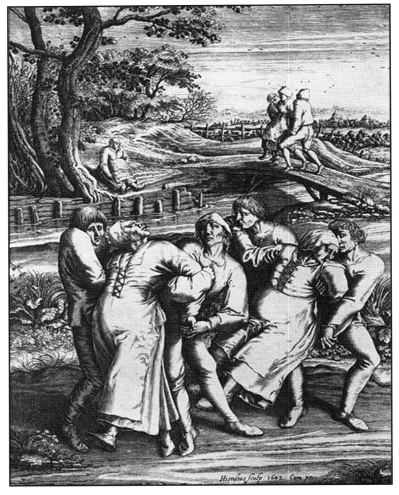

FIGURE 4–4. Epileptic seizure (Kupferstich von Heyden Hondius [1573–1649] nach einer Zeichnung von Pieter Brueghel der Ältere aus dem Jahre 1564: "Die Wallfahrt der Fallsüchtigen nach Meulebeeck" from public domain Wikipedia commons.)

may quickly spread to adjoining parts of the brain, causing the entire area to malfunction with involvement of the entire body. In tonic-clonic seizures, abnormal discharges may result in a temporary loss of consciousness and a "convulsion" characterized by severe muscle spasms and jerking throughout the body. The head may forcefully turn to one side, the teeth may clench, occasionally the tongue is bitten, and bladder control may be lost. Seizures usually last 1 to 2 minutes. Afterward, the individual may have a headache, be temporarily confused, and feel extremely tired. Usually, the person does not remember what happened during the seizure. Seizures come in gradations, some of which are mild and barely noticeable, others that are impossible not to notice. For the person who has never witnessed a seizure, the event can be startling and somewhat frightening, but for the most part they are not life threatening and certain first aid interventions can be implemented to prevent injury.

Seizures that accompany aphasia or other brain damage are not the norm, but at the same time, they are unexpected. One of my early supervisory errors (L.L.L.) involved failing to prepare a neophyte student clinician on the possibility of a seizure in a gentleman who was being evaluated by the new student in his very first visit to our clinic at the University of Colorado. About halfway into the evaluation, he had a tonic-clonic (grand mal) seizure, fell on the clinic room floor with a good deal of spasmodic contractions of the arms, legs, and muscles of the neck and face. The student clinician was so unprepared for this dramatic event that she bolted the room, left the clinic, and may still be loping along the front range of the hills of Colorado. I should have prepared her more adequately.

First aid for epilepsy is very simple. It keeps the person safe until the seizure stops naturally by itself. It is important for the public to know how to respond to all seizures, including the most noticeable kind—the generalized tonic-clonic seizure (Healthcare Magic, 2010).

When providing seizure first aid for generalized tonic clonic (grand mal) seizures, these are the key things to remember, according to the Epilepsy Foundation of America:

- Keep calm and reassure other people who may be nearby.
- Don't hold the person down or try to stop her movements.
- Time the seizure with your watch.
- Clear the area around the person of anything hard or sharp.
- Loosen ties or anything around the neck that may make breathing difficult.
- Put something flat and soft, like a folded jacket, under the head.
- Turn him or her gently onto one side. This will help keep the airway clear. Do not try to force the mouth open with any hard implement or with fingers. **It is *not* true that a person having a seizure can swallow his tongue.** Efforts to hold the tongue down can injure teeth or jaw (or you can injure a finger).
- Don't attempt artificial respiration except in the unlikely event that a person does not start breathing again after the seizure has stopped.
- Stay with the person until the seizure ends naturally.
- Be friendly and reassuring as consciousness returns.
- Offer to call a taxi, friend, or relative to help the person get home if she seems confused or unable to get home by herself. (Epilepsy Foundation, 2010)

There are numerous medical, physical, and emotional conditions that can be part of the package of the person with aphasia. A health care team with a primary care physician and medical and rehabilitation specialists are the usual team members and they must communicate and collaborate to implement the very best and most appropriate care for the person with aphasia.

Assessment

Aphasia is not very well understood by the general public. Usually if someone has a stroke or other type of brain damage that result in aphasia, a friend or family member will be the first to recognize that something is wrong. "He's not making sense. He doesn't understand me. He's saying the wrong words and can't seem to put a sentence together" are the first impressions that may be created and reported by those around for the emerging puzzling signs of aphasia. It isn't unusual to hear family members report that the person appears to have an emotional crisis or is "out of his mind." Some report that they thought their loved one "regressed to childhood or baby talk," or "seems to have something wrong with his tongue." All of these first impressions could not be further from the real cause, but they are understandable misimpressions by a lay public that is very unaware of the typical characteristics of aphasia. First responders who are called to give emergency care may be the first to recognize that the person is aphasic. They usually are much more in touch with the typical signs of stroke and aphasia and the jumbled words of the newly aphasic person will be red flags that signal possible damage to the brain. The physician who examines the individual for his or her brain injury will be next in line to recognize that the muddled communication is related to neurologic damage. Frequently this is a neurologist. The physician typically performs tests that require the individual to follow commands, answer questions, name objects, and converse (National Institute of Deafness and Other Communication Disorders: NIH, 2010). Once the person is medically and neurologically stable, if the physician suspects aphasia, the person is often referred to a speech-language pathologist who will conduct a comprehensive examination of the person's ability to communicate, including careful assessment of all of the modalities of speech and language (Figure 4–5). Production of speech, comprehension of speech, reading, writing, gesture, and all the subtle avenues of human communication will be explored to determine what is impaired and what is intact and how these impairments influence the person's life.

The purpose of any assessment of neurogenic communication disorders is to answer questions and provide information in five crucial areas (Figure 4–6). In aphasia, the reasons for appraisal (gathering information) and diagnosis (attaching a label to the interpretation of the findings) include the following:

- to identify the presence of aphasia
- to determine the severity of aphasic signs and symptoms and their impact on life participation and activities
- to target goals for communication therapy
- to document progress during treatment

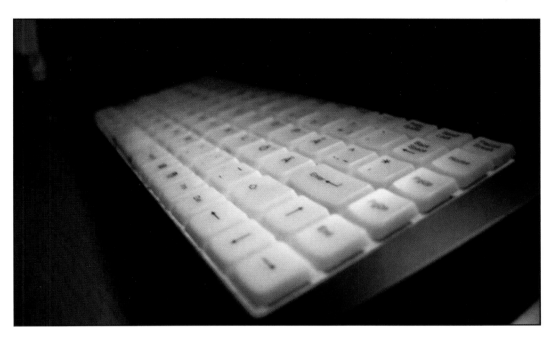

FIGURE 4–5. Keyboard.

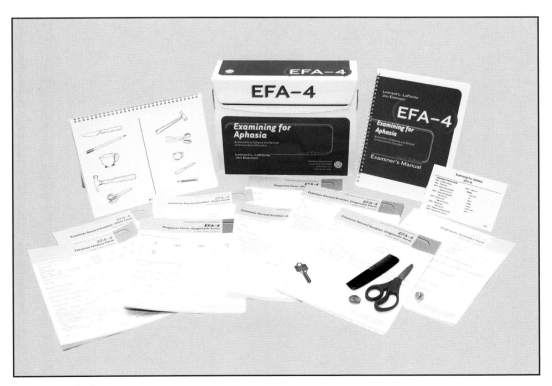

FIGURE 4–6. EFA-4.

■ to inform and counsel persons with aphasia, their families, and social support networks and to inform physicians, medical personnel, and health care reimbursement agencies

A considerable number of organized assessment instruments have been developed for determining the nature and extent of aphasia (Table 4–1). Most of these pay some attention to principles of psychometric testing and measurement, but too many are rather homemade, clinically based collections of materials that may miss or overlook important aspects of careful evaluation. Assessment instruments fall into several categories. Some are screening measures, some are comprehensive diagnostic tests that attempt to determine the type and severity of aphasia, some are measures oriented to determining daily life or functional communication, and some are measures of specialized or ancillary cognitive or language functioning. All of the above measures depend on careful and trained strategies for observing, determining, categorizing, and interpreting communication activities. There is no objective, technologically advanced measure of imaging the human brain and determining the precise aspects of language that are affected. We learn about aphasia by listening to people talk, listen, and express themselves across the modalities or channels of human interaction. These observations are most valid if they are organized, if they sample enough communication tasks, and if they are related to the language activities necessary for living, learning, and loving.

Available tests of aphasia include the following. This list is intended to be representative and not exhaustive and more detailed references to aphasia tests

Table 4–1. Tests of Aphasia

Test	*Purpose*
Boston Diagnostic Test of Aphasia (BDAE)	Comprehensive, Diagnostic
Examining for Aphasia-4 (EFA-4)	Comprehensive with Short Form
Western Aphasia Battery (WAB)	Comprehensive, Diagnostic
Porch Index of Communicative Ability (PICA)	Comprehensive, Diagnostic
Communicative Activities of Daily Living (CADL)	Functional, Pragmatic
Comprehensive Aphasia Test	Comprehensive
Psycholinguistic Assessment of Linguistic Processing in Aphasia (PALPA)	Comprehensive, Linguistic
Functional Assessment of Aphasia (ASHA-FACS)	Functional, Pragmatic
Reading Comprehension Battery for Aphasia (RCBA)	Reading Assessment
Kentucky Aphasia Test (KAT 1, 2, 3)	"Clinician friendly"
Boston Naming Test	Special naming test

can be found in the aphasia texts by Byng, Swinburn, and Pound (1999), Ball and Damico (2007), Davis (2007), La-Pointe (2005), Spreen and Risser (2003), Whitworth, Howard, and Webster (2005), and Worrall and Frattali (2000).

Aphasia Treatment

Mrs. Oglethorpe may recover completely from her aphasia. Mr. Thumper and most people who suffer brain damage with resulting aphasia may have to live with it and adjust their lifestyle for the rest of their lives. Early recovery or (sometimes called *spontaneous recovery* or *physiologic restitution*) is the best possible but not the most likely course of recovery. Speedy and relatively complete recovery also occurs following what is called *a transient ischemic attack* (TIA), a type of stroke or CVA in which the blood flow to the brain is temporarily interrupted but quickly re-established. During a TIA, language abilities may return in a few hours or a few days. TIAs, however, are not all good news, for people who suffer single or multiple TIAs are at much greater risk for a full blown completed stroke. A TIA is a "warning stroke" or "ministroke," and recognizing and treating TIAs can reduce the risk of a major stroke. There is a tendency to ignore TIAs as full recovery occurs and language and life are restored, but to ignore them is an invitation to disaster. The huge brain attack is lurking around the corner and the underlying vascular or blood supply problem that caused the TIA can be treated medically, and the big stroke bullet can be dodged. Most strokes are not preceded by TIAs. However, of the people who have had one or more TIAs, more than a third will later have a major stroke. TIAs are important in predicting *if* a stroke will occur rather than *when* the big one will hit. They can occur days, weeks, or even months before a major stroke. In about half the cases, the stroke occurs within one year of the TIA. If anyone you know (Grandma Bertha, Uncle Bud) has complained of the temporary disruption of vision, memory, speech, arm or leg numbness, weakness, or paralysis with subsequent full recovery, get them to medical treatment to try to rectify the underlying vascular condition and prevent the bogeyman of a major stroke. It should be taken seriously and not minimized or dismissed.

For most cases of aphasia, however, language recovery is not as simple or as complete. Although many individuals with aphasia, even the aphasia caused by a major stroke, experience a period of partial spontaneous recovery (in which some language abilities return over the span of a few days to a month after the brain injury), some amount of aphasia typically remains. In these cases, communication therapy is helpful. Recovery usually continues at a moderate pace even several years after the onset of aphasia, but informed therapy would never wait until spontaneous recovery runs its course. Most aphasiologists believe that the most effective treatment begins early in the recovery process. Some of the factors that influence the amount of improvement include the exact etiology or cause of the brain damage, the area of the brain that was damaged, the extent of the brain injury, and the age and health of the individual. Additional factors that can affect the prognosis for recovery include motivation, handedness, and educational level, as well as the type, quality, and intensiveness of the therapy. New and useful treatment strategies based on theories of brain plasticity, revamping of brain architecture, and synaptogenesis (creating or fostering new neuron connections) are emerging as exciting modes of behavioral and medical intervention (Moss Resourcenet.2010).

Aphasia therapy strives to improve an individual's ability to communicate by helping the person use remaining abilities, re-establish language abilities as much as possible, compensate for language problems, and learn alternative methods of communicating. Treatment may be offered in individual or group settings. Individual therapy focuses on the specific needs of the person. It must be customized to the precise needs, desires, and abilities and goals of each highly individual person (Moss Resourcenet, 2010). That is why workbooks and computerized programs cannot be the entire or even the principal medium of aphasia therapy. A live, motivated, well-prepared human clinician is the best form of behavioral individual therapy because online, real-time decisions are made relative to judgments of language adequacy; reinforcements, diversions, and human interaction are made in each and every session of quality aphasia therapy. It is important as well to track therapeutic progress by frequent reassessment or even session-by-session plotting of communication change (LaPointe, 1991).

Group therapy offers the opportunity to use new communication skills in a comfortable setting. Elman's book on group therapy is an efficient and well-documented chronicle of the benefits of group therapy (Elman, 2006). Stroke clubs or regional support groups formed by individuals who have had a stroke, or by rehabilitation professionals who deal with stroke and aphasia, are available in most major cities. The CONNECT program in the United Kingdom (http://www.ukconnect.org/), the University of Queensland aphasia groups in Australia (http://www.shrs.uq.edu.au/cdaru/aphasiagroups/index.html), the Aphasia Institute in Canada (http://www.aphasia.ca/about/index.html), and the Aphasia Center of California (http://pages.sbcglobal.net/stevenfry/index.html) are model examples of organizations that embrace group support and treatment for aphasia. These organizations offer information, a chance to socialize with others who have stroke, and the chance for individuals with aphasia to try new communication skills. Stroke clubs or support groups can help give the individual, caregivers, and family members the opportunity to adjust to the avalanche of life changes that accompany stroke and aphasia. Family involvement is a crucial component of aphasia treatment so that family members can learn not only the best way to communicate with their loved one but also the means to ward off the threat of devastating identity change that can accompany a life-changing medical crisis (Shadden & Koski, 2007).

Speech-language pathologists are frequently asked by other health care professionals and by family members how they can best communicate with persons with aphasia. Among the many suggestions are those presented in Table 4–2.

The Sociology of Aphasia

Social approaches to aphasia rehabilitation are a relatively recent and refreshing trend in aphasia intervention. Older approaches stuck quite close to an impairment-based medical model of treatment. Prior to the advocacy of aphasiologists such as Sarno (1981) and Holland (1980), little attention was paid

Table 4–2. How to Talk to People With Aphasia

- Simplify language by using short, uncomplicated sentences. But no baby-talk, please.
- Repeat the content words or write down key words to clarify meaning as needed.
- Maintain a natural conversational manner appropriate for an adult.
- Minimize distractions, such as a blaring radio, or the rehearsal of a tap-dancing tango music troupe.
- Include the person with aphasia in conversations. Don't refer to him or her in the third person or as if he or she were not present.
- Ask for and value the opinion of the person with aphasia, especially regarding family matters. Incorporate the person's desires into the goals of rehabilitation.
- Encourage any type of communication, whether it is speech, gesture, pointing, or drawing.
- Avoid correcting the individual's speech.
- Allow the individual plenty of time to talk.
- Encourage independence. Don't wipe the drool from the side of the mouth or cut his or her steak unless that was done before the stroke or is requested.
- Help the person become involved outside the home. Seek out support groups such as stroke clubs.

to communication in context or daily life activities that aphasia derailed. Most aphasia treatment was based on stimulus-response linguistic tasks. These days, interventionists are recognizing the ecology of communication and extending treatment venues to participation in communication activities of everyday life. This change in emphasis also has resulted in more attention being paid to the psychosocial issues of aphasia (Elman, 2005; Holland, 2007; LaPointe, 2002, 2003; 2005; Lyon, 1998). Coping with chronic conditions and the psychosocial elements of the illness experience is now given more notice in aphasia. In the later part of the 20th century, aphasiologists began addressing quality of life issues and social models of aphasia. The World Health Organization's evolving models of rehabilitation resulted in aphasi-

ologists developing a life participation approach to aphasia (LPAA). LPAA is a philosophy that places value and emphasis on reengagement in life, focuses intervention targets on communication activities of everyday life, and increases participation in the social milieu of a person with aphasia (Elman, 2005). This is a refreshing breeze that has been too long in coming and can be integrated very well with the more traditional approaches to stimulus-response impairment based treatment.

Efficacy and Effectiveness of Aphasia Treatment

As elegantly detailed by Holland et al. (1996), and the monumental work by Wertz et al. (1986), the field of aphasia treatment research is well beyond asking and answering the question of general treatment efficacy. The literature is rich with both group studies and single subject studies that provide evidence that treatment does improve language ability and quality of communicative life (Thompson, 2006). This is not to say that our work is over or that we can rest on our laurels, as further work detailing the effects of certain treatments for certain language deficits is needed. Systematic and orderly replication of established treatment outcomes also is necessary to enhance the carryover of findings, especially into the ecologically valid world of everyday communication. In addition, important unanswered issues regarding aphasia treatment remain. Among these are: When is treatment most effective? How often should treatment be provided? What interventions work best for specific language modality problems? Which language intervention strategies are most cost effective? Which pharmaceutical supplements maximally enhance communication change? The answers, my friend, are not blowing in the wind, but are emerging in the fertile minds of future aphasiologists. Progress toward answering these questions clearly has been made and will continue as the clinical science of aphasiology becomes increasingly sophisticated.

Research on Aphasia

Aphasia research is exploring new ways to evaluate and treat aphasia as well as to further understanding of the function of the brain. Good scientific inquiry dictates that we pursue levels of explanation and levels of application. Brain imaging techniques have been a revolution in our understanding of brain function during disease and normal functions (Figure 4–7). As with many innovative technologies, the ambition has sometimes outpaced the refinement of appropriate methodologies, but there is no denying that neural imaging continues to evolve and will continue to define brain function, determine the severity of brain damage, and shed light on elegant and redundant areas of the brain for processing human communication. These procedures include PET (positron emission tomography), CT (computed tomography), and MRI (magnetic resonance imaging), as well as functional magnetic resonance (fMRI) that identifies areas of the brain being activated during activities such as speaking or listening.

The use of computers and emerging technologies to augment and compensate for language loss is being honed to unprecedented levels. Revolutionary new drugs administered shortly after some types of stroke are being investigated and used as ways to reduce the severity of aphasia. Medical and surgical approaches to reduce the impact of aphasia and other brain-based communication problems promise much, but the necessity of behavioral intervention by highly trained experts in human communication and its disorders will be around for generations to come. As one once remarked at a meeting of the annual Clinical Aphasiology Conference, we look forward to continued advances in the understanding and treatment of aphasia as solace to those who are destined to treat the thousands of persons who will experience aphasia in the future, including those future clinicians who will treat *us*.

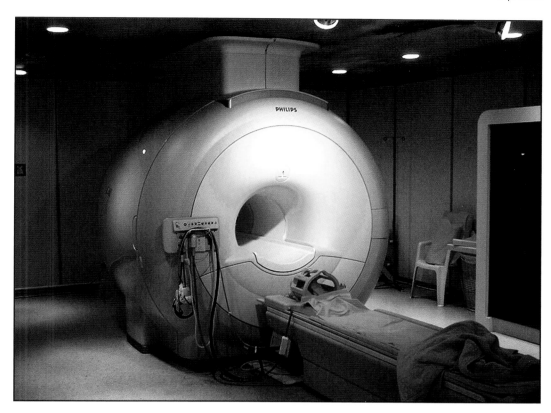

FIGURE 4–7. MRI scanner.

References

Ackerman, D. (2004). *An alchemy of mind: The marvel and mystery of the brain.* New York, NY: Scribner.

Brain statistics table. Retrieved May 4, 2005, from http://www.braininjurylawtexas .com/brain_statistics.htm

Ball, M. J., & Damico, J. S. (2007). *Clinical aphasiology: Future directions.* New York, NY: Psychology Press.

Byng, S., Swinburn, K., & Pound, C. (1999). *The aphasia therapy file.* Hove, East Sussex, UK: Psychology Press.

Elman, R. (2006). *Group treatment of neurogenic communication disorders: The expert clinician's approach.* San Diego, CA: Plural Publishing.

Epilepsy Foundation. (2010). *First aid.* Retrieved February 9, 2010, from http:// www.epilepsyfoundation.org/answer place/Medical/firstaid/

Davis, G. A. (2007). *Aphasiology: Disorders and clinical practice* (2nd ed.). New York, NY: Pearson.

Healthcare Magic. (2010). *First aid for seizures and epilepsy.* Retrieved February 9, 2010, from http://www.healthcaremagic.com/ articles/First-aid-for-seizures-and- epilepsy/7545

Holland, A. (1980). *Communication activities of daily living.* Austin, TX: Pro-Ed.

Holland, A. (2007). *Counseling in communication disorders: A wellness perspective.* San Diego, CA: Plural Publishing.

Holland, A., Fromm, D., DeRuyter, F., & Stein, M. (1996). Treatment efficacy: Aphasia.

Journal of Speech and Hearing Research, 39, S27–S36.

LaPointe, L. L. (1991). *Base-10 response form: Revised manual.* San Diego, CA: Singular Publishers.

LaPointe, L. L. (2002). The sociology of aphasia. *Journal of Medical Speech-Language Pathology, 10*(1), vii–x.

LaPointe, L. L. (2005). Preface to third edition. In L. L. LaPointe (Ed.), *Aphasia and related neurogenic language disorders* (p. xii). New York, NY: Thieme Medical Publishers.

LaPointe, L. L., & Eisenson, J. (2008). *Examining for aphasia* (4th ed.). Austin, TX: Pro-Ed.

Lyon, J. (1998). *Coping with aphasia.* San Diego, CA: Singular Publishing.

Moss Resourcenet. (2010). *Aphasia.* Retrieved February 9, 2010, from http://www.moss resourcenet.org/aphasia.htm

National Institute of Deafness and Other Communication Disorders: NIH. (2010). Retrieved February 9, 2010, from http://www.nidcd.nih.gov/health/voice/aphasia.asp

Neurologogy Channel. (2010). Retrieved February 10, 2010, from http://www.neurologychannel.com/seizures/index.shtml

Sarno, M. (1981). *Acquired aphasia.* New York, NY: Academic Press.

Shadden, B., & Koski, P. (2007). Social construction of self for persons with aphasia: When language as a cultural tool is impaired. *Journal of Medical Speech-Language Pathology, 15*(2), 99–106.

Spreen, O., & Risser, A. H. (2003). *Assessment of aphasia.* New York, NY: Oxford University Press.

Thompson, C. K. (2006). Single subject controlled experiments in aphasia: The science and the state of the science. *Journal of Communication Disorders, 39*(4), 266–291.

Wertz, R. T., LaPointe, L. L., & Rosenbek, J. C. (1989). *Aphasia: A clinical approach.* Austin, TX: Pro-Ed.

Wertz R. T., Weiss D. G., Aten J. L., Brookshire R. H., Garcia-Bunuel, L., Holland, A. L., . . . Brannegan, R. (1986). Comparison of clinic, home, and deferred language treatment for aphasia: A Veterans Administration cooperative study. *Archives of Neurology, 43,* 653–658.

Whitworth, A., Howard, D., & Webster, J. (2005). *A cognitive and neuropsycological approach to aphasia assessment: A clinician's approach.* Hove, East Sussex, UK: Psychology Press, Ltd.

Worrall, L. E., & Frattali, C. M. (2000). *Neurogenic communication disorders: A functional approach.* New York, NY: Thieme.

5

Nonfocal Brain Damage: Communication Disorders and a World of Other Problems

Leroy

Yeah. I know. The most embarrassing type of traumatic brain injury in the history of man. I was working on a construction site and had to, how you say, answer the call of nature. I was sitting there in a porta potty on our worksite where I worked on construction. We were building a bridge. Turned out to be a bridge to nowhere for me. I don't know how it happened; it was an accident I guess. I felt myself being lifted up . . . the whole porta potty . . . it had a cute name . . . something like Peter's Potties or Don's Johns or something. As it turned out a crane was lifting the portable toilets to load them to a higher spot near the top of the bridge. Well, they didn't know I was in it. And they dropped it. And not only did I really need to be hosed down when they found me, but I got a closed head injury out of it. Brain damage all over the place. My legs and arms don't work like they used to. My memory is shot. I can't work. I can't pay attention. My speech was goofed up for a long time. It's coming back pretty good now, but I still need lots of help. I used to be too embarrassed to tell people how it happened. Now it doesn't bother me as much. I just tell them I had a shitty accident.

Carl

Dementia is eating me alive. I was a college professor. I taught biochemistry and ran a laboratory with 15 people in it. How ironic. We were doing research on dendritic sprouting and looking for a possible cure for Alzheimer's and other dementias. So much for that research agenda. Too bad I couldn't have made a little faster progress. I noticed my memory skills starting to decline about three years ago. First, it was subtle things that everybody has problems with, forgetting names, missing meeting appointments, losing my keys about 4 times a week. Then I couldn't remember names of my family, and it started to affect my train of thought. Like right now. It's hard for me to string together a story. I can still get through the day, but I don't work anymore. In fact, now I even have trouble dressing myself and most of the time I just withdraw and don't care to talk to people. I go to the Tallahassee Memorial Hospital Adult Day Services Center. They help me a lot. We have interesting things to do every day and I think it is helping stem the tide a little. They have a real nice lady there who is kind to everybody. She treats us like family. She helps us pass the day and work on things that help our memory. She's also a real good piano player and has a voice like an angel. You should hear her sing Amazing Grace and Un bel di, vadremo. Puccini would be proud. I used to like opera, but now I'm relegated to Oprah. I can feel myself slipping.

Traumatic Brain Injury (TBI): What Is It? What Does It Look Like?

Traumatic brain injury (TBI) goes by several names, some less accurate than the more commonly accepted one that heads this section. It also is called closed head injury, acquired brain injury, or simply head injury. TBI occurs when a sudden trauma causes damage to the brain. Approximately 1.4 million Americans sustain head injuries each year, with associated costs estimated at $40 billion (Centers for Disease Control and Prevention, 2010). The bulk of these costs are attributable to cognitive and behavioral changes, yet these changes are not well understood because, in addition to overt damage to brain tissue and neurons, a condition called diffuse axonal injury (DAI) is a more subtle type of TBI brain pathology. DAI is widespread and difficult to pinpoint using standard brain imaging techniques. There are usually two contusion or bruise sites in a brain injury. One occurs at the primary site of the strike to the head and brain and is called the *coup* injury. The other is a rebound effect where the brain bounces off the inside of the skull opposite the site of the original blow. The damage here is termed the *contre coup* injury. The third characteristic related to the physics of brain injury involves shearing or twisting forces, and plays a role primarily in injuries that involve rapid and forceful movements of the head, such as in motor vehicle accidents. These unfortunate circumstances can cause rotational forces as in twisting whiplash-type injuries. Mother Physics can be cruel when it comes to how the brain is moved around.

More than five million Americans, approximately 2% of the population, currently live with disabilities related to brain injury. Males are more than twice as likely as females to experience a TBI, perhaps because of well-recognized gender traits of aggressiveness and testosterone-infused antics meant to impress females by engaging in risk-taking behavior. TBI is most common among adolescents (aged 15–24) and older adults (75 and older). It has been characterized as the *silent epidemic* because it appears to be underrecognized by both the general public as well as healthcare professionals. It may be silent, but its cost in both tragedy and effect on society is loud and strong.

The most common causes of TBI are motor vehicle collisions, falls, violence, and sports. Research has shown that approximately 85% of head injuries from bicycle accidents can be prevented with the use of helmets. Figure 5–1 is a breakdown of common causes of TBI from the United States Centers for Disease Control.

The aftermath of TBI can be temporary or long lasting. TBI can result when the head suddenly and violently hits an object, or when an object pierces the skull and enters brain tissue (NINDS: NIH, 2010). It can be caused by ramming the forehead into the dashboard of a Volvo, cracking the skull on the burl of a redwood tree after flying off a mountain bike, kissing the bottom of a swimming pool after a drunken dive from a balcony, or being beaten around the head

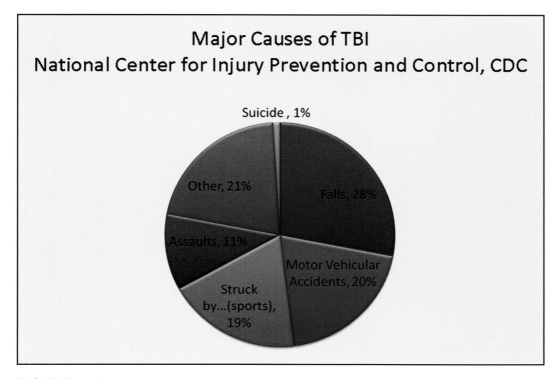

FIGURE 5–1. Causes of TBI.

with a hard salami. You name it. It most likely has caused traumatic brain damage somewhere, sometime. The annals of unusual causes of traumatic brain injury are weird and tragic and season medical case reports in journals worldwide. A failed suicide attempt by plunging a chopstick through the eye orbit is one of the most cringe worthy. Errant nail guns, screwdrivers, and even a strange case of TBI caused by a deer antler are on record. There are many more. Figure 5–2 is an x-ray of a traumatic brain injury caused by nails gone wild.

Symptoms of a TBI run the range from nearly undetectable to mild, moderate, or severe, depending on the extent and location of the damage to the brain. Loss of consciousness, (being "knocked out") even for a few seconds or minutes, is one of the clearest indications that the brain may have been affected by a crack to the head. A confusional state involving uncertainty about time, date, and location ("orientation times three" as it is called) and an episode of memory loss for the events surrounding the clout also are indicators of trauma to the brain.

A person with a mild TBI may remain conscious or may experience a loss of consciousness for a few seconds or minutes (NINDS: NIH, 2010). Other symptoms of mild TBI include headache, confusion, dizziness, blurred vision or tired eyes, ringing in the ears, bad taste in the mouth, fatigue or lethargy, a change in sleep patterns, behavioral or mood changes, and trouble with memory, concentration, attention, or thinking. Speech or language problems also may be evident and can affect either the motor speech system or language or both. A person with a moderate or severe TBI may show the same signs and symptoms, but also may have a headache that gets worse or does not go away; repeated vomiting or nausea; convulsions or seizures; an inability to awaken from sleep; dilation of one or both pupils of the eyes; imprecise speech; weakness or numbness in the extremities; loss of coordination; and increased confusion, restlessness, or agitation. Figure 5–3 depicts some of these noticeable indications of TBI.

The effects of TBI are widespread across the domains of physical changes, cognitive and behavioral changes, and speech, language, and swallowing difficulties. It has been said that the world of TBI is a microcosm ("small world") of all that we must know to assess and treat nearly everything motoric, communicative, and cognitive with which we deal. That inclusive world of signs and symptoms can be categorized under the following headings:

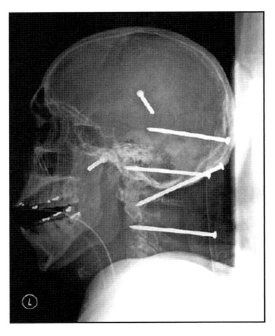

FIGURE 5–2. TBI from nails.

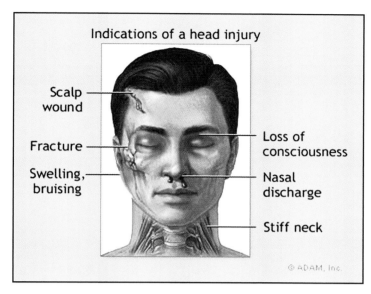

FIGURE 5–3. Indications of head injury (Copyright © Adam Images. Reproduced with permission.).

Physical Changes

- Impairment of the arms and legs
- Weakness
- Muscle coordination problems
- Full or partial paralysis
- Seizures (also called traumatic epilepsy)
- Changes in sexual functioning
- Ambulation (walking) problems
- Fatigue
- Head or facial disfigurement
- Swallowing problems, drooling
- Headaches
- Balance difficulties
- Sensory impairments (e.g., vision, hearing, taste, smell, touch, sense of body position or movement)

Cognitive Changes

- Shortened attention span
- Memory problems
- Problem-solving difficulties

- Poor judgment
- Partial or complete loss of reading and writing skills
- Language problems, including communication deficits and loss of vocabulary
- Inability to understand abstract concepts
- Difficulty learning new things

Communication Changes

Children or adults with a brain injury often have cognitive and communication problems that significantly impinge on their ability to enjoy acceptable quality of life or live independently. These problems vary depending on how widespread brain damage is and the location of the injury. Because the damage may be diffuse and both cortical and subcortical, all the signs and symptoms listed in the chapters on aphasia, right hemisphere syndrome, and swallowing come into play. It is indeed a microcosm.

- *Dysarthria(s)*—difficulty with the motoric control necessary to use and coordinate the movement subsystems of speech (respiration, phonation, articulation, resonance, prosody)
  - ☐ Imprecision of consonant and vowel sounds
  - ☐ Inadequate phonation with weak, soft loudness or pitch alterations
  - ☐ Poor speech breathing
  - ☐ Nasality and resonance imbalance
  - ☐ Muscles may be so weak or affected that the person is unable to produce sound or speak at all
- *Language problems* in semantics, syntax, phonology, and pragmatics, including
  - ☐ Both comprehension and production
  - ☐ Word retrieval and word finding
  - ☐ Word order and grammatical rule
  - ☐ Reading, writing, spelling
- *Social communication difficulty*, including:
  - ☐ taking turns in conversation
  - ☐ maintaining a topic of conversation
  - ☐ using an appropriate tone of voice
  - ☐ interpreting the subtleties of conversation (e.g., the difference between sarcasm and a serious statement)
  - ☐ responding to facial expressions and body language
  - ☐ keeping up with others in a fast-paced conversation

Individuals may seem hyperemotional (overreacting) or emotionally flat as a pancake. Most frustrating to families and friends, a person may have little to no awareness of just how inappropriately he or she is acting. In general, communication can be frustrating, unsuccessful, frightening, and full of surprises that surface periodically like little communicative creatures from the black lagoon.

Changes in Personality, Mood, and Behavior:

- Agitation, combativeness
- Depression and anxiety
- Low frustration tolerance
- Impulsivity
- Insensitivity to societal rules or values

Changes That Affect Academic Performance:

- Difficulty learning and remembering new things
- Trouble paying attention and staying focused
- Difficulty planning and following through with tasks

That is a wide, wide world of behavioral, medical, and academic disruption. TBI may be the most challenging single constellation of problems with which health professionals must deal. Add these issues to the backdrop of childhood and a developing nervous system and the tribulation is compounded.

The effects of brain injury in children can be especially challenging because the injury occurs to a developing brain that is being charged with the responsibility of learning tons of new things each day. Because the developmental processes continue after the injury, both previously learned skills and the development of future skills can be affected. Some students injured in early childhood may do relatively well until they reach middle or high school, when they are expected to demonstrate increasing competence and independence. The functions required at this level may not develop if the relevant areas of the brain have been damaged and are not developing normally. If a child or an elegantly tattooed and pierced teenager has been progressing adequately until then, both parents and educators may overlook the connection between the student's difficulties and the earlier brain injury. Students may be mistakenly identified as having attention deficit disorder (ADHD), behavior disordered, learning disordered (LD), or may simply be swimming upstream to keep up with academic demands. Because of the changing nature of ability and demands, students with TBI benefit from different strategies than those used for students with other diagnoses or disorders.

TBI: Blast Injuries

An old but resurgent cause of nonfocal brain-based disorder has reared its ugly head in the 21st century. Combat in Afghanistan, Iraq, and who knows wherever else has contributed to this new era of a unique pattern of wartime injuries (Figure 5–4). Gloriajean Wallace, an expert in neurogenic communication disorders at the University of Cincinnati, has chronicled this new and vicious type of blast injury (Wallace, 2006). The combat of this new century has brought not only Hummers, refined night vision technology, unmanned combat air vehicles, Star Trek-like high-power microwave (HPM) electronic pulses, and yet unrevealed methods of technologic brain-scrambling. Increasingly, the pattern of missile warfare exposes soldiers and civilian survivors of attacks to explosions that cause strong air-pressure "blasts." Multilevel injury from exposure to these detonations, referred to as "blast injury," has resulted in a complex constellation of impairments to the brain and other body organs. This multiorgan/multisystem involvement, known as "polytrauma," adds significant complexity to the medical and

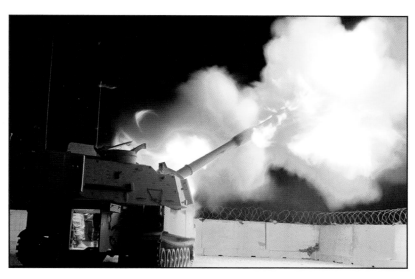

FIGURE 5–4. Potential cause of blast injury.

rehabilitation profile for individuals who survive blast injury. Figure 5–5 depicts a warzone emergency treatment of a blast injury (http://defense-update .com/images_new/eye_injury.jpg).

Medical speech-language pathologists (SLPs) are well prepared to provide services to patients with traumatic brain injury (TBI); aphasia; motor speech impairment; dysphagia; oral, facial, oral-pharyngeal, nasal-pharyngeal, and laryngeal trauma; and hearing loss. However, as Wallace (2006) points out in her comprehensive coverage of this new polypathology, medical SLPs are now faced with providing services to an increasing number of people who simultaneously may have some or all of these conditions. This vastly ups the ante and calls for increased cross-disciplinary collaboration.

The challenge in treating people with blast injury is in the area of triage, or judgments about prioritization and sequencing of assessment and treatment focus. This is no easy assignment. An understanding of blast injury basics provides clarity regarding the risk for polytrauma and the resulting communication and swallowing impairments that may be encountered by medical SLPs providing services to this population. Wallace (2006) contributes to advancing this understanding.

Blast Exposure

As Wallace (2006) explains,

> The term "blast injury" refers to injury from barotraumas caused by either an

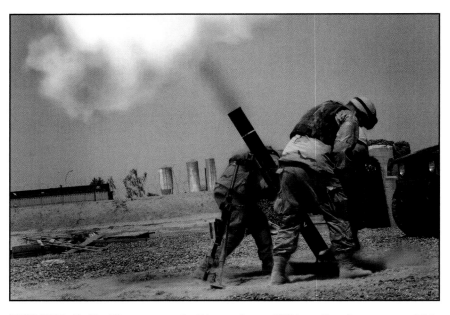

FIGURE 5–5. Blast wound. Photo from Wikimedia Commons. This image is a work of a U.S. Army soldier or employee, taken or made during the course of the person's official duties. As a work of the U.S. federal government, the image is in the public domain.

overpressurization or underpressurization of air over normal atmospheric pressure that affects the body's surface due to exposure to detonated devices or weapons . . . Air- and fluid-filled organs are especially susceptible to the overpressurization/underpressurization effects of blast waves, which cause the *primary effects* of blast exposure. Pulmonary barotraumas, tympanic membrane rupture and middle ear damage, abdominal hemorrhage, perforation of the globe of the eye, and concussion (TBI without physical sign of head injury) are some of the primary effects of blast exposure. *Secondary effects* of blast injury result from flying debris such as bomb fragments, and can result in eye penetration, open head brain injury. (p. 26)

and other penetrations of necessary and precious body parts.

The *tertiary effects* of blast injury result from the individual being thrown by the blast wind, and can cause fracture, traumatic amputation, closed and open brain injury, and many other problems. The *quaternary (or miscellaneous) effects* of blast injury is sort of a catch-all category, as Wallace (2006) explains, and refers to any other:

explosion-related injuries, illnesses, or diseases not due to primary, secondary, or tertiary mechanisms. These includes burns, crush injuries, closed and open head brain injury, angina, hyperglycemia, hypertension, and asthma and other breathing problems resulting from the inhalation of dust, smoke, or toxic fumes. (p. 27)

Blast injuries are not simple and our conferences and publications are devoting increasing attention to their management.

Our Role

Communication disorders resulting from blast injury can include it all, as Wallace has so aptly pointed out. Wallace (2006) further states how:

Cognitive communication impairments related to TBI, swallowing impairments, aphasia, motor speech impairment, oral and facial burns or other trauma, smoke inhalation and resulting laryngeal trauma, medical conditions requiring tracheotomy and ventilation, and hearing loss. Although the person is at risk for communication disorders in all these areas, TBI poses the greatest risk because it may be caused by all four mechanisms (primary, secondary, tertiary, and quaternary) of blast injury. (p. 28)

Reports are rampant on the Internet that improved medical technology now ensures that 90% of the wounded will survive and receive rapid and advanced medical attention. This is encouraging on the one hand, but on the other it assures that the rehabilitation mountains we face will be increasingly steep.

Blast injuries occur in the context of emotional trauma, and the loss of health and independence, bodily disfigurement, the polypathology that is experienced in warfare blast injuries place the individual at risk for a throng of psychiatric disorders, including post-traumatic stress disorder (PTSD) (Figure 5–6). As Wallace (2006) indicates, PTSD symptoms overlap the signs and symptoms of TBI; including "headache, dizziness, irritability, decreased concentration, memory problems, fatigue, visual disturbances, sensitivity to light and noise, judgment problems, anxiety, and depression. Similarities in the behavioral characteristics

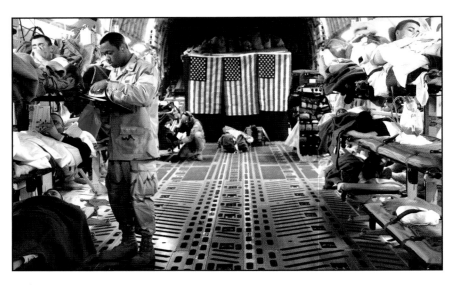

FIGURE 5–6. Evacuation of blast injury patients.

of people with TBI and/or PTSD can perplex the rehabilitation team's diagnostic assessment," and can make the road to recovery all the more treacherous. That path for individuals who have incurred blast injuries is a long and complicated one. "Medical SLPs must prepare to provide clinical services and to serve as community re-entry campaigners," (Wallace, 2006). The job does not end with assessment. Blast injury can be one of the most challenging rehabilitation puzzles we face. Even more so than "simple" TBI, it involves the world of all of the systems with which we deal. Any TBI is a genuine challenge. It takes dedication, up-to-date knowledge, and great motivation on the part of survivors, family, and health professionals to meet this challenge.

Dementia

Dementia (from Latin *de-* "apart, away" + *mens* [genitive *mentis*] "mind") is the progressive decline in cognitive function due to damage or disease in the brain beyond what might be expected from normal aging (Galvin, Pollack, & Morris, 2006). Although dementia is far more common in the geriatric population, it may occur in any stage of adulthood. As will be seen subsequently, in rare instances the cognitive decline apparent in dementia can be observed in childhood as well. Dementia is a nonspecific disorder syndrome (set of signs and symptoms) that may ravage thinking and other areas of cognition. The term *cognition* is sometimes slippery. Some experts define it very broadly, some narrowly. The mental process of *knowing* includes aspects such as awareness, perception, reasoning, judgment, and many other brilliant pieces in the mosaic of *knowledge*. Precious cognitive skills usually encompass all the everyday uses of memory (and there are many Ben & Jerry flavors of memory, including sensory memory, working memory, semantic memory, and episodic memory), attention, language, and problem solving. Cognition and higher level brain functions are complex and never simple. The scientific journal *Memory and Cognition,* for example, invites articles on the topics of the processes of human memory and learning, psycholinguistics, problem solving, thinking, decision making, and skilled performance. Cognition includes a salad bar of high-level brain functions, including the ability to learn and remember information; to organize, plan, and figure out the solutions to problems; to focus, maintain, and shift attention as necessary; to understand and use language; to accurately perceive the environment; to perform calculations; and to invent, construct, create, and enjoy things that separate us from the flatworms, oysters, and partridges.

Many classification schemes of the dementias can be found in the literature. These include (Freetipson, 2010):

- *Cortical dementia:* dementia where the brain damage primarily affects the brain's cortex, or outer layer. Cortical dementias tend to cause problems with memory, language, thinking, and social behavior.
- *Subcortical dementia:* dementia that affects parts of the brain below the cortex. Subcortical dementia tends to cause changes in emotions and movement in addition to problems with memory.
- *Progressive dementia:* dementia that gets worse over time, gradually interfering with more and more cognitive abilities.
- *Primary dementia:* dementia such as AD that does not result from any other disease.
- *Secondary dementia:* dementia that occurs as a result of a physical disease or injury.

Some types of dementia fit into more than one of these classifications. For example, AD is considered both a progressive and a cortical dementia. (Esiri, Lee, & Trojaowski, 2004).

Early Warning Symptoms and Late Warning Signs

In dementia, a wide variety of higher mental functions are changed and reduced with memory disruption being the hallmark.(Small, Fratiglioni, & Backman, 2001) In the later stages of dementia, affected persons may be disoriented in time (not knowing what day of the week, day of the month, month, or even what year it is), in place (not knowing where they are), and in person (not knowing who they are or others around them). This is the *disorientation times three* that was previously cited (Alzheimer's Association, 2010). The Alzheimer's Association (http://www.alz.org/index.asp) has a checklist of early warning signs of dementia. This list has been widely reproduced in the popular literature and has helped with early diagnosis of dementia and has helped dispel the idea that every little missed appointment or memory loss for someone's name is the beginning of dementia.

Ten Warning Signs

The following list has been used to mark the early warning signs of behavior that may need some follow-up by health care professionals. The advice usually is that, if several items on the list are checked, a doctor or other health care professional should be consulted for a complete evaluation of the person with the signs and symptoms (Better Health, 2010):

1. Recent Memory Loss That Affects Day to Day Functions

It is normal to forget meetings, work associates' names, or a friend's telephone number occasionally, but then remember them later. With dementia, Uncle Lester may forget things more often, or not remember them at all.

2. Difficulty Performing Familiar Tasks

Busy people multitask and can be so distracted from time to time that they may leave the parsnips and fava beans in the microwave and only remember to serve them when the meal has finished and people are picking their teeth. A person with dementia would be more likely to prepare a meal and not only forget to serve the exotic vegetables, but also forget he or she made them.

3. Problems With Language

Everyone has trouble finding the right word or name sometimes, but a person with dementia may forget simple words or frequently substitute inappropriate words, making sentences and conversation difficult to understand. Comprehension of language might also start to become a problem with difficulty understanding steps or sequences of directions.

4. Disorientation to Time and Place

It is normal to forget the day of the week or your destination for a moment. Most of us forget where we parked on occasion when coming out of the Costco big box store or Best Buy after scoping out the latest iteration of G-phones. A person with dementia can become lost on her own street, not knowing where she is, how she got there, or how to get back home to her little dog Fluffy.

5. Poor or Decreased Judgment

Dementia affects a person's memory and concentration or focused attention, and this in turn can affect judgment. Many activities, such as driving, require good judgment and when this ability is affected, the person will be a risk, not only to him or herself, but also to others on the road. A person with dementia may increase taking risky behavior such as crossing the street in the middle of the block with oncoming traffic, or pulling out in front of a speeding Vespa with an Italian talking on a mobile phone.

6. Problems With Abstract Thinking

Balancing a checkbook may be difficult for many of us. Sloppy accounting is widely distributed and has provided the reason for many a relationship stagger, but chronic and increasing problem solving and slovenly accounting can be more serious. Someone with dementia could forget completely what the numbers are and what needs to be done with them or when their new paycheck is deposited.

7. Misplacing Things

Anyone can temporarily misplace a wallet or keys. A person with dementia may repeatedly put things in inappropriate places, and get increasingly forgetful such as failing to remember to put the little fellow away after going to the toilet.

8. Changes in Mood or Behavior

We all experience mood swings. Someone with dementia can have rapid mood swings with greater peaks and valleys for no apparent reason. He or she may become confused, suspicious, or withdrawn.

9. Changes in Personality

People's personalities can change a little with age. But a person with dementia can become suspicious or fearful or apathetic and seemingly uncaring. He also may become disinhibited, overly familiar, and sometimes more touchy-feely than is customary.

10. Loss of Initiative

Many of us get increasingly sick and tired of doing dishes and housework, business activities, or obligatory brié and Chablis cocktail parties. Clam dip retains only so much allure after the 300th party. The person with dementia may lose interest in previously enjoyed activities, or become very passive and require cues prompting them to become involved. Television may become a passive provider of prolonged attention.

Dementia is not a specific disease and not all dementias are Alzheimer's disease. *Dementia* is a descriptive term for a collection of signs and symptoms that can be caused by a baffling array of disorders that affect the brain. In most cases, the signs and symptoms creep up on people. Another problem in diagnosis of dementia is the general misunderstanding of the cognitive changes that accompany normal aging. People with dementia have significantly impaired intellectual functioning that interferes with normal activities and relationships. Melvin can't play cards. Myrtle can still knit, but her mittens are of different sizes. People lose their ability to solve problems and maintain emotional control, and they may experience personality changes and behavioral problems

such as agitation, delusions, and hallucinations. Fritzi is much crabbier than usual and spits his orange juice onto the table because it has pulp and he likes it pulpless. Memory loss, however, is the hallmark of dementia. It is more than just misplacing the keys, but more like misplacing the car. Memory loss by itself, however, does not mean that a person has dementia. Physicians diagnose dementia only if two or more brain functions—such as memory, language skills, perception, or other cognitive skills including reasoning and judgment—are considerably impaired without loss of consciousness. On average, people with dementia from Alzheimer's disease live for 8 to 10 years after they are diagnosed. However, some people live as long as 20 years. Patients with AD often die of aspiration pneumonia (getting liquid or food into the airway and lungs) because they lose the ability to swallow late in the course of the disease.

Reversibility

Symptoms and signs of dementia can be classified as either reversible or irreversible, depending on the cause of the impairments. Unfortunately *non*reversible dementia is the norm with less than 10% of cases traced to causes that may be reversed with treatment. The most common reversible dementia is the cognitive change brought on by adverse reactions to medication. Older adults make up only 12% of the population, but they receive more than 30% of all prescriptions written in the United States. Unfortunately, as people age, natural changes within the body make adverse effects from medication more likely. More important, however, is the fact that older adults take an average of more than five prescription drugs and three over-the-counter drugs at the same time. In geriatric clinics, the most common cause of reversible dementia is an adverse medication reaction (Christensen & White, 2007).

Depression also is a reversible cause. A person is more likely to be suffering from depression than dementia if there is a history of psychiatric illness, a rapid onset of cognitive symptoms, difficulties with sleep, or a very rapid decline in the ability to perform everyday activities (Rabins, 1983) Because depression and dementia are difficult to distinguish, it requires careful medical management to discover if the cause of dementia is reversible. A number of medical conditions can lead to memory problems. These conditions include hormonal imbalances; infectious diseases including AIDS and syphilis; tumors of the frontal or temporal lobe of the cerebral cortex; normal-pressure hydrocephalus (caused by excess fluid in the brain); and deficiencies of certain vitamins, especially B12.

Causes

More than 50 etiologies or causes of dementia are recognized, with Alzheimer's disease being the most frequent (Mace & Rabins, 2008). These can be categorized under:

- Diseases that cause degeneration or loss of nerve cells in the brain such as Alzheimer's, Parkinson's, and Huntington's (Figure 5–7).
- Diseases that affect blood vessels, such as stroke, which can cause a disorder known as vascular or multi-infarct dementia (WebMD, 2010).
- Toxic reactions, like excessive alcohol or drug use.

- Nutritional deficiencies, like vitamin B12 and folate deficiency.
- Infections that affect the brain and spinal cord, such as AIDS dementia complex and Creutzfeldt-Jakob disease.
- Certain types of hydrocephalus, an accumulation of fluid in the brain that can result from developmental abnormalities, infections, injury, or brain tumors.
- Head injury—either a single severe head injury or longer term smaller injuries, as in boxers (sometimes referred to as *dementia pugilistica*).
- Illness other than in the brain—kidney, liver, and lung diseases all can lead to dementia.

Alzheimer's disease (AD) causes 50 to 60% of all dementias. Because AD cannot be diagnosed definitively until autopsy, many writers refer to it as either "dementia of Alzheimer's type" (DAT) or "probable Alzheimer's dementia" (PAD). Alzheimer's disease is the most common cause of dementia in people aged 65 and older (Figure 5–8). Gerontologists (health care professionals specializing in aging) believe that up to 4 million people in the United States are currently living with the disease: 1 in 10 people over the age of 65 and nearly half of those over 85 have AD. At least 360,000 Americans are diagnosed with AD each year and about 50,000 are reported to die from it. According to the Alzheimer's Association, every 71 seconds someone is diagnosed with the dementia associated with Alzheimer's disease in the United States. Current facts and figures about Alzheimer's disease are organized on a useful information Web site by the Alzheimer's Association (http://www.alz.org/national/documents/report_alzfactsfigures2008.pdf).

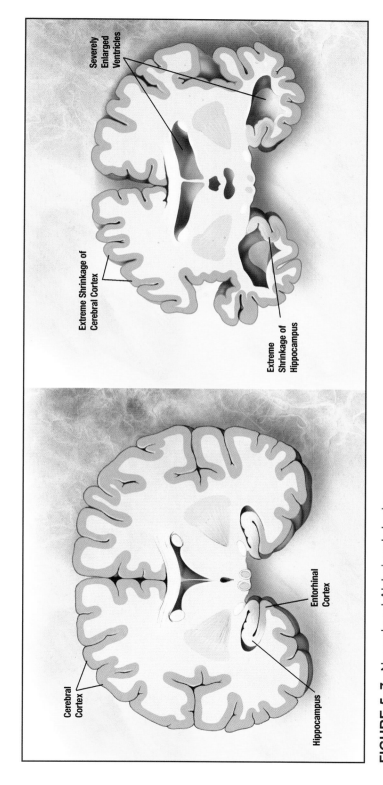

FIGURE 5–7. Normal and Alzheimer's brains.

Severely Enlarged Ventricles

Extreme Shrinkage of Cerebral Cortex

Extreme Shrinkage of Hippocampus

Cerebral Cortex

Entorhinal Cortex

Hippocampus

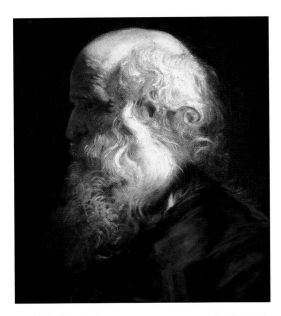

FIGURE 5–8. Aged person with Alzheimer's disease. (Study of the head of an old man, Peter Paul Rubens [Ulm 1610-1615]. Reprinted under the terms of the GNU Free Documentation License.)

In most people, signs and symptoms of AD appear after age 60. However, there are some early-onset forms of the disease, usually linked to a specific gene defect that may appear as early as age 30. AD usually causes a gradual decline in cognitive abilities over a span averaging 7 to 10 years. Nearly all brain functions, including memory, movement, language, judgment, behavior, and abstract thinking eventually are affected. AD is characterized by two abnormalities in the brain: *amyloid plaques* and *neurofibrillary tangles*. Amyloid plaques, found in the tissue between the neurons or brain cells, are unusual clusters of a protein called beta amyloid. Degenerating bits of brain cells may be part of these plaques. Neurofibrillary tangles are bundles of twisted filaments found within neurons. These tangles are largely made up of a

protein called *tau*. In healthy neurons, the tau protein helps the delivery and structure system of a healthy brain cell. However, in AD, tau is changed in a way that causes it to twist into pairs of filaments that collect into tangles not unlike a microscopic backlash of tangled line on a fishing reel.(MedicineNet, 2010). This disruption of the neuron's transport system may impair communication or synapses between nerve cells and cause them to wither and die (St. George-Hyslop, 2000).

Vascular Dementia

Vascular dementia is the second most common cause of dementia, after Alzheimer's disease. It accounts for up to 20% of all dementias and is caused by brain damage from cerebrovascular or cardiovascular problems (impaired blood circulation to the brain and/or heart), many times associated with strokes. Congestive heart failure (after all, the heart is a pump and is responsible for keeping the brain perfused with nourishment including oxygen and glucose-laden blood) also can be associated with dying neurons and emergent dementia. Vascular dementia also may result from certain genetic diseases, *endocarditis* (infection of a heart valve), or *amyloid angiopathy* (a process in which amyloid protein builds up in the brain's blood vessels, sometimes causing "bleeding" strokes). In some cases, vascular dementia may be diagnosed as "Alzheimer's" even though there eventually is no evidence of plaques or tangles in the wondrous neurons of the brain. My mother (LLL) got at least three diagnoses of "Alzheimer's disease" by three different physicians although time revealed that her encroaching dementia was indeed vascular and due to congestive heart failure and poorly functioning cardiac valves. The incidence of vascular dementia increases with advancing age and is similar in men and women.

Symptoms of vascular dementia occasionally begin suddenly, frequently after a stroke. A history of high blood pressure, vascular disease, or previous strokes or heart attacks raise warning flags for the development of vascular dementia. This vicious disease that claimed my mother's recent and short-term memory may or may not get worse with time, depending on whether the person has additional strokes or the condition of the precious, blood-carrying vascular system deteriorates. In some cases, symptoms may get better with time. When the disease does get worse, it often progresses in a stepwise manner, with sudden changes in ability. Unlike people with Alzheimer's, people with vascular dementia often maintain their more intact aspects of their personality and normal levels of emotional responsiveness until the later stages of the disease.

Several kinds or types of vascular dementia exist and they vary slightly in their causes and symptoms. One type, called multi-infarct dementia (MID), is caused by numerous small strokes in the brain. MID typically includes many damaged areas, called *infarcts*, along with wide-ranging injuries to the white matter (nerve fibers) of the brain (MedicineNet, 2010)

Because the damage in MID may affect isolated areas of the brain, the signs and symptoms can be limited to one side of the body or they may affect just one or a few specific functions, such as language. Neurologists call these "local" or "focal" symptoms, as opposed to the "global" or "diffuse" signs and symptoms seen in Alzheimer's, which affect many functions and are not restricted to one side of the body. (MedicineNet, 2010).

Although not all strokes cause dementia, in some cases a single stroke can damage the brain enough to cause dementia. This condition is called single-infarct dementia. Dementia is more common when the stroke takes place on the left side (hemisphere) of the brain and/or when it involves the hippocampus, that critical little seahorse-shaped brain structure that is so important for memory and acts as the "save as" button to convert short-term memories into long-term storage.

Another type of vascular dementia is called *Binswanger's disease*. This unusual form of dementia is characterized by damage to small blood vessels in the white matter of the brain (white matter is found in the inner layers of the brain and contains many nerve fibers coated with a whitish, fatty substance called myelin). Binswanger's disease leads to brain lesions, loss of memory, disordered cognition, mood changes, and all of the other mischief of dementia (MedicineNet, 2010).

Lewy Body Dementia

Lewy body dementia is similar to Alzheimer's but may progress more rapidly and is frequently characterized by hallucinations ("I see snakes!" "I hear Roy Orbison." "I see little pink cartoon bunnies!"). The word "hallucination" comes from Latin and means "to wander mentally." Hallucinations have been defined as the "perception of a nonexistent object or event" and "sensory experiences that are not caused by stimulation of the relevant sensory organs" (Bipolar, 2010).

In layman's terms, hallucinations involve hearing, seeing, feeling, smelling, and even tasting things that are not real. However, auditory hallucinations (hearing voices or other sounds that have no physical source) are the most common type. In Lewy body dementia, abnormal neurons or brain cells called Lewy bodies occur throughout widespread areas of the brain and cause the cognitive and perceptual disruption.

Frontal-Temporal Dementia

Frontal-temporal dementia (FTD) has a variant sometimes referred to as Pick's disease after a Czech neurologist (Pick, a Czech, was referred to punningly at an Academy of Aphasia meeting as a man who infrequently picked up a check). Fronto-temporal dementia is sometimes called frontal lobe dementia and describes a cluster of diseases characterized by degeneration of nerve cells, especially those in the frontal and temporal lobes of the brain. Unlike Alzheimer's, FTD usually does not include formation of amyloid plaques. In many people with FTD, there is an abnormal form of tau protein in the brain, which accumulates into neurofibrillary tangles. This disrupts normal cell activities and may cause the cells to die. In FTD, the brain cells of the frontal lobe (controlling emotions, mood, and thought) and temporal lobe (controlling speech, language, and memory) shrink or die. As a result, FTD is characterized by disturbances in speech/language, personality, and behavior.

Experts believe FTD accounts for 2 to 10% of all cases of dementia. Symptoms of FTD usually appear between the ages of 40 and 65. In many cases, people with FTD have a family history of dementia, suggesting that there is a strong genetic factor in the disease. The duration of FTD varies, with some patients declining rapidly over 2 to 3 years and others showing only minimal changes for many years. People with FTD live with the disease for an average of 5 to 10 years after diagnosis (Esiri, Lee, & Trojanowski 2004).

Because structures found in the frontal and temporal lobes of the brain control judgment and social behavior, people with FTD often have problems maintaining normal interactions and following social conventions. They may steal or exhibit impolite and socially inappropriate behavior, and they may neglect their normal responsibilities. Other common symptoms include loss of speech and language, compulsive or repetitive behavior, increased appetite, and motor problems such as stiffness and balance problems. Memory loss also may occur, although it typically appears late in the disease.

Language and Communication in Dementia

Language functioning may be relatively spared in the early stages of dementing diseases, but the good news is tempered by storm clouds on the horizon. Speech and language are likely to decline considerably in the mid to late stages. It is important to realize that most (although not all) dementia is not static but progressive and declines in behavior and function are expected. People with dementia often have difficulty with language expression, word fluency, and naming objects. Syntax and comprehension of language generally are preserved in the early stages; however, in the later stages, the storm clouds get closer and the impaired language front moves in. Speech may become halting due to word-finding difficulties. Names are lost or interchanged much more frequently. ("Tom! Lyell! No, Chickee! Put that accordion down and turn on the TV.") Greater difficulty speaking in full sentences is evident because of the great effort that is required to retrieve and order the right words. Writing skills may deteriorate, unless the person was a physician, in which case it was probably barely legible prior to the dementia. Speech comprehension may suffer during the end-stage of the disease with a decrease in responsiveness and failure to understand conversation and directions, especially if they are linguistically complex and rapidly presented (Bourgeois, 2010).

Approaches to Treatment

As mentioned earlier, some cases of dementia that are caused by identifiable medical conditions can be treated, fully or partly restoring, or drawing to a stop the decline of mental function. When dementia cannot be reversed, the goal of treatment is to make life as easy as possible for the person and the caregivers. For people with vascular dementia, doctors may prescribe medicines to lower high blood pressure and medicines for high cholesterol. These drugs cannot reverse existing dementia, but they may prevent future strokes and heart disease that can lead to further brain damage.

The American Speech-Language-Hearing Association (ASHA) has formulated guidelines for treatment (http://www.asha.org/docs/html/PS2005-00118.html). It is the position of this association that speech-language pathologists (SLPs) play a primary role in the screening, assessment, diagnosis, treatment, and

research of cognitive-communication disorders, including those associated with dementia. Given the growth in the number of older adults in the United States, the high incidence and prevalence of dementia in this population, and the negative impact of dementia on cognitive-communication abilities, appropriate assessment and intervention are critical and speech-language pathologists have a crucial role on the treatment team. Bourgeois (2010) presents many principles of treating the cognitive-communicative disturbances of dementia and details specific strategies that have an evidence-based rationale for their use. The Academy of Neurological Communication Sciences and Disorders (ANCDS) and the *Journal of Medical Speech-Language Pathology* have published guidelines and details on the scope of practice for treating people with dementia. Many clinical studies on communication treatment of dementia and the range of other neurologically based communication disorders are archived on the Web site of the Clinical Aphasiology Conference (http://www.ancds.org/; http://www.clinicalaphasiology.org/. The *Journal of Medical Speech-Language Pathology* can be accessed at the following website (Journal of Medical Speech-Language Pathology http://www.cengage.com/community/jmslp).

In addition to cognitive-communication problems, swallowing disorders often are present in persons with dementia. SLPs have a primary role in the screening, assessment, diagnosis, treatment, and research of swallowing disorders associated with dementia.

If the cause of dementia cannot be treated, the doctor will work with the person and caregivers to develop a plan to make life easier and more comfortable. Care plans may include tips to help the person be independent and manage daily life as long as possible. Education of the family and other caregivers is critical to successfully caring for a person with dementia. The life of a caregiver for one who has dementia is not easy. It has been characterized as "the longest funeral" and "36-hour day" (Mace & Rabins, 2008). Caregivers need support, counseling, information, and respite. Our Tallahassee Memorial HealthCare Adult Day Services center is a great example of the type of respite day care. Not only does this allow caregivers and families to work during the day and provide breathing space from the around the clock care necessary, but it also is a caring, warm, familylike environment that provides stimulation and learning. Pet therapy, music and art therapy, memory book training, field trips, visitors with reptiles, and the occasional Oktoberfest accordion player in lederhosen provide a swathe of brain and life stimulation. This is a model of a caring and stimulating environment. The guardianship and empathy of Ms. Corinne, Ms. Sheila, and others provide a place that is safe and invigorating. It and the Adult Day Care centers like it are a godsend to clients with dementia and their families unlike treatments utilized in past ages (Figure 5–9).

As dementia gets worse, memory, judgment, and the ability to make and carry out plans (executive function) may decline either gradually or sometimes precipitously. Depending on the type of dementia and the portions of the brain affected, the person's behavior may become out of control; the person may become angry, agitated, or combative. Swinging the fist or slap attempts are not unknown. The person may wander and become lost. These problems can make it difficult for family members

or others to continue providing care at home. The family may have to face the difficult decisions involved in consideration of whether to place the person in a care facility that has a dementia unit. These are not easy decisions and the health care team of professionals can help with them (Shulz, 2000).

Future

Researchers are working around the clock to develop new drugs for Alzheimer's disease and other types of dementia. Many researchers believe a vaccine that reduces the number of amyloid plaques in the brain ultimately might prove to be the most effective treatment for AD. Researchers also are investigating possible methods of gene therapy for dementia. In one case, researchers used cells genetically engineered to produce nerve growth factor and transplanted them into monkeys' forebrains. The transplanted cells boosted the amount of nerve growth factors in the brain and seemed to prevent degeneration of acetylcholine-producing brain cells in the animals. This suggests that gene therapy might help to reduce or delay symptoms of the disease. Researchers now are testing a similar therapy in a small number of patients. Other researchers have experimented with gene therapy that adds a gene called *neprilysin* in a mouse model that produces human beta amyloid. They found that increasing the level of neprilysin greatly reduced the amount of bad brain parts in the mice and halted the amyloid-related brain degeneration. They now are trying to determine whether neprilysin gene therapy can improve cognition in mice. One might not think of mice as having a full deck of cognitive skills, but watching a

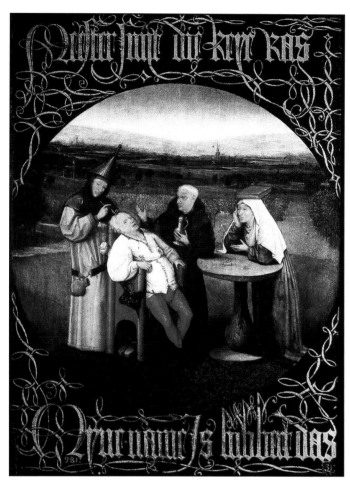

FIGURE 5–9. Trepanation old print. (*Das Steinschneiden* by Hieronimus Bosch, 1500. Public domain at Wikimedia Commons.)

few of the old Tom and Jerry cartoons might convince us otherwise. Gene therapy has been politicized in the United States, and countries such as Australia and Sweden which seem to have less political intrusion into research agendas seem to be ahead of the United States in some aspects of gene therapy development. Research at our university and at other centers throughout the world are working every day on issues of brain plasticity, neuronal and dendritic sprouting, and creating new, healthy archi-

tecture of this amazing, three-pound, squishy mass that controls all we are and all we want to be.

There is still a long way to go, but some of the diseases and conditions that cause nonfocal brain damage are experiencing rapid technological advances regarding understanding, diagnosis, and treatment. We can only hope that the coming generations will experience breakthroughs that allow humane and effective intervention for these terrible brain-based disorders.

Childhood Dementia

Childhood dementia? It seems like an oxymoron, such as "deafening silence," "plastic glass," or "vegetarian meatballs." Dementia most commonly affects adults and is most prominently associated with aging, but it *can* also occur in children (Figure 5–10). For example, infections and poisoning can lead to dementia in children, adolescents, or adults. Dementia essentially is a gradual loss of cognitive skills and memory beyond what would be expected by normal development or aging. It is surprising that it can happen in childhood but, tragically, it can. Several disorders normally unique to children can cause rapid or gradual decline in memory, cognitive skills, and even motoric performance in young people. These rare conditions are reviewed in several pediatric neurology textbooks, included in the classic text by Swaiman, Ashwal, & Ferriero (2006). Several of these distinctive conditions have recently come to light and a clearer picture of their characteristics is emerging. Conditions that can cause dementia in childhood include:

- Niemann-Pick disease
- Batten disease
- Lafora body disease

Childhood Dementia and Niemann-Pick Disease

Niemann-Pick disease is a group of inherited disorders that affect metabolism and are caused by specific genetic abnormalities. Children with Niemann-Pick disease cannot properly utilize cholesterol and other body chemicals. Therefore, excessive amounts of cholesterol accumulate in the liver and spleen and excessive amounts of other chemicals accumulate in the brain and can then contribute to brain dysfunction (Nunn, Williams, & Ouvrier, 2002)

Symptoms and signs of Niemann-Pick disease may include:

- Dementia
- Confusion and disorientation
- Problems with learning and memory.

Niemann-Pick disease usually begins in young school-age children but it also may appear during teenage years or early adulthood. The cognitive decline seen in this tragic disease leads to some of the same cognitive disruptions in memory and thinking that are seen in dementia in older people.

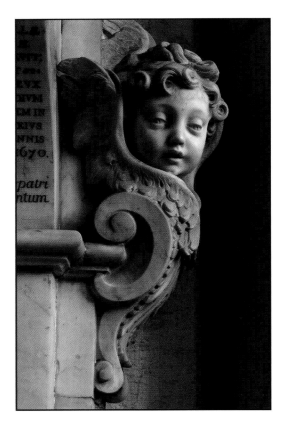

FIGURE 5–10. Cherub.

Batten Disease and Childhood Dementia

Batten disease is a fatal, hereditary disorder of the nervous system that begins in childhood. Symptoms of Batten disease are linked to a buildup of substances called lipopigments in the tissues of the body including the brain. Early signs of Batten disease include:

- Personality and behavior changes
- Slow learning
- Motoric clumsiness and stumbling

Over time, children who contract Batten disease suffer a decline in mental and cognitive skills and may develop seizures and progressive loss of vision and gross motor skills.

The progression of Batten disease is tragic and inevitable. In nearly all cases, these children will develop childhood dementia and become blind and bedridden. The disease frequently results in death in the late teens or early 20s.

Childhood Dementia and Lafora Body Disease

Lafora body disease is a rare genetic disease that causes seizures, rapidly progressive dementia, and movement and fine motor problems. These problems usually begin in late childhood or early adolescence. Children with Lafora body disease have microscopic structures called Lafora bodies in the brain, skin, liver, and muscles. Most affected children die within 2 to 10 years after the onset of abnormal signs and an accurate diagnosis.

A number of other childhood disorders that are equally tragic and rare can include symptoms of childhood dementia. So childhood dementia is not a mis-

nomer or an oxymoron. It can be caused by a number of rare genetic or metabolic diseases that alter thinking, memory, and other cognitive skills just as the dementia usually seen in much older people.

Summary

A number of nonfocal diseases and disorders that affect diffuse and widespread areas of the brain can wreak havoc with speech, language, thinking, and swallowing. TBI and dementia are a couple of the most common and most dreadful. Speech-language pathologists and other members of the rehabilitation team are prepared to bring maximal degrees of normalcy into these shattered lives.

References

Alzheimer's Association. (2010). Retrieved February 13, 2010, from http://www.alz.org/index.asp

Better Health. (2010). Retrieved February 13, 2010, from http://www.betterhealth.vic.gov.au/bhcv2/bhcarticles.nsf/pages/Dementia_diagnosis_and_early_signs

Bipolar. (2010). *Hallucinations.* Retrieved February 13, 2010, from http://bipolar.about.com/cs/faqs/f/faq_hallucinate.htm

Bourgeois, M. (2010). Dementia. In L. L. LaPointe (Ed.), *Aphasia and related language disorders* (4th ed.). New York, NY: Thieme Medical Publishers.

Centers for Disease Control. (2010). *TBI.* Retrieved February 13, 2010, from http://www.cdc.gov/ncipc/tbi/TBI.htm

Christensen, M., & White, H. (2007). Dementia assessment and management. *Journal of the American Medical Directors Association, 8*(3), e89–e98.

Esiri, M. M., Lee, M., & Trojanowski J. Q. (2004). *The neuropathology of dementia* (2nd ed.). Cambridge, UK: Cambridge University Press.

Freetipson. (2010). Retrieved February 13, 2010, from http://www.freetipson.co.uk/healthcare/dementia/different_kinds_dementia.html

Galvin J. E., Pollack, J., & Morris, J. (2006). Clinical phenotype of Parkinson disease dementia. *Neurology, 67*(9): 1605–1611.

Mace, N. L., & Rabins, P. V. (2008). *The 36-hour day: A family guide to caring for persons with Alzheimer disease, related dementing illnesses, and memory loss in later life* (4th ed.). Baltimore, MD: Johns Hopkins University Press.

MedicineNet. (2010). *Dementia.* Retrieved February 13, 2010, from http://www.medicinenet.com/dementia/page2.htm

NINDS, NIH. (2010). *TBI.* Retrieved February 13, 2010, from http://www.ninds.nih.gov/disorders/tbi/tbi.htm

Nunn K., Williams K., & Ouvrier, R. (2002). The Australian childhood dementia study. *European Child and Adolescent Psychiatry, 11*(2), 63–70.

Rabins, J. (1983). Reversible dementia and the misdiagnosis of dementia: A review. *Hospital and Community Psychiatry, 34,* 830–835.

Shulz, R. (2000). *Handbook on dementia caregiving: Evidence-based interventions for family caregivers.* New York, NY: Springer.

Small, B. J., Fratiglioni, L., & Backman, L. (2001). Canaries in a coal mine: Cognitive markers of preclinical Alzheimer disease. *Archives of General Psychiatry, 58*(9), 859–860.

Swaiman, K. F., Ashwal, S., & Ferriero, D. M. (2006). *Pediatric neurology: Principles and practice* (4th ed.). Philadelphia, PA: Mosby.

St. George-Hyslop, P. H. (2000). Piecing together Alzheimer's. *Scientific American, 283,* 76–83.

Wallace, G. L. (2006). Blast injury basics: A guide for the medical speech-language pathologist. *ASHA Leader, 11*(9), 26–28.

WebMD. (2010). *Alzheimers.* Retrieved February 13, 2010, from http://www.webmd.com/alzheimers/guide/alzheimers-dementia

6

Right Hemisphere Syndrome

When the Right Goes Wrong . . .

Frances Begay is a 38-year-old woman who lives in Chinle, Arizona. She is an American Indian and was born in Gallup, New Mexico and has lived much of her life on the Navajo Nation, in northern Arizona and New Mexico in the United States. She left her home area to attend boarding school and to study nursing in Phoenix. She has two daughters, ages 5 and 8, and worked for 10 years as a surgical nurse in a large hospital. Two years ago she had a "thromboembolic cerebrovascular accident," a stroke that damaged the right cerebral hemisphere of her brain. For several weeks after the cerebrovascular accident (CVA), she was hospitalized and left with difficulty moving her left arm and leg; with what the physician called "slurred speech"; and with difficulty reading and writing. Two years later, and after a brief period of physiotherapy and speech rehabilitation, she can walk and talk, but has a strange complex of complaints, many of which she believes are taken only half seriously by her family and some health care professionals.

As Frances puts it, "I still have trouble recognizing people. It's like I can see the details of their faces, but I can't hook it up with who the person is. Some of these I should really know. My husband said I even had trouble recognizing him right after my stroke. My speech is better, but I have trouble with long conversations, and if someone gives me directions in long sentences, forget it. I have trouble seeing things, also. Maybe I need new glasses. When I read to my girls—we're reading them stories of Navajo legends about Coyote and Spider Woman—some of it I skip or I get lost following the lines. Sometimes my family says I act strange. My old aunt says I might have some bad ghosts around me and I need to go to a sing, or a healing ceremony with sand paintings. She says this will restore hózhó, the Navajo sense of balance or harmony. I'm ready to try the old ways. I can't go back to work like this. I get lost. I can't find my way around buildings. I can't sing. My voice is flat. My emotions are different. My husband tells me I'm rude, and I interrupt and don't listen to him. I don't get people's meanings from their speech or facial expression. I really can't comprehend long, important conversations or paragraphs in books. My attention and memory are terrible. These are all such covered problems. They're not visible. People don't understand them. But they are driving me nuts. I wish someone could explain all of this to me and my family. I wish someone would help me."

Introduction

Frances Begay has some of the classic signs and symptoms of right hemisphere syndrome (RHS). Presumably, people like Frances have suffered right cerebral hemisphere brain damage as long as they have endured the slings and arrows of neuropathology, or damage to the nervous system. About as many people have strokes to the right hemisphere of the brain as have strokes to the left hemisphere, but one would never know it by the numbers registered in rehabilitation programs. Nearly 700,000 people will have a new or recurrent stroke each year in the United States, and more than 4 million people survive and still carry the effects of stroke. Because about half of the figures presented above can be expected to result in right hemisphere damage (RHD) and right hemisphere syndrome (RHS), it is easy to appreciate that this is a significant health and rehabilitation issue. It affects old and young, educated and uneducated, fit and unfit, rich and poor, male and female. A prime minister is as vulnerable as a street cleaner. Yet right hemisphere syndrome is thought by

some to be a neglected and relatively undiagnosed aspect of stroke (Foerch et al., 2005). Foerch and colleagues examined data from a prospective multicenter hospital stroke registry, including over 20,000 patients with stroke or transient ischemic attack, and found a remarkable difference in the rate of diagnosis of left-hemisphere and right-hemisphere stroke events. Why is right-brain stroke so unnoticed? The disproportionate diagnosis was greatest in those least severely affected; suggesting that perceived severity or significance of symptoms and signs is the dominant factor. The major behavioral asymmetry between the brain hemispheres is the lateralization of speech and language functions; specifically the left-hemispheric dominance of language functions. Probably patients, their families—and their physicians—might be more likely to recognize a disturbance of speech or language from left-hemisphere stroke than the much subtler perceptual and behavioral effects seen in right hemisphere syndrome. Although the disturbances are not as apparent and dramatic in RHS, they can be crucially disruptive to leading a normal life. This chapter draws back the veil on some of these nuances.

Historical Perspective

Damage to the left cerebral hemisphere creates obvious, dramatic, and tragically debilitating conditions that can be recognized by nearly anyone. Right hemisphere damage is veiled, subtle, and sneaky. As is almost universally recognized, much more research and clinical attention in higher cortical dysfunction has been directed toward the more apparent disturbances that accompany left hemisphere damage. In fact, in one of his many writings about unique and interesting cases of neurologic aberration, the gifted writer and neurologist Oliver Sacks (1995) suggested that, indeed, the entire history of neurology and neuropsychology can be viewed as the investigation of the left hemisphere. This is quite apparent in early and even some contemporary writings on the right hemisphere. The role of the right cerebral hemisphere is characterized in the literature as being "minor," "spare," "subdominant," "mute," and even "subservient to the Czar" of the left hemisphere. Yet people continue to be stricken with and endure the disability of right hemisphere syndrome, and, I will argue, continue to endure the medical and rehabilitative neglect of their subtle, not so subtle, and puzzling perceptual, cognitive, and communication disruptions. This is a most neglected, underdiagnosed, and underappreciated set or cluster of behavioral higher cortical deficits, but careful examination reveals that these deficits translate to very genuine altered life participation and activities that have a significant impact on perceived quality of life. Those of us who have labored in the vineyards of clinical rehabilitation of people with cortical damage rec-

ognize oft-quoted comments by family and professionals. We hear these comments so frequently; they are almost like familiar songs we have heard before. In aphasia, we commonly hear, "He understands everything you say. He just can't talk." For people afflicted with apraxia of speech, we hear, "I know what it is, but I just can't say it." In right hemisphere syndrome, the refrain is a bit different. We hear from family and fellow medical professionals, "He talks . . . but he isn't the same."

Historically, we see relatively few references (compared to the "other" hemisphere) to the disturbances of the right hemisphere (Figure 6–1). The British neurologist John Hughlings Jackson (1874) wrote cogently about many topics and was one of the first to give credence

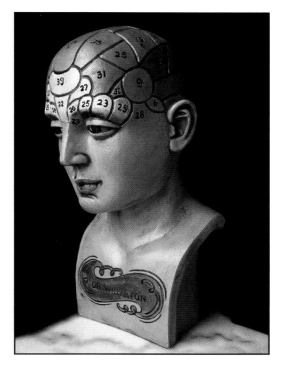

FIGURE 6–1. Phrenology head. Public domain at Wikimedia Commons.

to the somewhat different role of the right hemisphere (Figure 6–2). In 1874 he suggested that the two hemispheres have different functional roles. The left, he suggested, mediates verbal activity and the right was devoted to visuoperceptive, visuospatial, and visuoconstructive tasks. This stance was not generally accepted at the time, but gained broader acceptance in the 1940s when clinical insights were gained from vast numbers of head-injured war veterans. More contemporaneously, others, including the British neurologist MacDonald Critchley (1962), the neurolinguist Ruth Lesser (1978), and the late American aphasiologist Jon Eisenson (1984) noted that right hemisphere lesions could, in fact, produce subtle linguistic deficits. Eisenson suggested the right hemisphere was involved in super- or extraordinary language functions. Critchley stated that the

right hemisphere indeed has a role in language, and Lesser reported that the right hemisphere damaged subjects she had tested were worse than non-brain-damaged subjects on a semantic discrimination task. The old phrenology heads that inaccurately associated bumps on the head with human behaviors and brain functions were all the vogue for many years in the early 1800s.

Causes of Right Hemisphere Damage

Just as for all of the disruptions of speaking, understanding, thinking, and perceiving that are related to brain damage, a variety of diseases and conditions can create RHS. A cartwheel somersault from a motorcycle that fractures the

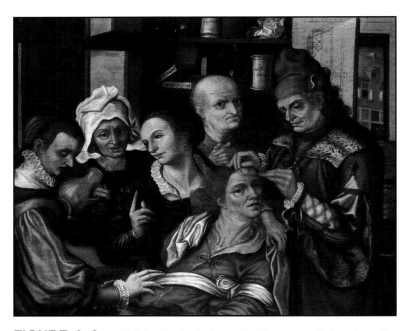

FIGURE 6–2. Old Master Painting. (*A Surgeon Extracting the Stone of Folly*, Pieter Huys, 1545–1577. Public domain at Wikimedia Commons.)

skull and damages neurons (brain cells); a brain-penetrating bullet from a handgun; an errant arrow from a drunken archer; a bathtub fall with a nasty head bump on the toilet; a whap on the head with a cricket or baseball bat; and a self-induced suicide attempt by poking a chopstick through the orbit of the eye all are documented types of brain damage that have been caused by trauma, direct insult to brain tissue. The category of **traumatic brain injury (TBI)** is one of the most frequent causes of nervous system damage in people aged 15 to 24 years. A significant number of TBIs also are seen in two other demographic age categories, toddlers ages 1 to 3 years and the elderly, ages 75 years and older. The last two age groups are susceptible to falls that injure the brain. We can expect to see many more people with TBI as in the texting while driving victim of Figure 6–3.

The leading cause of brain damage and RHS is stroke or **cerebrovascular accident (CVA)**. Additional details on causes of damage to the brain are covered in detail in the chapter in this book on Aphasia, but a review is presented here. "Cerebro-" refers to the brain; "vascular" refers to the blood supply; and "accident" refers generally to something going awry with the brain-blood supply. The term "accident" in CVA actually is a bit confusing, as it is easily mixed up with the traumatic brain injury (TBI) category, which is associated with so many forms of vehicular, shooting, and falling accidents. In fact, cerebrovascular accident (CVA) is no accident at all, but the result of underlying conditions that can interrupt the blood supply to brain tissue (Figure 6–4). When that happens, and life-giving nutrients in the bloodstream are prevented from nourishing brain cells for more than about 4 minutes, permanent death of brain cells can occur. The most frequent causes of blood supply interruption are blood clots (thromboses)

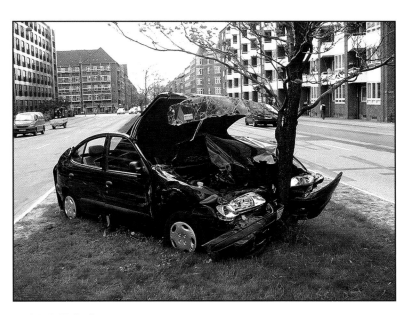

FIGURE 6–3. Crash. Public domain at Wikimedia Commons.

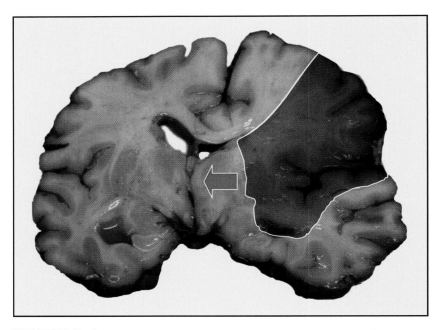

FIGURE 6–4. Brain with a stroke (cerebrovascular accident).

that develop and dam the stream of blood; or clots that break off and move with the current upstream until they reach impassable vessels. These moving clots are called *emboli* (plural). One moving clot is an *embolism*. For all practical purposes, it is very difficult for medical specialists to discern if a CVA was caused by a moving or nonmoving blood clot, so it is not at all unusual to see the terms combined in reports of brain damage. *Thromboembolic* is the term used in these cases, and it would not be unusual to read a medical report of a hospitalized survivor of a CVA that says, "This 72-year-old ballerina suffered a right cerebral hemisphere thromboembolic CVA in the middle cerebral artery." That means that the unfortunate dancer had either a moving or nonmoving interruption to the blood vessels that are distributed in the middle-exterior region of the right cerebral hemisphere of her brain. No doubt the dance would

be tragically interrupted if damage was similar to that shown in Figure 6–4.

Aside from these two categories of brain damage (TBI and CVA), there are a number of other ways that the brain can go bad. Infections of viruses or bacteria can cause damage to the brain. The HIV-AIDS virus can attack brain tissue as can a variety of other **infectious diseases** or agents. *Toxins* or poisons also can get into the blood supply and damage brain cells. A wide variety of recreational drugs ("ecstasy" and a lot of others) can leave the user with more than a euphoric "high" but also permanently damaged brain cells. A study in the United States has provided the first direct evidence that chronic use of methylenedioxymethamphetamine MDMA, popularly known as "ecstasy," causes brain damage in users. Using advanced brain imaging techniques, the study found that MDMA harms neurons that release serotonin, a brain chemical thought to play an important role in regulating memory and other functions. In another study, researchers found that heavy MDMA users have memory problems that persist for at least 2 weeks after they have stopped using the drug. Both studies suggest that the extent of damage is directly correlated with the amount of MDMA use (Mathias, 1999). Another well-known and widely used neurotoxin (brain poison) is alcohol, and the long-term effects of alcohol use are well documented in the brain damage literature. Perhaps the drinking salute should not be "Cheers," or "Bottoms up," but "Have a pint. Kill some neurons."

Another category of brain damage is that of *neurodegenerative diseases*. This category includes hundreds of rare and not-so-rare conditions such as Alzheimer's disease (Figure 6–5), Parkinson disease, amyotrophic lateral sclerosis (ALS), multiple sclerosis (MS), and Huntington's disease. These conditions can kill brain cells, sometimes rapidly, sometimes over a span of decades. They can affect many different parts of the nervous system. Some of them seem to attack motor or movement systems, some of them target the cerebral hemispheres and can cause dementia, with severe memory loss. Some types of brain damage compromise the very human behaviors of attending, thinking, planning, perceiving, emoting, communicating, and just acting cool and having a good time as in Figure 6–6.

So it should be clear that brain damage can come from many sources. The brain is an intricate network of billions of interconnected neurons and networks that allow all of our pleasures of daily life. It is responsible for our abilities to taste a Devonshire strawberry tart, to plan a holiday at the Matamanoa Resort in Fiji, to carry out the dust bin, to sing to our parakeet, to listen to a classic Fawlty Towers routine ("Don't mention the war . . . "), to figure out how many U.S. dollars are necessary to purchase a Hong Kong vegetarian lunch of tarot mock fish and tofu chicken, and to whisper words of appreciation for the selflessness of a soul mate. It is also a tapestry that can come unraveled, and when the unraveling is located in the

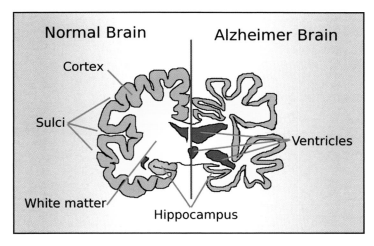

FIGURE 6–5. Normal brain and brain demonstrating Alzheimer's disease.

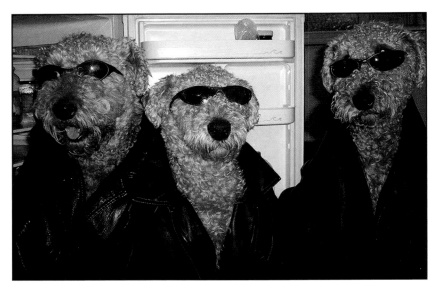

FIGURE 6–6. Cool dogs.

right cerebral hemisphere a remarkable and strange conglomeration of signs, symptoms, and characteristics can ensue (Figure 6–7). It is to those specific and strange deficits that we now turn.

Characteristic Deficits in Right Hemisphere Syndrome (RHS)

As one peruses the growing literature on right hemisphere damage, it becomes apparent that researchers and clinicians report a diversity of language and language-related perceptual and cognitive disturbances. The most frequent complaints appear to be neglect of visual half space; affective and emotional deficits; and cognitive and subtle communicative deficits. Oliver Sacks described the strange case of "Dr. P." in *The Man Who Mistook His Wife for a Hat* (1985). Dr. P was a music professor or teacher with a cerebral tumor in the posterior region of

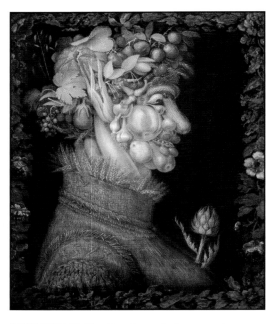

FIGURE 6–7. Garden of signs and symptoms. (*The Gardener*, Giuseppe Arcimboldo, 1590s. Public domain on Wikimedia Commons.)

his right hemisphere. Not only did he mistake his wife for a hat (which could be a socially punishing mix up), but he was characterized as presenting unusual visual neglect and recognition problems; the inability grasp the theme or gist of pictures with preserved elaborate focus on the details; and a startling prosopagnosia, or facial recognition problem. The wonderful crafter of evocative language, Oliver Sacks, also has rhapsodized about the lost world of music that occasionally is due to malfunction of the right cerebral hemisphere.

Tompkins (1995), Beeman and Chiarello (1998), Myers (1999), and Blake (2005) each have produced a comprehensive review of right hemisphere impairment in cognition and communication. Myers characterizes a "typical" description of right hemisphere syndrome as including the following features:

- Adequate communication in superficial conversation or discourse
- Flatness of voice and affect
- Perceptions by listeners of inattention, insensitivity or rudeness, poor language pragmatics (frequent interruptions; little eye contact).

Brownell and his colleagues (1995) propose that the right hemisphere may be less focally organized than the left and that the primary underpinnings of the reported deficits in RHS are fundamental impairments in perception, attention, and integration. These base disturbances have the capability of creating a garden of cognitive and communicative disabilities all of which can affect life quality. Behavioral management can address many of these disturbances. Although we await definitive efficacy data on clinical interventions, a growing literature attests to the principles and specific strategies of behavioral intervention. The effectiveness of these interventions is increasingly strengthened by care-

fully controlled case studies and by empirical intervention research. Both Tompkins (1995) and Myers (1999) catalog many of these principles and outcomes of behavioral intervention. The brain in the bottle is slowly revealing its secrets (Figure 6–8).

This "garden" of perceptual, cognitive, and communicative disruption in RHS has led to what some might portray as an overgrowth of attempts to classify and categorize them (see Figure 6–7). Myers, in *Aphasia and Related Neurogenic Language Disorders* (LaPointe, 1997), used a classification system of linguistic deficits, extralinguistic deficits, and nonlinguistic deficits to try to capture the richness of RHS. Her subsequent writing (Myers, 1999) has abridged this classification scheme somewhat.

In this chapter we advance another scheme of classification of RHS. We believe the signs, symptoms, and characteristics of right hemisphere dysfunction

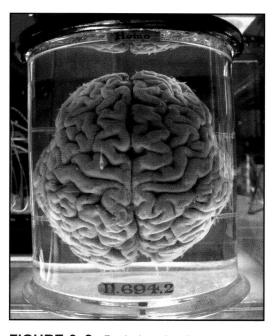

FIGURE 6–8. Brain in a bottle.

can be encapsulated by the following three primary categories:

1. Visual-perceptual disorders
2. Primary communication-cognition effects
3. Complex communication-cognition effects

Visual-Perceptual Disorders

Visual-perceptual disorders are among the most frequently mentioned set of deficits associated with RHS. Given the role of the right in all kinds of visual tasks, as well as its role in attention, it is not surprising that manifestations in visual performance occur after stroke or other cerebral pathology. These difficulties occasionally clear early through physiologic restitution, but all too frequently they do not. Typical complaints from hospital personnel include, "She is leaving all the food on half of her tray." Although aspects of neglect are sometimes difficult to uncover, they are of more than just academic interest. Quality of life may be altered by observed and reported difficulty with:

■ Responding to people and objects to the left of midline
■ Failure to attend to the left part of the body during self-care (grooming, bathing, eating, dressing)
■ Movement or recognition of the left limbs
■ Navigating hallways and passageways
■ Reading the left portions of printed material
■ Using margins during writing
■ Following films, theater, or television
■ Localizing sounds.

The visual-perceptual problems of RHD are not simply a matter of neglect or inattention to the *left* side of body midline. Visual neglect has been reported to occur in 30 to 60% of those who suffer right hemisphere damage. Although it may clear, it may last for several months or even years. Some survivors of RHD have persistent neglect that can be demonstrated for the duration of life. Neglect is far more prevalent on the left, but it can occur to the right as well, and occurs in left hemisphere damage occasionally but frequently may be masked by coexisting aphasia. In fact, lesion sites creating visual neglect include frontal and parietal cortex, basal ganglia, internal capsule, and thalamus. In addition, neglect can occur across modalities and, although most common in vision, it has been reported for auditory, tactile, and olfactory stimuli. To the surprise of some, neglect can be reflected in motoric leftward movements. The following three figures present illustrative examples of visual-perceptual neglect or inattention across a series of tasks that are frequently requested during assessment. Figure 6–9 is an attempt by a woman with visual neglect to copy pictures of a clock, a house, and a tree. Figure 6–10 is a line cancellation task completed by a man with visual neglect. Notice the neglect of drawing cancellation lines on the left side of the paper. Figure 6–11 is a tracing of eye movements made by a woman with visual neglect as she explores a picture. Notice that most of the movements are confined to the right half of the visual space.

In addition to visual neglect, "face blindness" (prosopagnosia) is a less common, but debilitating condition as well. It results in social, pragmatic, and identity problems, and frequently has

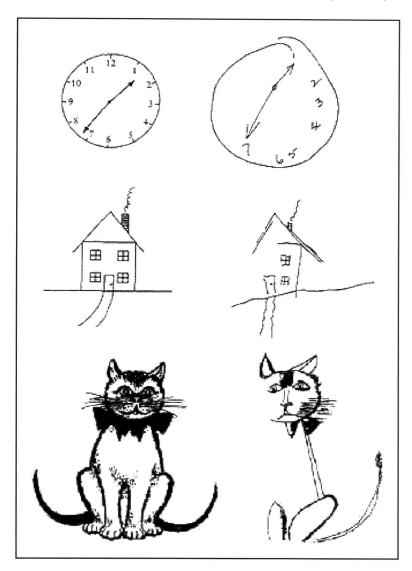

FIGURE 6–9. Visual neglect copying.

been diagnosed as a psychiatric condition. The fusiform gyrus, an area of the brain important for visual functions, has been linked with dissociation of the neural centers that link emotionality and visual pattern recognition and is a site of damage linked with this strange inability to recognize faces, even of those who are close friends or family.

Figure 6–12 presents areas of the brain associated with facial recognition.

It is difficult for someone without the condition of prosopagnosia to visualize what it is like. To have difficulty piecing together the elements of a very familiar face (even one's wife or child) and not be able to make sense of it or interpret meaning from it must be a

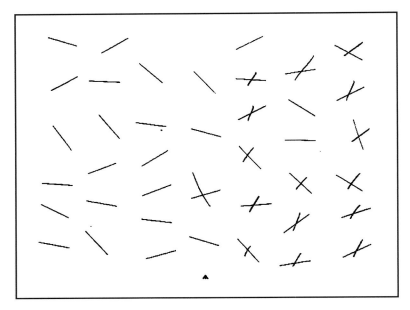

FIGURE 6–10. Line cancellation task (Instructions: "Strike through all of the lines that you can see.")

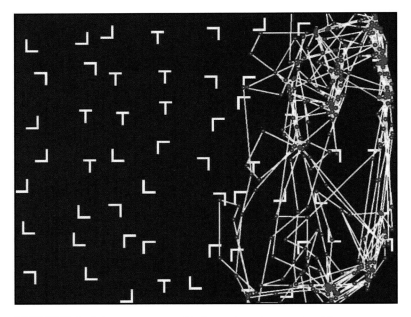

FIGURE 6–11. Evidence of left neglect in eye tracking.

strange and devastating condition. The fusiform gyrus is an area of the brain that helps associate facial memories with meaning. When it is damaged, as with Oliver Sacks' Dr. P, the remarkable condition of prosopagnosia can be the result.

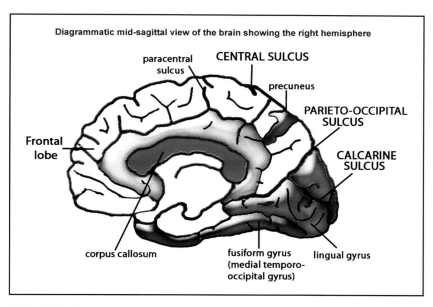

FIGURE 6–12. Fusiform gyrus. Areas of the brain associated with face recognition problems.

People with RHS also have difficulty with visuo-constructive tasks, such as copying block designs, making patterns or forms with toothpicks, assembling jigsaw puzzles, or doing visuo-constructive manipulations in their "mind's eye." And the mind's eye can be fooled. As you look at Figure 6–13 and move your head closer to and farther from the figure you get the remarkable perception of movement. Visual reconstruction in the mind's eye is an unheralded little appreciated skill. For example, most of us can visualize in our mind what a bicycle looks like. Most of us probably would call to mind a side view of a bike with saddle or seat, handlebars, and two wheels with a view of the spokes. A visuo-constructive manipulation would be required, however, if the instructions were, "Now visualize and describe the bicycle from the rider's point of view." This type of perceptual-constructive revisualization is very difficult for some-

one with RHS. So is map reading, map-folding (difficult for some of us without RHS as well), maze tracing, and following trails or paths in a prescribed manner. Reconstructing directions in one's head ("How do you get from the hair dresser's shop to the Blind Hairy-Nosed Wombat Pub?") is problematic as well, and is the reason that so many people with RHS get lost, wander about hospital wards, or can't find their way home from simple trips to do errands. This has been called "topographic disorientation" and is a common observation and complaint in RHD.

Primary Communication-Cognition Effects

In contemporary models of higher cortical function and dysfunction, it is becoming increasingly recognized that the relationships among various cognitive domains and language are less than

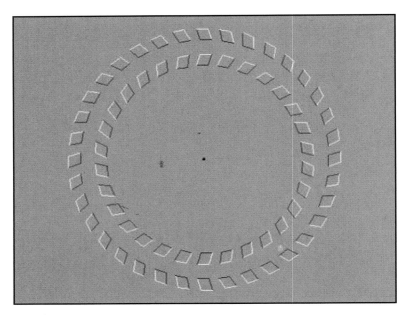

FIGURE 6–13. Visual illusion. Move your head closer. Watch it move.

clear. We know that such cognitive domains as attention and memory not only support linguistic processing, but also may be critically interwoven with it. Research efforts in our laboratories at Florida State University and at the University of Queensland have focused on issues of cognitive resource allocation, the effects of distraction, and dual task paradigms on linguistic processing, and the development of ways to separate or identify cognitive influences on language. In RHS, we see not just the subtle visual problems outlined above, but, increasingly, disruption of primary language and cognitive functions. Of course, these effects may not be as obvious or dramatic as is traditionally seen in the aphasias of left hemisphere damage, but careful assessment can reveal some very genuine problems that create trouble with communication and cognition not apparent in the premorbid state. Joanette, Goulet, and Hannequin (1990)

were among the first to catalogue the verbal problems in persons with right hemisphere problems. These primary communication-cognition effects are evident in:

■ attention and memory,
■ reading,
■ writing,
■ verbal fluency and naming,
■ narratives, and
■ comprehension.

Attention and Memory

The parameters of the control of information processing and the varieties of disruption of these cognitive processes are legendary. In RHD, current research efforts are attempting to clarify the nature of disruptions of sustained attention, focused attention, and divided attention on language processing. The right hemisphere plays an important role in attention, and the arousal system so necessary for forms of attention seems quite lateralized to the right.

The orientation of attention across spatial boundaries may account for the visual neglect syndromes we see. Right hemisphere frontal lobe areas are important for maintaining attention; hence, sustained attention or vigilance can be difficult tasks as well. Selective attention also has been attributed to right hemisphere function. These cognitive effects can impact a wide range of interactive behaviors and may play a role in the wandering concentration and pragmatically inappropriate behavior we observe in such things as poor eye contact during conversational discourse.

The memory parameters of working memory, episodic and autobiographic memory, and long-term memory appear to be differentially affected across subjects with RHS and are the focus of a good deal of clinical research in laboratories and hospitals around the world.

Reading

Appreciation and interpretation of printed letter strings is another basic process frequently disrupted in RHS. This may be the influence of visuoperceptive problems or of the person's difficulty in integrating and piecing together parts of a printed narrative into a cohesive whole. The person with RHS may get lost reading long newspaper or magazine articles and fail to extract or get the sense of meaning from printed material. Of course, in the assessment of language of adolescents and adults, it is important to use age-appropriate material. There is nothing quite so demeaning as asking a former professor of creative writing to read "Cinderella," "The Three Little Pigs," or stories about puppies, balloons, and ice cream birthday parties. Reading is an activity whose value varies considerably across people. One of my former patients, who was diligently working on reading exercises I had prepared, reminded me, "You know, Mister, I never have finished a whole book. I like to look at the funny papers, but I don't want to work so hard at this reading stuff, 'cause I'm just going to go sit by the river with my brother."

On the other hand, there is a legendary anecdote about the effects of stroke on the life a famous neurologist who suffered severe reading impairment. His biggest disappointment, according to one of his former students, was the sentiment "The world's library was closed to me, as if with seven seals."

Writing

Writing can be affected by neglect, cohesion, and integration, or in other subtle ways that are the result of myriad cognitive-perceptual disruptions seen in RHS. These effects can be evident in cursive writing, block printing, or in longer attempts to write letters or narratives. Writing short or overlearned material, such as a signature, days of the week, or short sentences, may not reveal the underlying deficits of writing. Story retelling or rewriting is a good way to get an idea of RHS writing impairment. By telling a story, and then asking a person to retell it or rewrite it, the examiner or clinician has a better idea of what the intended story is supposed to be about. Effects on writing may be uniquely observed in written forms of Asian languages such as Japanese, Korean, Chinese, and other languages whose written form is based on idiographic presentation. Because the right hemisphere is so involved in visuospatial and visuoconstructive tasks, the demands of a pictographic-based written language may be uniquely affected.

Verbal Fluency and Naming

A common way of testing the naming and word retrieval capacity of people who have had brain damage is to ask them to write or say as many examples of a certain category as they can in a set time. For example, write all the names of animals you can think of in one minute. This task is sometimes called category naming fluency or semantic generative naming. It may be tested as well by asking a person to name all of the words they can think of in one minute that begin with certain letters (such as F, A, or S) or all the countries or vegetables they can name in one minute. For example, for some of our research on generative naming, we used such categories as *Units of Time, Relatives, Four-Footed Animals, Colors, Parts of the Human Body* (some interesting responses), and *Articles of Clothing*.

Narratives

Narratives are stories that are told or written. There is a set story framework expected by listeners for the different types of narratives we use. Orientation to people or places in the story is important, as is proper sequence and tying together of elements of it, along with a story ending or conclusion. The confused storytelling in RHS results in specific problems for the listener. These include specific problems such as:

- Poor topic maintenance, shifting around from topic to topic
- Failure to observe turn-taking rules; poor sharing of floor dominance; too much interrupting

- Poor or limited initiation of conversational exchange
- Repetition and reiteration of the same thoughts
- Difficulty shifting topics
- Poor recognition of facial expression and body language cues
- Poor monitoring of output (naughty or inappropriate topics); insensitivity to the speaker (e.g., "I can see your nose hairs wiggle when you talk.")

Stories may be too long, not well tied together from sentence-to-sentence, or slower in RHS. This may be evident in different types of narrative discourse such as **procedural discourse** ("Tell me how you make a peanut butter and tuna sandwich.") or **narrative discourse**, ("Tell me what you did on your holiday in Bosnia.").

Comprehension

Some language comprehension tasks are easy ("Please saddle the rhinoceros.") and some are much more layered and complex ("If you've completed your tango, roll up your left sleeve, place the fork next to the small yellow bird, throw the vehicle in reverse, and dance with the lady with the hole in her stocking"). In RHS, comprehension generally is intact for relatively simple, one-step, conversational commands. It gives the appearance of being unaffected by the brain damage. However, when a person with RHD is overloaded with language length and complexity, or given three-stage commands that tax memory, comprehension may suffer.

So a person with right hemisphere damage may have far fewer obvious problems of language disruption than his hospital ward mate with aphasia, but four areas of language function may reveal impairment. These include *verbal fluency and naming difficulty*; problems in producing both *procedural and narrative discourse*, subtle difficulty with *writing and reading*, and *failure to comprehend complex, lengthy material*.

These are the *primary communication-cognition effects* seen in RHS, and it takes careful detective work to assess them properly and uncover how they are affecting the person's interactions with others.

Complex Communication-Cognition Effects

The complex communication-cognition effects of the third prime category of dysfunction in RHS require even more careful assessment strategies to uncover them. These problems may be revealed by difficulties with the following:

- Inference, relevance, and literality;
- Interpretation of body language and facial expression;
- Adhering to conversational rules;
- Producing and comprehending socially appropriate humor, emotions, and social pragmatics.

Inference, Relevance, and Literality

People with RHS cannot seem to handle some of the subtle or complex elements of language. Several studies including work done by Myers (1997) and by Brownell and colleagues (2004) cited earlier have demonstrated that inference (i.e., the process of drawing things together and arriving at an inferred conclusion) is difficult. They can see the trees, and even the bark on the trees, but they cannot appreciate the forest. Details are meticulously recited but the theme, the gist, the overarching inference about the essence of a scene or experience is not fully appreciated. When one of our

clients with RHS was told a story related to a house fire in the neighborhood, he was unable to infer what was going on from just the details of the description. For example, he was told, "A fire truck came screaming up right across the street from my house on Bayview Drive. Firefighters jumped out of the truck, hooked up hoses and ran into the house, and smoke was pouring out of a second floor window. What do you suspect was going on in the house?" The very typical response, devoid of inference or patching the pieces of the story together was, "How am I supposed to know? I wasn't in the house." When pressed and prompted with "Smoke pouring out the window? Firefighters running in the house with hoses? What would you guess is going on?" the reply was similar. "I don't know. I was not in the house. How could I know?"

Similarly, when shown emotion-laden pictures, a person with RHS will recite the details of what is seen, but be reluctant or refuse to infer further. For a picture of a mother comforting a crying little girl at graveside, with people in black clothing dabbing their eyes next to a casket, a patient with RHS described the scene as, "A mother and a little girl . . . crying. People standing around. A large oblong box . . . looks like a minister or priest . . ." When prompted with "How do you think the people feel? What is going on here?" the reply was, "Just a lot of people around a hole in the ground with a box. I don't know how they feel."

These are prime examples of both failure to appreciate or comprehend the emotionality or gist of a scene, as well as a reluctance to speculate or infer the essence of what the scene depicts. It also has elements of disruption of emotionality, a condition that has been frequently described in RHS.

Abstraction, inference, and derived relevance are very high-level cognitive-linguistic operations, and they can be altered in RHS. When asked to produce the name of a picture of a cigarette alongside a cup and saucer of coffee, a patient replied, "I don't smoke. I don't drink coffee; I drink tea. And only Earl Grey."

These disruptions of abstraction can create genuine problems in the subtle language operations necessary to comprehend, appreciate, and produce metaphor ("His love for the chicken was a storm of confusion."), sarcasm ("Why don't you eat the entire inventory of the Pizza Hut?"), or indirect meaning ("Is it cold in here or is it me?").

Interpretation of Body Language and Facial Expression

The right hemisphere seems to have responsibility for deriving the interpretation of body language and the emotive aspects of facial expression as well. Facial expressions can go a long way in communicating emotions and nonverbal messages. Louis Armstrong demonstrates remarkable and delightful facial expression in Figure 6–14. Most of our facial expressions are more subtle and we become adept at associating meaning with them. But not people with right hemisphere syndrome. Families of people with RHS complain that, "They don't get it. They don't understand when I'm kidding, or for that matter when I'm surprised or upset. If I smile or frown when I say something, they don't get the added facial expression. Plus, they don't seem to be able to produce emotionally colored language like before. I can't tell whether they are serious, sad, overjoyed, or frightened by the tone of voice. It's all kind of flat."

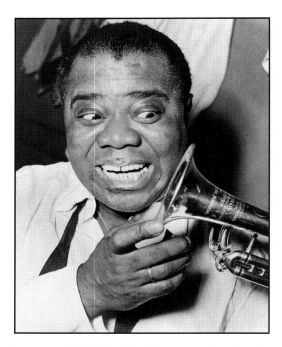

FIGURE 6–14. Facial expression. Louis Armstrong. From Library of Congress Prints and Photographs Division. New York World-Telegram and the Sun Newspaper Photograph Collection. http://hdl.loc.gov/loc.pnp/cph.3c27235.

Adhering to Conversational Rules

Rules that govern the interplay of conversation exist. Some of these rules, which largely go unstated, yet are learned by all of us, fit under the rubric of language *pragmatics*, or the *use* of language in social situations. Although some people without brain damage have trouble with the finer points of language pragmatics as well, people with RHS may have noticeable and annoying habits of excessive conversation dominance, interruption, or failure to read the signs of turn taking in conversational discourse. Until one stops and thinks about it, we may not be aware that the drama of this subtle interplay of conversational pragmatics is performed every time we talk to someone at length. For example, the following cues relative to giving up one's turn in a conversation have been researched carefully in normal speakers as well as in people with brain damage.

Turn-Yielding Cues. Turn-yielding cues are used by speakers to let the listener know that the speaker has finished what she intended to say; and that someone else may now speak. The display of a turn-yielding cue does not *require* the listener to take the floor; she may remain silent or let the speaker know that there is no immediate desire to take over. If the turn-taking mechanism is operating the way it should, the listener will take her turn in response to a turn-yielding cue emitted by the speaker, and the speaker will immediately yield

A number of turn-yielding cues have been identified reliably in conversation. Five are verbal or paralinguistic and can be picked up by simply paying attention and listening. These include:

- *Intonation:* the use of subtle pitch differences at the end of a meaningful clause. We signal intent to yield the floor with manipulations of our voices. It takes some practice to begin to identify these pitch differences, but we all use them and respond to them. We also use drops in pitch and/or loudness to signal we're done.
- *Drawing out a final syllable:* inserting a drawl-like durational increase of the vowel in a final syllable (e.g., "... give me the caaaash").
- *"Sociocentric" sequences:* the appearance of stereotyped expressions, for example: "but ah," "you know," "you know what I'm saying."
- *Syntax:* the completion of a grammatical clause involving a subject-predicate combination. The identification of this

cue takes some linguistic sophistication, but a phrase such as, "... so I took the 3 million and I bought a yacht." not only is a clear turn-yielding cue, but also may be an outright conversation stopper.

- *Gesture:* another turn-yielding cue involves gesticulation and therefore is transmitted via the visual channel. We can do this by use of our hands, releasing eye contact, or a head nod or change of facial expression.

There are an equal number of cues that indicate that the speaker wants to talk, not yield. We raise our chins slightly; we raise our eyebrows; we gesture; sometimes we rather overtly say, "Would you take a breath, please? I have something I would like to insert in your small Shakespearean epic of a monologue."

All of these rules of the pragmatics of language use, especially in conversational discourse, might be altered by brain damage; and seem to be particularly vulnerable to right brain damage. But notice how discreet they are. It takes a trained observer and examiner to discern these violations of conversational rules, and the behaviors associated with them are not nearly as overt or dramatic as the word-retrieval and grammatical errors of left hemisphere damage. No wonder the families of people with RHS report, "She's not the same. I don't know what it is, but she's different. Hard to communicate with her."

Producing and Comprehending Socially Appropriate Humor, Emotions, and Social Pragmatics

Humor is an important part of social interaction and communication. Surely, there are broad individual differences in appreciation of and production of humor, but it remains one of the cross-cultural mainstays of communicative interaction. Someone once said that it is one of the noblest and most enjoyable forms of human communication, and is the shortest distance between two people. RHD, however, can affect humor in strange ways. The right hemisphere has important links to the brain's limbic system, a system intimately related to emotion. Laughter, smiling, quipping, clever repartee, or outright joke telling are manifestations of appreciation and production of humor and this marvelous link between people can be scratched and broken in RHS. Sometimes this problem with humor takes the form of socially inappropriate comments ("Well, Preacher, I guess I'll go drain my lizard, if you get what I mean.") Another type of alteration of humor is the supposed "gallows humor" exhibited by those with RHS. This has been reported as a disproportionate response to slapstick humorous situations that depict someone either endangered or injured. Slipping on a banana peel, falling down a stairwell, getting cart wheeled by a bull, all appear to be hilariously funny to some people with RHS, although responses to other types of humor seem to be diminished.

The 1940s and 1950s films of the Three Stooges regularly screened on television even today in the United States and elsewhere, are notorious examples of painful, violent, endangerment humor that are broadly slapstick and usually involve someone getting crowned, pinched, poked in the eye, or slapped around. These are exactly the types of situations that seem to be appreciated by those who exhibit "gallows humor," and someone once suggested that perhaps showing Three Stooges films would be a good way to screen for abnormal humorous reactions in RHS (Figure 6–15).

Social pragmatics and inappropriateness of social topic are also observed in RHS. Female clinicians have complained about patients in therapy situations who cannot seem to focus on the appropriate tasks at hand, but instead persist with questions and comments that are socially out of place. "Are you married? Do you have a boyfriend? Do you enjoy sex at the carwash?" are types

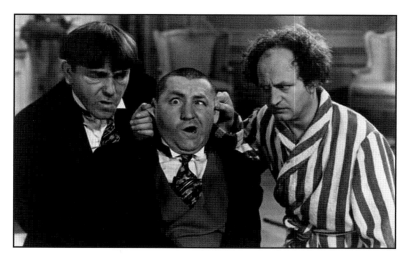

FIGURE 6–15. "Gallows" humor. Three Stooges.

of inappropriate comments that have been parried and diverted by clinicians. It takes clinical experience and skill to deal with these situations and channel them into more productive therapeutic paths, but good clinicians learn quickly that it is not necessarily a moral or ethical issue but a part of the condition and disease, just as is unfiltered swearing in some people with brain damage.

Another extraordinary aspect of social pragmatics that can be observed in RHS is a problem with what some researchers have called **theory of mind (ToM)**. This is a complex cognitive-perceptual difficulty that is manifested by seeing situations from another person's point of view. Theory of Mind has been characterized, as the ability to infer others' mental states, such as their beliefs, knowledge and desires, and many cognitive neuroscientists believe it is a central cognitive capability that underlies our ability to engage in social interaction. In a typical ToM test, a person is presented with a short story or a picture sequence in which the central story character is not aware of certain changes in the environment (in the story). So the story character comes to form a false belief. The task is to identify whether this belief will then lead to unintended or unexpected consequences. For example, presenting a picture series, or even better, a video or film of the following sequence of events may test this facility:

1. Mr. Fawlty comes into the kitchen with Manuel and sees a goat cheese and fresh basil pizza on the table.
2. Mr. Fawlty asks Manuel to put the pizza in the refrigerator; and watches as Manuel does so. Mr. Fawlty and Manuel then leave the room.
3. Polly enters the kitchen; discovers the pizza in the refrigerator; and

removes it and puts it in the oven. She leaves.
4. Mr. Fawlty re-enters the kitchen. Where does he look for the pizza?

The correct answer is: "In the refrigerator," because Mr. Fawlty does not know that Polly moved the pizza to the oven. If the response is "In the oven," this indicates that the person being tested has difficulty conceptualizing that Mr. Fawlty really does not know the actual location of the pizza.

When these types of ToM tasks are assessed, two control questions are usually asked as well, a reality question and a memory question.

The *reality question* is, "Where is the pizza really?" This is to make sure the person being assessed had paid attention to the transfer of the pizza from the refrigerator to the oven. The *memory' question* is, "Where was the pizza in the beginning?" This is designed to make sure the person being assessed had not forgotten where Manuel had put the pizza at the beginning of the scenario. Typically, several of these scenarios are presented in order to see if a pattern of difficulty emerges.

Individuals with right-hemisphere damage following a stroke often display difficulties on ToM tests; people with left-hemisphere damage typically do not. Measurement of theory of mind has been a particularly attractive research topic for those interested in the development of cognition in children. The acquisition of a mature "theory of mind" is a major achievement of the preschool years. Questions remain about the development of social understanding, but it is clear that, at a certain age, children begin to get it. The understanding that other persons have things going on in their minds (knowledge and beliefs different from one's own), and that those beliefs can be true or false is a major breakthrough in a child's ability to see the world through others' eyes. In fact, the disorder of autism has been linked to a failure to develop theory of mind, although a good deal of controversy can be spotted in the literature on this topic. The role brain damage plays in acquired deficits of ToM remains to be fully explored, but researchers such as Brownell and his colleagues (Winner, Brownell, Happe, Blum, & Pincus, 1998) are attempting to discover it. Difficulty with ToM remains one of the challenges and may well emerge as one more puzzling, unusual cognitive and communication effects of damage to the right brain.

Strange But True: Rare and Unusual Effects of RHS

One of the fascinating things about studying the brain and behavior generally, and the right brain specifically, is the number of even more unusual and rare conditions that continue to pop up in the medical and neuropsychology literature. The following examples are perhaps extraordinary, and no doubt one would have to experience contact with large numbers of people with right brain damage to encounter them, but they illustrate further what a bewildering wonder is the human brain, and the tragic and curious behaviors that can arise from damage to it. These conditions reside in the strange border zone of neuropsychiatric conditions and have been misinterpreted and perhaps misdiagnosed for years. Evidence is accumulating that these conditions indeed can be attributed to right brain damage.

Capgras Syndrome

This facial recognition or misidentification syndrome has been called "the delusion of doubles." One can readily see that it is related to the facial recognition problem described earlier, but with one important difference. Jean Marie Joseph Capgras, a French neuropsychiatrist, first described the condition in 1923 (Ellis, 1994). It is the perception or belief that emotionally linked associates (family, close friends) are doubles or imposters. Recent evidence has linked it to damage of the neuroanatomic pathways responsible for emotional reaction to familiar visual stimuli.

Autoscopic Disorder

Another misidentification syndrome linked to right brain damage is autoscopic disorder. This is the strange disorder in which a patient perceives and believes that *he saw himself*. People with right brain damage have reported self-sightings on the street in a crowd; in a shopping mall; or in buildings where a large number of people were gathered. In the medical literature, autoscopic disorder has been associated with migraine, infection, epilepsy, and particularly with brain tumors in the frontal-parietal lobe of the right cerebral hemisphere (Krizek, 2000).

Gourmand Syndrome

One of the most unusual conditions associated with right brain damage is found in the case reports of several patients who appeared to be left with a changed, and unusual craving for gourmet dining. The writers describe these patients as people who were not unusually interested in food or gourmet dining prior to suffering right brain stroke. After the stroke, and extending well into the recovery period over a span of months, these unusual food cravings continued. One case report detailed an example of a craving for, " . . . date trees and lamb roast with couscous and mint tea, the Moroccan way . . . " Another individual with the so-called gourmand syndrome continued his cravings for fine dining to the point of becoming the restaurant critic for the local newspaper.

These are the common and uncommon disruptions of cognitive and communication behaviors that are rarely revealed by standardized aphasia tests or language batteries. To observe these disorders, one must design specialized tasks or conduct careful in vivo observation of social interactive behavior. Myers (1999), Tompkins (1985), Brownell and Joanette (1993), Halper, Cherney, and Burns (1993), and Brownell, Gardner, Prather, and Martino (1995), and Blake (2005) illustrate examples of many of these RHS behaviors. Families are at a loss to explain the "changed" person they must deal with and frequently these perceived changes are the result of the array of characteristics presented in the preceding paragraphs.

Assessment and Rehabilitation: Some General Principles

Assessment of RHS is not the same as assessment for aphasia. The standardized aphasia batteries that have been used for years cannot be directly translated to the problems of the right hemisphere. Blake (2005) presents some guidelines for assessment. Few standardized approaches exist for evaluation of RHS and experienced clinicians use a more general evaluative format to understand the disorder. The foundation of any good assessment of a neurogenic communication-cognitive disorder is a careful history and appropriate observation and interpretation of behavior. Usually, an audio or video recording of an interview can serve as an introductory basis for deciding what else to assess. This recorded interview should include open-ended questions about the individual's personal history; orientation to time, place, and self; awareness of aspects of the disorder; specific deficits; and a picture narrative. From this recorded foundation, a clinician can explore deficits in more detail with specific subtests or evaluation strategies that are appropriate to the person interviewed and consistent with the time available.

Several commercially available measures of right hemisphere function are available including the RICE-R (Halper, Cherney, Burns, & Mogil, 1996); the Mini-Inventory of Right Brain Damage (Pimental & Kingsbury, 1989); and the Right Hemisphere Language Battery (Bryan, 1989). Tompkins et al. (1998) reviewed strategies in functional outcome assessment of RHS and analyze many of the complex issues involved in how these myriad disturbances impact daily life. Recently, the Montreal Examination of Communication has been published in several languages and offers a detailed approach to evaluation of right hemisphere damage

At Florida State University we rely on specially constructed language and cognitive tasks supplemented by a rich array of computerized measures. The computerized assessment packages allow standardized assessment of reaction time and speed of information processing. A number of cognitive domains are addressed including speed of processing in milliseconds, recognition and working memory, form discrimination, and sustained and divided attention.

Intervention and treatment for the consequences of right hemisphere brain damage have been slow in arriving. As Blake (2005) has remarked studies of treatment strategies and efficacy are lacking in RHS. Rehabilitation specialists such as speech-language pathologists, occupational therapists, and psychologists not only have encountered territorial professional overlap among team members, but also have discovered that reimbursement for RHS from insurance and third-party payers is difficult to accomplish and sustain. Halper and Cherney (1998) address the history of intervention for the behavioral sequelae of right brain damage in a helpful review. They rightly point out that treatment strategies are in their infancy, and that a major issue is whether or not improvement on selected tasks generalizes to daily life. Sometimes, if the treatment targets the development of compensatory strategies, the impairment still exists, but a person can learn tricks and techniques to circumvent the problem. In one of the earliest studies to address treatment of right hemisphere effects, LaPointe and Culton (1969) presented a case report of successful learned compensation by a man with RHS.

Halper, Cherney, and Burns (1996) outline a number of approaches and tasks for right brain damage. Their tasks address the areas of attention, perception, memory, orientation, pragmatics,

and higher level cognition (organization, reasoning, judgment, and problem solving). Within each of these areas, they present long- and short-term functionally based objectives and an array of procedures to guide the practicing clinician. They correctly point out that many of these procedures need to be addressed by empirical research so that we can firm up our support of evidence-based practice with RHD. As with so much of our behavioral treatment, we still need to address the issues of appropriate candidates for treatment; the timing of intervention; the most efficient and efficacious approaches; and the clinical significance and social validation of any gains that are realized. In the meantime, people with RHS need help, and an increasing corpus of innovative approaches is evident in the rehabilitation literature. Computerized programs available for intervention and treatment include programs that address remembering names, inferential naming, auditory and visual instructions, hierarchical attention training, visual and auditory memory span, and word memory and discrimination.

All of these clinical management measures are behaviorally based. An important point cannot be overstressed, particularly considering the history of relative neglect of treatment of RHS. That point is that these subtle and not so subtle effects on the quality of life of people with RHS can and should be addressed within the framework of contemporary models of rehabilitation science. These people should not be denied treatment or relegated to low priority status for intervention just because their signs and symptoms are less obvious than people with aphasia or because the identification of RHS is fairly recent. Life participation and activity models of disability can be used to guide careful construction of behavioral treatment paths.

Frances Begay needs to have her concerns and cares taken seriously. Rehabilitation science professionals have a growing array of means to help her, and it is time that her problems are recognized, discriminated, met with appropriate referral, addressed, and understood. She deserves to have her life restored with a sense of hózhó, the Navajo concept of balance and harmony (Figure 6–16). As in the intricate weaving of a Navajo rug, the brain is a remarkable tapestry of patterns. We owe it to Frances to learn as much as we can about these patterns in order to help her when her weaving is in disarray.

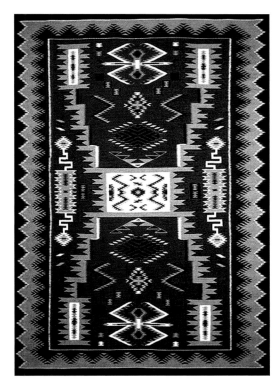

FIGURE 6–16. Navajo rug. Public domain on Wikimedia commons.

References

Ardilla, A. (1984). *Right hemisphere: Neurology and neuropsychology* (Monographs in Neuroscience). London, UK: Routledge Press.

Beeman, M., & Chiarello, C. (Eds.). (1998). *Right hemisphere language comprehension: Perspectives from cognitive neuroscience.* Mahwah, NJ: Lawrence Erlbaum.

Blake, M. L. (2005). Right hemisphere syndrome. In L. L. LaPointe (Ed.), *Aphasia and related neurogenic language disorders.* New York, NY: Thieme.

Brownell, H. (2004). Right hemisphere language and communication function in adults. In R. D. Kent (Ed.), *MIT encyclopedia of communication disorders* (pp. 386–388). Cambridge, MA: MIT Press.

Brownell, H. H., & Joanette, Y. (1993). *Narrative discourse in neurologically impaired and normal aging adults.* San Diego, CA: Singular Publishing Group.

Brownell, H. H., Gardner, H., Prather, P., & Martino, G. (1995). Language, communication, and the right hemisphere. In H. S. Kirshner (Ed.), *Handbook of neurological speech and language disorders* (pp. 325–349). New York, NY: Marcel Dekker.

Côté, H., Payer, M., Giroux, F., & Joanette, Y. (2007). Towards a description of clinical communication impairment profiles following right-hemisphere damage. *Aphasiology,* http://www.informaworld.com/smpp/title~content=t713393920~db=all~tab=issueslist~branches=21 - v2121(6 - 8), 739–749.

Critchley, M. (1962). Speech and speech loss in relation to the duality of the brain. In V. Mountcastle (Ed.), *Interhemispheric relations and cerebral dominance* (pp. 208–213). Baltimore, MD: Johns Hopkins University Press.

Eisenson, J. (1984). *Adult aphasia.* Englewood Cliffs, NJ: Prentice-Hall.

Ellis, H. (1994). The role of the right hemisphere in Capgras delusion. *Psychopathology, 27,* 177–185.

Foerch, C., Misselwitz, B., Sitzer, M., Berger, K., Stienmetz, H., & Neumann-Haefelin, T. (2005). Difference in recognition of right and left hemisphere stroke. *Lancet, 366*(9483), 392–393.

Halper, A., & Cherney, L. R. (1998). Cognitive-communication problems after right hemisphere stroke: A review of intervention studies. *Topics in Stroke Rehabilitation, 5*(1), 1–10.

Halper, A., Cherney, L. R., Burns, M. & Mogil, S. I. (1996). *The RIC evaluation in right hemisphere dysfunction-revised (RICE-R).* Gaithersburg, MD: Aspen.

Jackson, J. H. (1874). On the nature of the duality of the brain. Reprinted in J. Taylor (Ed.), *Selected writings of John Hughlings Jackson* (Vol. 2., pp. 129–145, 1932). London, UK: Hodder & Stoughton.

Joanette, Y., Goulet, P., & Hannequin, D. (1990). *Right hemisphere and verbal communication.* New York, NY: Springer.

Krizek, G.O. (2000). Is Doppelgänger phenomenon a result of right hemisphere brain injury? *Psychiatric Times, 17*, 10.

LaPointe, L. L. (1997). *Aphasia and related neurogenic language disorders.* New York, NY: Thieme.

LaPointe, L. L., & Culton, G. L. (1969). Visual-spatial neglect subsequent to brain injury. *Journal of Speech and Hearing Disorders, 34*, 82–86.

Lesser, R. (1978). *Linguistic investigations of aphasia. Studies in language disability and remediation.* New York, NY: Elsevier.

Mathias, R. (1999, November). Research notes. *NIDA Research News, 14*(4), 1–3.

Myers, P. S. (1999). *Right hemisphere damage: Disorders of communication and cognition.* San Diego, CA: Singular Publishing Group.

Myers, P. S., & Mackisack, E. L. (1990). Right hemisphere syndrome. In L. L. LaPointe (Ed.), *Aphasia and related neurogenic language disorders* (pp. 177–195). New York, NY: Thieme.

Regard, M., & Landis, T. (1997). Gourmand syndrome: Eating passion associated with right anterior lesions. *Neurology, 48,* 1185.

Sacks, O. (1985). *The man who mistook his wife for a hat.* New York, NY: Simon & Shuster.

Sacks, O. (1995). *An anthropologist on Mars.* New York, NY: Vintage Press.

Sacks, O. (2007). *Musicophilia: Tales of music and the brain.* New York, NY: Alfred A. Knopf.

Tomkins, C.A. (1995). *Right hemisphere communication disorders: Theory and management.* San Diego, CA: Singular Publishing Group.

Tompkins, C. A., Lehman, M. T., Wyatt, A. D., & Schulz, R. (1998). Functional outcome assessments of adults with right hemisphere brain damage. *Seminars in Speech and Language, 19,* 303–321.

Winner, E., Brownell H., Happe F., Blum A., & Pincus D. (1998). Distinguishing lies from jokes: Theory of mind deficits and discourse interpretation in right hemisphere brain-damaged patients. *Brain and Language, 62,* 89–106.

7

Acquired Aphasia in Childhood

Case 1—Hemorrhagic Stroke

Brett was an 11-year, 7-month-old right-handed boy when he experienced an intracerebral (within the brain) hemorrhage. He initially presented with a left-sided headache, right facial and limb weakness, and intermittent violent movements of his left limbs. On arrival at hospital, his reflexes were normal and pupils equal. Brett lost consciousness soon after admission. A computed tomographic (CT) scan performed on the day of onset indicated a large hemorrhage in the left temporo-parietal subcortical region. There was considerable mass effect causing a midline shift of the brain toward the right (Figure 7–1).

A left frontal craniotomy (hole cut in the skull) was also performed on the day of admission to hospital to enable evacuation of the hematoma (blood clot) to relieve pressure on Brett's brain. The

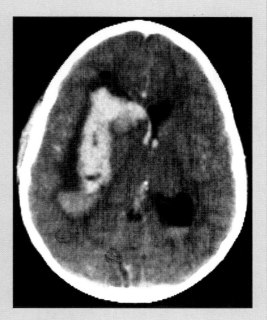

FIGURE 7–1. Case 1: CT scan showing a large hemorrhage in the left temporo-parietal subcortical region.

stroke experienced by Brett left him with a severe expressive and receptive aphasia, dysarthria, and right hemiplegia. Brett showed a gradual increase in his consciousness, mobility, and speech up to his discharge from hospital at two months postonset. However, his severe language impairment persisted and was still evident when assessed at the Centre for Neurogenic Communication Disorders Research at three years, six months postonset. Although a comprehensive language assessment conducted at that time showed that Brett exhibited general depression in all language areas, his major language problems fell in the areas of confrontation naming, auditory comprehension, repetition, expressive syntax, oral reading, reading comprehension, and spelling. As will be evident from materials provided later in this chapter, Brett's language profile differs in two major ways to classical descriptions of the clinical features of acquired childhood aphasia. First, recovery from acquired childhood aphasia was once thought to be excellent and almost complete. Brett, however, remained severely language impaired many years after his stroke. Second, although acquired childhood aphasia is commonly described as being of a nonfluent type, Brett demonstrated persistent problems in both the expressive and receptive (e.g., auditory comprehension difficulties) aspects of language. The persistent nature of Brett's language disorder may have been related to the extensive nature of the brain damage caused by his stroke.

Case 2—Closed Head Injury

Sara, a 9-year-old right-handed schoolgirl was admitted to hospital following a horseback riding accident. Unfortunately for Sara, her horse named "Topper" was startled when hit on the side of the head by a stone thrown by a passing lawn mower causing him to rear and throwing Sara to the ground hitting her head. Although Sara did not suffer any loss of consciousness immediately following the accident, she was unresponsive to commands. On admission to hospital, Sara was described as irritable and thrashing about and her eyes were deviated to the left. A CT scan performed shortly after admission was normal with the exception of a fracture of the skull in the left occipital region. At 1 day after trauma, Sara appeared to recognize her mother, but made no attempt to communicate. During the following 24 hours rapid deterioration occurred to a state of deep coma. A repeat CT scan at this stage demonstrated right cerebral edema (swelling) with compressed ventricles. Sara was electively ventilated and paralyzed until 1 week after trauma. By 9 days postaccident, Sara could open her eyes and follow simple commands. Two weeks after the accident, Sara was described as bright and enjoyed watching television; however, she did not initiate communication and failed to respond socially. Based on a comprehensive language assessment and analysis of her conversational skills at 4 weeks postaccident, Sara was diagnosed with only a high-level language deficit affecting both her verbal fluency and word-retrieval abilities as well as her higher level comprehension skills.

Her performance on a standard aphasia battery was within normal limits. It also was apparent from the conversational analysis that Sara had difficulty interpreting jokes in any more than a literal sense and also demonstrated difficulty understanding complex instructions, with frequent repetitions required. Overall, Sara's case is typical of the majority of children with a closed head injury in that she recovered basic communicative competency within a very short period after the injury. Despite the rapid recovery of her speech and language abilities, however, she continued to show subtle high-level language deficits, a feature also typical of the majority of children with closed head injury. Such subtle deficits are particularly significant in terms of the child's long-term integration into school and social environments.

Case 3—Brain Tumor

At the age of 6 years, 8 months Jane underwent investigations for symptoms of ataxia, lethargy, and vomiting. Her symptoms had been present for 2 to 3 months. A CT scan revealed a large tumor in the midline of Jane's cerebellum (Figure 7–2). Diagnostic tests identified the tumor as a solid cerebellar astrocytoma. Surgery was performed and the tumor completely removed. No radiotherapy or chemotherapy was required. Jane underwent a largely uneventful postoperative recovery; however, she did experience some difficulty at school and was reported by her teachers as having difficulty keeping up with her peers. A comprehensive language assessment carried out 3 years, 5 months postsurgery showed that Jane performed within normal limits on most tests of general language function. However, Jane's performance on tests of high-level language abilities was below average. In particular, she was unable to interpret and manipulate language of the level required in order to understand ambiguous sentences, make inferences, or recreate sentences. In addition, her performance on the Boston Naming Test was indicative of a mild naming impairment.

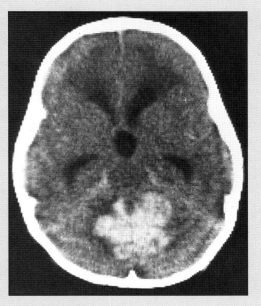

FIGURE 7–2. Case 3: CT scan showing the presence of a midline cerebellar astrocytoma.

Introduction

Childhood language disorders usually are divided into developmental and acquired disorders. Most clinicians and researchers use the term "developmental language disorder" to describe language problems that are present from the initial stages of language development. The cause (etiology) of developmental language disorders in the majority of cases is unknown and, therefore, are said to have an idiopathic origin. Developmental language disorders, however, also may occur secondary to other conditions such as peripheral hearing loss, mental retardation, cerebral palsy, child autism, or environmental deprivation.

Acquired childhood language disorders, in contrast, result from some form of brain damage suffered by the child after a period of normal language acquisition. The brain damage, in turn, can result from a variety of causes, including head trauma, cerebrovascular accidents, brain tumors, infections, and seizure disorders. This chapter focuses on acquired childhood language disorders in terms of their clinical features, and etiology. Discussion of developmental language disorders such as those occurring in association with cerebral palsy is not included.

Clinical Features of Acquired Childhood Aphasia

Traditional Description of Acquired Childhood Aphasia

Although during the period extending from the first descriptions of acquired childhood aphasia in the late 1800s (e.g., Bernhardt, 1885; Freud, 1897) to the late 1970s relatively few studies attempted to define the nature of acquired aphasia in childhood, a traditional description of the condition did emerge. According to the traditional view, the primary features of acquired childhood aphasia are as set out in Table 7–1.

The stated rarity of acquired childhood aphasia appears to be based largely on the observation that children who exhibited aphasia following brain injury often were reported in early studies to show rapid recovery of language skills. For example, Bernhardt (1885) stated that childhood aphasia was not rare, but because the aphasia was of a transient nature and rarely permanent, it often was not reported, thereby reducing the perceived incidence of the condition.

Another characteristic of the traditional description of childhood acquired aphasia is a period of mutism immediately postonset. This was described as the chief characteristic of acquired childhood aphasia by some early researchers (e.g., Alajouanine & Lhermitte, 1965). Certainly mutism frequently is reported as an early symptom of acquired childhood aphasia. When present, the period of suppressed spontaneous speech may last from a few days to months. Hécaen (1983) carried out a retrospective study involving 56 children with acquired aphasia ranging from 3.5 to 15 years of age, with brain lesions resulting from a variety of etiologies including trauma, tumor, and hematoma. Hécaen found mutism to be the predominant clinical symptom in the initial stage postonset, occurring in 47% of his group of children with acquired aphasias.

Following the period of mutism, when speech returns, there often is a period during which the aphasic child is unwilling to speak. This period also

Table 7–1. Clinical Features of Acquired Childhood Aphasia According to the Traditional View

- The condition is rare and transient in nature with most affected individuals exhibiting good recovery
- The condition is characterized by an initial period of mutism (suppression of spontaneous speech) that may last days or months
- When speech returns the aphasia is of a nonfluent, motor-type aphasia
- Features characteristic of fluent-type of aphasia (e.g., auditory comprehension deficit, jargon, paraphasic errors) occur only rarely and are absent in the majority of cases
- Presence of simplified syntax (telegraphic expression)
- Hesitations
- Impaired naming abilities
- Presence of disturbances in reading and writing (primarily in the early [acute] stage postonset)
- A concomitant dysarthria is present in most cases

has been described as representing a loss or reduction of "speech initiative" (Hécaen, 1976, 1983). Increased incentives and encouragements are required in this period to get children to produce even the few words they are capable of producing. Alajouanine and Lhermitte (1965) offered a purely psychological reason for the presence of mutism in children with acquired aphasia. They proposed that the suppression of spontaneous speech might be the result of a psychological reaction experienced by the children in response to their inability to communicate. Alajouanine and Lhermitte (1965) noted that children tend toward isolation, refusal, and silence in response to conflict or difficulties. Furthermore, these authors also observed that the unwillingness of aphasic children to speak after speech returns is similar to the behavior of normal children when faced with a difficult problem they cannot solve and wish to put aside.

Other features of acquired childhood aphasia reported in earlier studies include telegraphic speech (speech output resembles someone reading a telegram), simplified sentence production, hesitations, and dysarthria. Although, according to the traditional view, expressive language problems are common in acquired childhood aphasia and that the aphasia is of a nonfluent, motor-type, there has been considerable debate concerning the presence of deficits typical of fluent-type aphasia (e.g., auditory comprehension difficulties). Many investigators have noted that paraphasias, logorrhea, and jargon are rare, or in the majority of cases absent. Likewise, by far the majority of early researchers in this field considered impairments in auditory comprehension to be a rare occurrence in children with acquired aphasia.

Another characteristic of acquired childhood aphasia noted to be present, particularly in the early stages postonset, is a naming deficit or poverty of lexical stock (Alajouanine & Lhermitte, 1965; Collignon, Hécaen, & Angerlerques, 1968). In some cases, this deficit has been reported to persist long term, often being explicitly mentioned in the affected child's school reports (Hécaen, 1976). Hesitations also have been noted in the speech of children with acquired aphasia, possibly reflecting the presence of either word-finding difficulties or, alternatively, dysarthria.

The presence of a "reading disorder" was frequently documented among the characteristics of acquired childhood aphasia by early researchers, although details of the nature of the so-called reading problem were not provided. Likewise, a writing deficit also is a commonly reported feature of acquired childhood aphasia and, indeed, has been described as one of the most persistent and most variable of all the symptoms of acquired childhood aphasia (Hécaen, 1976).

Contemporary Descriptions of Acquired Childhood Aphasia

In the past, acquired childhood aphasia was considered rare, but when it did occur it was thought to be characterized by an initial period of mutism followed by a nonfluent, motor-type of language impairment with no accompanying comprehension deficit or other features of a fluent-type of aphasia. Furthermore, the condition was regarded as being transitory in nature, with affected individuals making a good recovery. In more recent years, and especially since the 1980s, many of these earlier held views of acquired childhood aphasia have been challenged.

It is now recognized that acquired childhood aphasia is not as rare as pre-

viously thought, and despite the rapid recovery seen in some cases, 25 to 50% of children who experience acquired aphasia still have aphasic symptoms 1 year postonset (Satz & Bullard-Bates, 1981). It is the latter children in particular who require the services of a speech-language pathologist. Furthermore, although acquired childhood aphasia appears to be predominantly a nonfluent aphasia, this pattern of language disturbance is by no means invariant, and fluent aphasia does occur in some cases. In particular, a number of publications in more recent years have documented the occurrence of an initial fluent aphasia in children with neurologic impairment (e.g., Van Hout & Lyon, 1986), and although the majority of early studies stressed the apparent absence or rarity of receptive speech disorders such as paraphasias, and so forth, more recent studies have documented the occurrence of these features in the spontaneous speech of children with acquired aphasia (Van Hout & Lyon, 1986). Some researchers have suggested that the traditional description of acquired childhood aphasia is more commonly observed in children less than 10 years of age, whereas older children tend to present more like adult aphasics in whom the language disorder may be of a nonfluent or fluent type.

In summary, clinically the aphasia pattern observed in cases of acquired childhood aphasia appears in most cases to resemble that of a nonfluent aphasia. Often, there is an initial mutism followed by a period of reduced speech initiative together with a reduced lexicon, simplified syntax, hesitations, and dysarthria. Disturbances in reading and writing also are common. Variations to this pattern of language disturbance, however, do exist, and fluent aphasia does occur in some cases. At this time, it is unknown whether the variations in the manifestations of acquired childhood aphasia are related to either age/maturation mechanisms or age-independent factors such as lesion size, lesion site, etiology, or time postonset of the disorder.

Acquired Childhood Aphasia of Different Etiologies

The general clinical features of acquired childhood aphasia described previously are largely based on the findings of studies that included aphasic children with a variety of underlying etiologies including trauma, vascular lesions, tumors, infections, and convulsive disorder. As well as influencing the prognosis for recovery of language function in cases of acquired childhood aphasia, there is some evidence that the etiology also has an important influence on the type of aphasia that is exhibited. It is no longer possible to assume that the effects of slow-onset lesions (e.g., tumors) on language are the same as those of rapid-onset lesions (e.g., cerebrovascular accidents and head trauma). Furthermore, children who have suffered traumatic head injuries characteristically exhibit expressive language deficits and typically show good recovery. In cases of acquired childhood aphasia following vascular lesions, the prognosis for recovery is poorer and the aphasic symptoms more variable and more persistent. In addition, although acquired childhood aphasia can be caused by a similar range of disorders of the nervous system as adult aphasia, the relative importance of each of the different causes to the occurrence of language disturbances in children differs from the situation seen in adults. For instance, although in

peacetime cerebrovascular accidents are the most common cause of aphasia in adults, the most common cause of acquired childhood aphasia is traumatic brain injury. Consequently, instead of describing the linguistic skills of groups of children with acquired aphasia resulting from different causes, as has occurred in the past, there is a need to examine the clinical features of the acquired childhood aphasia associated with each etiology separately.

Acquired Childhood Aphasia Following Vascular Disorders

Acute hemiplegia of childhood is a term used by many pediatricians and neurologists to describe the sudden onset of hemiplegia in children. A wide variety of vascular diseases of the brain, including both occlusive and hemorrhagic disorders, have been described under this heading.

Idiopathic Childhood Hemiplegia

The most commonly reported and dramatic syndrome resulting from an ischemic stroke in childhood is idiopathic childhood hemiplegia. This syndrome involves the sudden onset of hemiplegia as a result of a unilateral brain infarct of unknown origin and can affect children from a few months of age up to 12 years of age. Females are affected more than males in a ratio of about 3 to 2.

The cause of idiopathic childhood hemiplegia has been argued for many years and a variety of possible causes proposed including: polioencephalitis, encephalitis, venous thrombosis, demyelination, epilepsy, and occlusion of the internal carotid artery. Although there appears to be some agreement that arterial occlusion is the most common cause of idiopathic childhood hemiplegia, the reason for the occlusion is less certain. In some reported cases, neither angiography nor postmortem examination was able to demonstrate the presence of vascular lesions, suggesting that in these cases an embolus may have temporarily blocked a cerebral artery and then later broken up before the angiogram was taken or the postmortem performed.

Other Vascular Occlusive Disorders in Childhood

A number of other vascular occlusive disorders peculiar to childhood also can cause strokes in children. These disorders include: vascular disease associated with congenital heart disease, arteritis (inflammation of an artery) of various types, sickle cell anemia, vascular occlusion associated with irradiation of the base of the brain, Moyamoya disease, and strokes associated with homocystinuria and Fabry's angiokeratosis.

Ischemic strokes (i.e., stroke resulting from blockage of a blood vessel) associated with congenital heart disease occur most frequently in the first 2 years of life, corresponding to the stage when congenital heart disease has its greatest frequency (6 per 1,000 live births).

Various types of arteritis, including that associated with lupus erythematosus and occurring secondary to infections in the tonsillar fossa and lymph glands in the neck, also have been reported to cause ischemic stroke in children. Lupus erythematosus is a diffuse inflammatory disease that involves the kidneys, skin, hematologic system, the central nervous system, and occasionally the liver. It is more common in females than males with a ratio of 10 to 1. Although the average onset is around 30 years of age, symptoms can occur in the first decade of life. Hemiplegia secondary to cerebral arteritis, which is either transitory or permanent, occurs in approximately 5% of patients with lupus erythematosus.

Both arterial and venous occlusions leading to cerebral infarction have been observed in children with sickle cell disease, an inherited blood disorder. Likewise, cerebral infarcts have been reported subsequent to cobalt radiation of the base of the brain for treatment of a variety of neoplastic disorders in children.

Another vascular disorder of childhood that may cause vascular occlusion of the internal carotid artery is Moyamoya disease. Patients with this condition present with headache, seizures, strokelike episodes, visual symptoms, and mental retardation as well as, in some cases, a movement disorder, a gait disturbance, and/or speech deficit. Typically, the symptoms are bihemispheric. Moyamoya disease is characterized by the presence of a network of fine blood vessels at the base of the brain. The etiology of Moyamoya disease is uncertain; however, it is possible that several types of arterial disease in childhood may lead to Moyamoya.

Complications of certain hereditary metabolic diseases also occasionally cause occlusive vascular disease in children. Two such conditions include homocystinuria and Fabry's disease. Both of these conditions result from enzyme deficiencies and both, among other effects, may cause structural damage to the blood vessels leading to thrombosis.

Brain Hemorrhage in Childhood

Spontaneous intracranial hemorrhage (bleeding from a ruptured blood vessel) is much less common in children than in adults. Two major types of cerebral hemorrhage occur in childhood: one type occurs secondary to hematologic diseases such as leukemia, sickle cell disease, hemophilia, and thrombopenic purpura; the second type occurs secondary to vascular abnormalities such as arteriovenous malformations, although only approximately 10% of arteriovenous malformations cause hemorrhage or other problems in childhood.

Few studies of acquired aphasia occurring secondary to vascular disorders in children have been reported in the literature. The studies that have been published, however, suggest that the pattern of language symptoms is similar to that seen in cases of adult aphasia of vascular origin.

Overall, the lack of studies dealing specifically with acquired childhood aphasia following vascular disorder means that little is known about the prognosis for recovery from acquired aphasia in children with vascular origin. Some authors, however, have reported that children with acquired aphasia of vascular origin recover language less well than those with aphasia resulting from traumatic head injuries.

Acquired Childhood Aphasia Following Traumatic Brain Injury (TBI)

Performance on Formal Language Tests

Contrary to the traditional view that children make a rapid and full recovery from TBI, over the past two decades, a number of studies have documented the existence of persistent language deficits subsequent to severe TBI in children. Areas of language function reported to be deficient in children following TBI include: verbal fluency, object naming, word and sentence repetition, and written output.

The most comprehensive series of studies to document the language abilities of children with TBI using tests developed for pediatric application was reported by Jordan and colleagues (Jordan, Cannon, & Murdoch, 1992; Jordan & Murdoch, 1990, 1993, 1994; Jordan, Ozanne, & Murdoch, 1988). Jordan et al. (1988) assessed the language abilities of a group of 20 TBI children, between 8 and 16 years of age, at least 12 months postinjury using the Test of Language Development series and the Neurosensory Center Comprehensive Examination for Aphasia (NCCEA). They found the TBI group to be mildly language impaired when compared to the language abilities of a group of age- and sex-matched, non-neurologically impaired controls. In particular, these investigators identified the presence of a specific deficit in naming in the TBI group. The linguistic impairment exhibited by the TBI children studied by Jordan et al. (1988), was similar to that reported to occur following TBI in adults in that the children with TBI also presented with a "subclinical aphasia" characterized by dysnomia. Jordan et al. (1988) concluded that, in contrast to the traditional view that the immature brain makes a rapid and full recovery following traumatic injury, TBI in children can produce long-term and persistent language deficits. In a follow-up study of the same group of children with TBI 12 months later, Jordan and Murdoch (1990) observed that the naming deficit had persisted while verbal fluency abilities had deteriorated.

The high-level language functioning of a group of 11 children with severe TBI was assessed by Jordan, Cremona-Meteyard, and King (1996). Their findings indicated that the children with severe TBI had a lesser ability to create sentences with reference to social stimuli and a reduced ability to interpret ambiguous or figurative expressions than a group of matched controls. Jordan et al. (1992) investigated the linguistic performance of a group of mildly head-injured children in adulthood but failed to identify any persistent linguistic deficits for this group even in the very long term. In contrast, however, Jordan and Murdoch (1994) were able to identify late linguistic sequelae from 10 to 34 years following severe TBI sustained during childhood. It would appear, therefore, that children with mild TBI may be relatively spared in terms of persistent linguistic deficits when compared to their severely TBI counterparts, although marked variability in linguistic outcomes is evident within the severe TBI group.

Therefore, contrary to the long-held view that children make a rapid and full recovery from TBI, a number of studies reported over the past two decades have documented the existence of persistent language deficits subsequent to severe TBI in childhood. In particular, studies of language function after pediatric TBI have shown that expressive oral language skills, including verbal fluency and naming to confrontation, are most consistently compromised, whereas receptive language is less impaired and tends to recover earlier after injury. The observed language impairment often is characterized initially by reduced verbal output or, in its most severe form, mutism, which is following in the longer term by subtle high-level language deficits. Subclinical language disturbance, as reflected in impoverished verbal fluency, dysnomia and decreased word finding ability, is consistently reported in the literature. Frank aphasia, however, occurs in only a very small proportion of children suffering from TBI, if at all. The pattern of language impairment reported subsequent to childhood TBI, therefore, is similar in many ways to that reported in the literature relating to adult TBI.

Acquired Childhood Aphasia Associated With Brain Tumors

Intracerebral tumors are a recognized cause of acquired aphasia in children. Neoplasms of the posterior cranial fossa (i.e., those involving the cerebellum, pons, fourth ventricle, and cisterna magna) occur more frequently in children than supratentorial tumors. Cerebellar astrocytoma is the most common type of posterior fossa tumor in childhood, occurring most frequently in children between 5 and 9 years of age. Fortunately, cerebellar astrocytomas are also highly curable and have an excellent prognosis following surgical removal. Next to cerebellar astrocytoma, medulloblastoma is the most frequent tumor type involving structures within the posterior cranial fossa in children. Generally, these latter tumors involve children at a younger age than do cerebellar astrocytomas, their maximum incidence being with the age range of 3 to 7 years. Although cerebellar astrocytoma and medulloblastoma initially may present in a similar manner, the prognosis of these two tumors types is quite different. Although astrocytoma has a very favorable prognosis, medulloblastoma has a poor prognosis for recovery. The third most frequently encountered tumor of the posterior cranial fossa is the ependymoma. These neoplasms grow from the floor of the fourth ventricle and affect children of a similar age to medulloblastoma, and like the latter tumor type, ependymoma has a poor prognosis with a high proportion of tumors recurring after surgical removal.

Considering their location in the central nervous system, it would not be expected that posterior fossa tumors would cause language problems. A number of secondary effects, however, are associated with these tumors, which can, in some cases, lead to language deficits. Many posterior fossa tumors either originate from or invade the fourth ventricle of the brain. As a result, hydrocephalus may occur following obstruction of the flow of cerebrospinal fluid. Subsequent compression of the cerebral cortex could lead to dysfunction in the central speech-language centers. In addition, radiotherapy administered after surgical removal of posterior fossa tumors to prevent tumor spread or recurrence has been reported to cause aphasia in some adults and intellectual deficits in some children. Furthermore, the negative effects of radiotherapy have been reported to appear as delayed reaction, so that any associated language deficit may only appear in the long term.

Given that tumors located in the posterior cranial fossa represent the most common form of brain tumors in children, research conducted in the area of linguistic deficits resulting from treatment and/or surgery following childhood tumor has had its focus particularly on those located in that region of the brain (Hudson & Murdoch 1992a, 1992b; Hudson, Murdoch, & Ozanne, 1989; Murdoch & Hudson-Tennent, 1994). In fact, the most extensive investigations of the language abilities of children treated for posterior fossa tumors to date have been carried out by Murdoch and colleagues. The aforementioned researchers found that these children performed significantly below their peers on both receptive and expressive language tasks. Results of these studies (e.g., Hudson & Murdoch, 1992b) indicated that these chil-

dren might not be competent language users when compared to their matched controls. Areas of impairment included auditory comprehension, oral expression, and in particular reduced higher level language abilities, with deficiencies in understanding and manipulating complex, abstract language structures (Hudson & Murdoch, 1992a).

Acquired Childhood Aphasia Following Infection

Infectious disorders of the central nervous system are recognized as a significant cause of acquired childhood aphasia. Van Dongen, Loonen, and van Dongen (1985) reported that of 27 children with acquired aphasia referred to their clinic over a 4-year period, 15% had a history of infectious disease. Similarly, Van Hout, Evrard, and Lyon (1985) noted that 38% of their child cases with acquired aphasia had an infectious disorder.

Although the brain and its membranous coverings can be infected by the same range of microorganisms as other organs of the body, in the majority of cases of acquired childhood aphasia with infectious disease reported in the literature, the infectious disorder involved has been herpes simplex encephalitis. As a result of the destructive nature of the lesions associated with infectious disorders, and in particular herpes simplex encephalitis, the language disorder associated with this disease tends to be more severe than in acquired aphasia resulting from other causes. Van Hout and Lyon (1986) reported a case of Wernicke's aphasia in a 10-year-old boy subsequent to herpes simplex encephalitis. Their subject exhibited a number of features atypical of the usual descriptions of acquired childhood aphasia in that he exhibited symptoms such as a severe comprehension deficit, neologistic jargon, logorrhea and anosagnosia, the latter two features in particular usually being described as lacking in aphasic children. Van Hout and Lyon (1986) attributed the severe language disorder exhibited by their subject to the destructive bilateral damage to the temporal lobes caused by herpes simplex encephalitis.

Acquired Childhood Aphasia Associated With Convulsive Disorder

The first cases of acquired childhood aphasia with convulsive disorder was reported by Landau and Kleffner in 1957. Landau-Kleffner syndrome, also known as acquired epileptic aphasia, appears to result from a heterogeneous group of conditions with variable etiologies. Onset has been reported to occur between the ages of 2 to 13 years with the majority of children experiencing their first loss of language function somewhere between 3 and 7 years of age. Most authors agree that males are affected twice as often as females.

Acquired epileptic aphasia is characterized by an initial deterioration of language comprehension followed by disruption of the child's expressive abilities. In some cases, the onset of language deterioration is abrupt whereas in others the language disturbance develops gradually. Comprehension may be totally lost or reduced to understanding only short phrases and simple instructions. Often, due to the reduced comprehension ability, the presence of a hearing loss is suspected in the early stages of the disorder and many of the subjects initially are thought to be deaf. However, in the majority of cases, their audiograms are within normal limits. In association with the reduction in comprehension, the spontaneous speech of the child also changes.

In most reported cases of expressive language, impairments succeed the onset of auditory comprehension deficits, with either a progressive loss of vocabulary and/or phonological disturbances. Expressively, the child may become mute, use jargon or produce odd sounds, exhibit misarticulations, inappropriate substitution of words, and anomia, or resort to gestures and grunts. Unlike acquired childhood aphasia following focal unilateral lesions, in Landau-Kleffner syndrome, jargon aphasia with paraphasia and neologisms often are observed before the complete loss of language function that may last several months or even years. Over the course of the condition, the degree of language impairment often fluctuates, with periods of transient recovery after the introduction or change of an anti-epileptic drug. Preceding, co-occurring with, or following the language deterioration, there may be a series of convulsive seizures. The cause of acquired epileptic aphasia is unknown.

Summary

Although it has long been believed that acquired aphasia in children is primarily of the nonfluent type, in recent years this belief has been challenged by studies which have demonstrated that fluent aphasias can be observed in children if language examination is carried out in the early stages postonset. In addition, there is now evidence to suggest that the type of aphasia resulting from brain damage in children varies according to the underlying etiology.

Clearly there is a need for more research to further elucidate the specific clinical features of each of the speech-language deficits associated with the various neurologic disorders that may cause acquired childhood aphasia.

References

Alajouanine, T., & Lhermitte, F. (1965). Acquired aphasia in children. *Brain, 88,* 653–662.

Bernhardt, M. (1885). Ueber die spastiche cerebralparalyse im kindersatter (hemiplegia spastica infantalis), nebst einem excurse uber: aphasie bie kindern. *Archiv für Pathologische Anatomie und Physiologie und für Klinische Medecin, 102,* 26–80.

Collignon, R., Hécaen, H., & Angerlerques, G. (1968). A propos de 12 cas d'aphasie acquisc chez l'enfant. *Acta Neurologica et Psychiatrica Belgica, 68,* 245–277.

Freud, S. (1897). *Infantile cerebral paralysis.* Coral Gables, FL: University of Miami.

Hécaen, H. (1976). Acquired aphasia in children and the ontogenesis of hemispheric functional specialization. *Brain and Language, 3,* 114–134.

Hécaen, H. (1983). Acquired aphasia in children: Revisited. *Neuropsychologia, 21,* 581–587.

Hudson, L. J., & Murdoch, B. E. (1992a). Chronic language deficits in children treated for posterior fossa tumour. *Aphasiology, 6,* 135–150.

Hudson, L. J., & Murdoch, B. E. (1992b). Language recovery following surgery and CNS prophylaxis for the treatment of childhood medulloblastomas: A prospective study of three cases. *Aphasiology, 6,* 17–28.

Hudson, L. J., Murdoch, B. E., & Ozanne, A. E. (1989). Posterior fossa tumours in childhood: associated speech and language disorders post-surgery. *Aphasiology, 3,* 1–18.

Jordan, F. M., Cannon, A., & Murdoch, B. E. (1992). Language abilities of mildly closed head injured children 10 years post-injury. *Brain Injury, 6,* 39–44.

Jordan, F. M., Cremona-Meteyard, S., & King, A. (1996). High-level linguistic disturbances subsequent to childhood closed head injury. *Brain Injury, 10,* 729–738.

Jordan, F. M., & Murdoch, B. E. (1990). Linguistic status following closed head injury: A follow-up study. *Brain Injury, 4,* 147–154.

Jordan, F. M., & Murdoch, B. E. (1993). A prospective study of the linguistic skills of children with closed head injury. *Aphasiology, 7,* 503–512.

Jordan, F. M., & Murdoch, B. E. (1994). Severe closed head injury in childhood: Linguistic outcome into adulthood. *Brain Injury, 8,* 501–508.

Jordan, F. M., Ozanne, A. E., & Murdoch, B. E. (1988). Long-term speech and language disorders subsequent to closed head injury in children. *Brain Injury, 2,* 179–185.

Landau, W. M., & Kleffner, F. R. (1957). Syndrome of acquired aphasia with convulsive disorder in children. *Neurology, 10,* 915–921.

Murdoch, B. E., & Hudson-Tennent, L. J. (1994). Differential language outcomes in children treated for posterior fossa tumours. *Aphasiology, 8,* 507–534.

Satz, P., & Bullard-Bates, C. (1981). Acquired aphasia in children. In M. T. Sarno (Ed.), *Acquired aphasia* (pp. 75–93). New York, NY: Academic Press.

van Dongen, H. R., Loonen, M. C. B., & van Dongen K. J. (1985). Anatomical basis of acquired fluent aphasia in children. *Annals of Neurology, 17,* 306–309.

Van Hout, A., Evrard, P., & Lyon, G. (1985). On the positive semiology of acquired aphasia in children. *Developmental Medicine and Child Neurology, 27,* 231–241.

Van Hout, A., & Lyon, G. (1986). Wernicke's aphasia in a 10 year old boy. *Brain and Language, 29,* 268–285.

8

Motor Speech Disorders in Adults: Dysarthrias and Apraxia of Speech

Jason is sitting in a therapy room talking about his workout regimen. He is a young man of 22, with a sleeveless shirt to show off his "guns." He is enrolled part-time as a student at a local university where he also attends speech therapy. When he talks, the reason for speech therapy becomes clear. He is difficult to understand. In fact, listening to him and understanding requires a good bit of concentration on the part of the listener. His speech rate is slow; he stops occasionally to adjust his palatal lift prosthesis, which sometimes rattles in his mouth. "It needs an adjustment," Jason says. He also must work very hard to coordinate breathing and speech, getting a few words out then pausing to take another lengthy breath for a few more words. On his neck is a telltale scar, indicating that, at one time, a machine had to do the breathing for him.

Jason is the classic picture of a young person whose life was dramatically changed after a motor vehicle accident. When asked to tell his story, Jason reflects . . .

Three years ago . . . I went to a party . . . and got really drunk . . . then decided to drive home . . . 30 miles. I made it 29 . . . when I passed the officer . . . (makes a car steering motion) I went off . . . hit three trees . . . going 90 miles an hour (another big breath). I was lucky he was there . . . it was the middle of the night . . . I never would have made it . . .

Such is the story for many of the people we work with. An accident, a disease, a stroke, can change life in an instant. So many of the things that were once taken for granted—the ability to speak clearly, to breathe without effort—are now a constant challenge. Communication/speech is so integral to everything we do, and when it becomes difficult to produce clearly, what a dramatic change it makes to the overall quality of a person's life.

Introduction

In reading through these chapters and the many individual stories about brain-based communication impairments, you have learned more about the complexities of communication. We hope that your interest as a future clinician has been piqued by the fascinating array of neurogenic disorders, even though your heart aches for the suffering those individuals experience (welcome to the world of allied health). Throughout this process, you probably began to develop an appreciation for the differences between speech and language. They are inextricably linked, yet can be differentially affected by damage to the brain. The previous chapters of this textbook were devoted primarily to those disorders of language and cognition (aphasia, disorders of a nonfocal nature, and right hemisphere dysfunction) that deal with the organization, formulation, and social rules of communication. What you will find in the following chapters is a review of impairments that relate purely to the motor execution of speech (i.e., muscle capability, motor plan). A motor speech impairment indicates problems with one or more aspects of

the speech mechanism as reviewed in Chapter 2. Just to remind you,, those component systems include respiration, phonation, resonance, and articulation. The speech difficulties experienced by a person with a motor speech impairment fall into one of two categories: some type of disruption in (1) the speech musculature or (2) the motor plan that arrives from the brain, which directs the muscles how to move. These categories each carry a specific diagnosis:

Dysarthria: A group of neurologic speech disorders resulting from abnormalities in the strength, speed, range, steadiness, tone, or accuracy of movements required for control of the respiratory, phonatory, resonatory, articulatory, and prosodic aspects of speech production.

Apraxia of Speech: A neurologic speech disorder reflecting an impaired capacity to plan or program sensorimotor commands necessary for directing movements that result in phonetically and prosodically normal speech. (Duffy, 2005, p. 5)

When you consider the following excerpt from the definition of dysarthria, " . . . abnormalities in the strength, speed, range, steadiness, tone or accuracy of movements . . . " you can derive that this definition is really referring to the status of the speech musculature, something about the muscles of the speech mechanism is causing a problem with the coordination and execution of speech. On the other hand, the definition for apraxia makes no mention of how speech is produced, but how it is planned or programmed. Therefore, although both are considered motor speech disorders, they are two distinctly different problems.

Scope of the Problem

In Chapter 3, we learned that 49 million Americans have a communication disorder. That number reflects both developmental (problems you are born with) and acquired (a problem that occurs after normal development of speech/language has occurred) causes. An extensive study of acquired communication disorders in over 14,000 cases that occurred in the Department of Neurology Mayo Clinic from 1987 to 1990 and 1993 to 2001 revealed that roughly 41% suffered from motor speech disorders (Dufy, 2005). Based on that number, it is probably safe to say that you will encounter an individual with a motor speech disorder at some point in your practice as a speech-language pathologist. It is just as likely that currently you may know someone who has motor speech impairment, perhaps a friend of the family with Parkinson disease, or a neighbor who was in a car accident, or a grandparent who suffered a stroke.

Definition

From the above definition of the dysarthrias as a "group of disorders," it becomes obvious that there is more than one type of dysarthria. In the late 1960s, a group of master clinicians (Darley, Aronson, & Brown, 1969a, 1969b) suggested that dysarthria, which up to that point was only differentiated from aphasia and perhaps apraxia of speech, actually seemed to contain several subtypes. Their careful analysis of over 200 patients with dysarthria led to six specific types (flaccid, spastic, ataxic, hyperkinetic, hypoki-

netic, and mixed), classified by common lesion sites as well as unique characteristics of motor (muscle) performance.

Dysarthria

Flaccid Dysarthria

Flaccid dysarthria is named for the nature of the muscle in those who suffer from this diagnosis. Flaccidity means a lack of muscle firmness or tone so muscles will appear to be somewhat floppy or droopy. The general lack of tone in the muscles is also known as hypotone (hypo- meaning less than optimal) and it can be an indication of muscle weakness. A look at Figure 8–1 reveals characteristics of flaccid paralysis. The individual in Figure 8–1 has a condition Bell's palsy, which is a flaccid paralysis of the hemiface (half the face). Notice the droopiness or sagging of the structures surrounding the eye, nose, and mouth on the right side of the individual's face. Another example of the condition (Bell's palsy) is seen in Figures 8–2A through 8–2E. Notice that, in this case, the condition is less obvious when the facial structures are at rest. When the structures are functioning, however, you can see that movement is compromised and the weakness becomes more apparent.

In Chapter 1, you learned about the general organization of the nervous system into the central nervous system (CNS) and the peripheral nervous system (PNS). As a reminder, the CNS contains the brain and spinal cord, and the PNS is composed of the cranial and spinal nerves that arise primarily from the brainstem and spinal cord. Flaccid

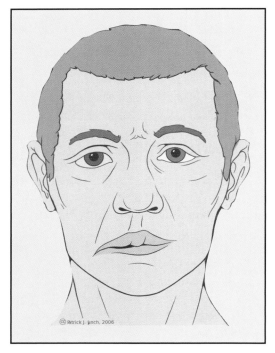

FIGURE 8–1. An illustration of Bell's palsy, paralysis of the facial nerve (cranial nerve VII). From Wikimedia Commons. Patrick J. Lynch; illustrator; C. Carl Jaffe; MD; cardiologist Yale University Center for Advanced Instructional Media Medical Illustrations by Patrick Lynch, generated for multimedia teaching projects by the Yale University School of Medicine, Center for Advanced Instructional Media, 1987–2000. Patrick J. Lynch (http://patricklynch.net), Creative Commons Attribution 2.5 License 2006.

In Chapter 2, the structures of the speech mechanism were reviewed, including the respiratory, phonatory, and resonance systems and the articulators. Flaccid dysarthria can affect just one, a combination of, or even all of the systems that contribute to speech. The systems that are affected are dependent on where the damage lies in the PNS. Seven of the twelve cranial nerves in the PNS contribute in some way to speech production. Functionally, these nerves provide sensation and movement to those structures responsible for phonation (larynx), resonance (soft palate or velum), and the articulators (lips, teeth, hard palate, jaw, and tongue). It is easy to imagine, then, that damage to these nerves would result in problems with speech execution, making individuals who suffer from flaccid dysarthria difficult to understand (unintelligible). Although there are many speech characteristics that can fall under the umbrella of flaccid dysarthria, those most frequently noted are hypernasality, imprecise articulation, breathy voice quality, and shortened utterances.

With your knowledge of the cranial nerves, let's analyze these symptoms (Appendix 8-A). Hypernasality means "too much nasal resonance." You have learned from this text that resonance has to do with the movement of the velum or soft palate. You also know that the velum typically is elevated to seal off the nasal passages so that, for most speech sounds, sound resonates and airflow passes through the oral cavity, *not* the nasal cavity. Thus, hypernasality must mean that the velum is not doing its job effectively and allowing too much sound and airflow to pass through the nasal cavity. Simply put, the sound resonating in the nasal passages when it should not distorts the sound. In addi-

dysarthria is a result of damage to the PNS. More specifically, flaccid dysarthria is present following damage to the cranial nerves that are involved in speech and/or the spinal nerves that supply the respiratory system. Table 8–1 contains a listing of the cranial nerves that contribute to speech production. In reviewing this list, you should recognize that these cranial nerves are responsible for a large portion of the sensory and motor function of speech execution.

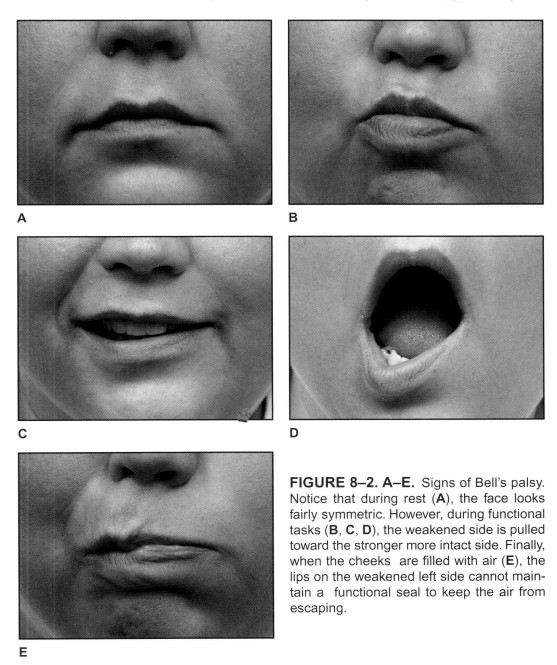

FIGURE 8–2. A–E. Signs of Bell's palsy. Notice that during rest (**A**), the face looks fairly symmetric. However, during functional tasks (**B**, **C**, **D**), the weakened side is pulled toward the stronger more intact side. Finally, when the cheeks are filled with air (**E**), the lips on the weakened left side cannot maintain a functional seal to keep the air from escaping.

tion, the airflow traveling through the nasal cavity detracts from the airflow that is needed in the oral cavity to accurately articulate many of the speech sounds. All this occurs when there is damage to the motor portion of cranial nerve X or vagus, which supplies the velum.

Imprecise articulation indicates a problem with the function of the articulators, specifically, those articulatory

Table 8–1. Cranial Nerves That Contribute to Speech Production

Cranial Nerve	Name	Motor/ Sensory Mixed	Primary Function for Speech
V	Trigeminal	Mixed	Facial sensation (S) Jaw movement (M)
VII	Facial	Mixed	Oral cavity (S) Facial expression (M)
VIII	Auditory	Sensory	Hearing and balance
IX	Glossopharyngeal	Mixed	Pharyngeal sensation (S) Pharyngeal movement (M)
X	Vagus	Mixed	Laryngeal sensation (S) Phonation, Velar elevation (M)
XI	Spinal-Accessory	Motor	Head and shoulder movement
XII	Hypoglossal	Motor	Tongue movement

structures that are dynamic or moveable (lips, jaw, and tongue). In order to produce intelligible speech at a normal rate (around 140 words per minute), the articulators must move rapidly and with a great deal of precision. If they are not able to, the rate of speech production will slow and the precision or crispness of speech will be affected. The cranial nerves that are implicated for the movable articulators include trigeminal, facial, glossopharyngeal, vagus, spinal accessory, and hypoglossal (see Table 8–1). I am sure that you notice another nerve that is included in the table that is not listed here. Although not directly involved with the innervation (nerve supply) to the articulators, cranial nerve eight (vestibulocochlear) also is important because it is the auditory nerve, and hearing speech does influence how it is produced.

Another of the primary features of flaccid dysarthria is a breathy vocal quality. The quality of the voice has to do with phonation. A breathy vocal quality is an indication of excessive air leaking through the glottis (the space between the folds). In the case of flaccid dysarthria, excessive air goes through the glottis due to incomplete closure during voicing, likely secondary to the hypotone and weakness in the laryngeal musculature. In some individuals, there may be bilateral weakness of all the muscles of phonation and in others only one side may be affected by weakness (paralysis).

A number of possible etiologies (causes) may lead to flaccid dysarthria. Traumatic injuries, which may be secondary to everyday accidents involving the head and neck, inadvertent injury during surgeries to the neck, and motor vehicle accidents that place a great deal of stress on the brainstem area, all could contribute to damage to the PNS affecting speech (Freed, 2000). Flaccid dysarthria also may be present following a stroke. The type of stroke would have to be very specific, however. In Chapter 3, you learned about strokes that occur in the brain. In order to impact the PNS, the stroke would have to occur in the brainstem. Remember that the majority of cranial nerves originate along the brainstem so a stroke (whether ischemic or hemorrhagic) in this location likely would have a direct impact on the adjacent cranial nerves (see Figure 1–16).

Disease is another potential cause of flaccid dysarthria. There are conditions or diseases that directly impact the PNS. Several examples include Guillain-Barré syndrome, myasthenia gravis, and muscular dystrophy. The common theme to all etiologies that result in flaccid dysarthria is that they somehow impact the PNS.

tone and weakness can make it difficult to move structures (Figure 8–3); in extreme cases, tight contractures caused by spasticity can lead to changes in the structure. This phenomenon can and does occur in the speech musculature as well. As a result, the most salient speech features of spastic dysarthria are imprecise articulation, reduced pitch and stress variation, and harsh vocal quality, implicating primarily the articulatory, phonatory, and respiratory systems. Although some degree of hypernasality may be present, resonance typically is not one of the primary problems for individuals with spastic dysarthria.

Spasticity, then, is a condition that could affect all subsystems of the speech mechanism although it is likely that

Spastic Dysarthria

Spastic dysarthria, like flaccid dysarthria, is named for the nature of the muscle impairment present in this condition. Spasticity in muscle refers to *hypertone*, or excessive muscle tone. So, whereas the muscles in flaccid dysarthria are lacking tone or floppy, muscles in an individual with spasticity have increased tone. An understanding of spasticity is important here. People may think of increased muscle tone, or tight muscles, indicate strength (aren't tight muscles what we would all like to have?). For the "buff" people working out at the gym, that may be the case. In the situation of spasticity, however, increased tone should not be equated with strength. Instead, spasticity exists in muscle after there has been bilateral damage to the motor pathways in the brain. Therefore, although spastic muscles are tight, they are not strong. In fact, they more typically demonstrate weakness. The combination of increased

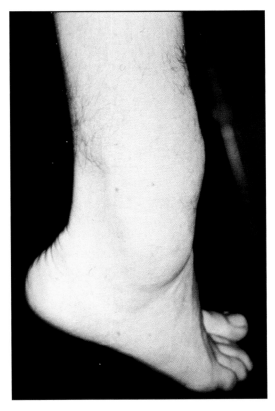

FIGURE 8–3. Spasticity in the lower limb.

some aspects will demonstrate more impairment than others. Unlike flaccidity, however, the effects of spasticity will impact the entire system. For example, if phonation is impaired by spasticity, then muscles in the entire system will demonstrate the effects of increased or hypertone. In flaccid dysarthria, you might see just one aspect of phonation (one vocal fold) demonstrate weakness in a system that otherwise functions well. Because one of the primary features of spastic dysarthria includes imprecise articulation, it is clear that the increased tone has a direct impact on the articulatory system. Restricted movement of the articulators from the spasticity leads to difficulty in making full articulatory contacts and difficulty with the rapid movements required to transition between sounds. These restrictions translate directly to imprecision and a slowed rate of speech. The inaccuracy that occurs will affect all speech: consonants as well as vowels.

Phonation is another speech system often affected by spastic dysarthria. In fact, the phonatory characteristics may differentiate spastic dysarthria from other dysarthrias, as many of the dysarthrias also include imprecise articulation and slowed rate. Spasticity affects the intrinsic laryngeal musculature exactly in the manner you would expect. The excessive tightness of muscles leads to tight adduction (hyperadduction) of the vocal folds. The result is the perception of a "strained" vocal quality. The tightness in the musculature also impacts the muscles that are responsible for changing vocal pitch. Thus, individuals with spastic dysarthria tend to have little pitch variation or intonation in their speech (monotone).

Now let's consider the respiratory system. Remember that the respiratory system never rests, breathing is necessary 24/7; thus, those muscles are continuously working. Tight muscles of the respiratory system can limit the amount of movement for breathing, resulting in shallow breaths. Shallow breaths will certainly impact speech (fewer words per breath, reduced stress patterns) but also may compromise gas exchange (oxygenation of the blood and tissues). If this restricted movement occurs over a long period of time, it can actually change the shape of the rib cage, which will contribute even more to limitations in movement. Because you understand that respiration is akin to the power source that drives speech production, then you know that with more shallow breaths there is less air pressure to generate voice and shape into speech. Therefore, when spasticity affects the respiratory system, the result will be reduced breath support for speech resulting in short utterances, low volume, reduced stress patterns, and less air pressure for generating speech sounds.

Etiologies that lead to spastic dysarthria include any condition or injury that results in bilateral brain damage. Remember that, in order to demonstrate spasticity, damage has to occur in the motor pathways in both left and right hemispheres. The usual culprits are stroke (most likely a second stroke as it has to occur in both hemispheres), a lack of oxygen to the brain (anoxia), traumatic brain injury, multiple sclerosis, and the list goes on. Although this list looks diverse in the type of injury, the common thread is the diffuse nature of brain injury that occurs. Widespread injury, such as what occurs with traumatic brain injury or anoxia, most certainly will include both hemispheres. Conditions like stroke or multiple sclerosis, on the other hand, can impact smaller, more discrete areas, but if they occur in both hemispheres, spasticity can result.

Ataxic Dysarthria

Another of the dysarthrias is called ataxic dysarthria. Ataxic dysarthria is named for the condition of *ataxia*, which is defined as a general lack of coordination in muscle movements. In Chapter 1, you learned about the cerebellum, a structure that is located at the back and below the cerebral hemispheres. The cerebellum is "highly connected" to motor pathways on several levels. First, there are connections to and from the cerebral hemispheres, there is proprioceptive feedback from the speech mechanism, connections with the brainstem, and interaction with the basal ganglia. Functionally, the cerebellum helps to coordinate and refine motor movements, an activity that actually sounds much simpler than it really is.

Let's consider an example. On a late spring day, you come in from a hot, steamy walk around campus and make what of course would be your first stop, the refrigerator for a nice cold beverage. You approach the refrigerator and reach out for the handle. Instead of slamming your hand into the door of the fridge, you slow your movements so that you grasp the handle with just the right amount of force. Then you open the door and look inside. Once you spy the object you want, you once again reach forward to grasp the can/bottle. Now, chances are you won't knock the can or bottle over in your attempt to pick it up. Instead, your hand slows to a stop just as you reach the object and you will grasp it with just enough force to keep it contained in your hand as you pull it from the fridge. This describes such an easy task, something we do every day without even considering how difficult it is. At each phase of movement, there is a great deal of planning, refining, coordinating, and smoothing movement so that the end result occurs without incident. The cerebellum is the structure that facilitates and oversees this process in its entirety. More specifically, the cerebellum assists with the timing, degree, and coordination of motor movement. Consequently, damage to the cerebellum will result in movements that are halting, jerky, and lacking in precision and timing, with a general lack of coordination that affects entire movements.

The movements just described are ataxic in nature. Following cerebellar damage, ataxic characteristics will be seen across all motor systems of the body, those responsible for walking (ambulation), standing, speech, or any motor activity that you might attempt. Another example of ataxia is in the speech of individuals who are inebriated. Excess alcohol is toxic to the cerebellum and its effects, although transient (short-term) are presented as ataxia. The speech of individuals who have ataxic dysarthria has been described as similar to "drunken" speech. The distinguishing features of ataxic dysarthria then, relate to the irregular movements that can occur within the speech mechanism. In particular, the articulatory system demonstrates the most salient features of ataxic dysarthria.

When disruptions in the articulatory timing and force of movement are present, the production of consonants, vowels, and the transitions between them are uncoordinated. Consequently, the precision we have discussed as necessary for intelligible speech is sorely lacking. Instead, the articulators tend to overshoot or undershoot their placement targets, sounds may be prolonged, distorted, or possibly even omitted altogether. Another important feature is that the pattern of imprecision is not always predictable. An example can be seen in one of the common assessment tasks, diadochokinetics. In this task, speakers are asked to produce a syllable (usually /puh/, /tuh/, or /kuh/; see Chapter 11 for a full description of this task) as accurately and rapidly as possible. Performance on this task in a "normal" system yields approximately 5 to 7 repetitions per second (Tomblin, Morris, & Spriestersback, 2000). An individual with flaccid or spastic dysarthria would perform much slower but the productions would be steady and rhythmic. However, an individual with ataxic dysarthria would have productions that vary. They might produce two syllables slowly followed by three rushed and one prolonged syllable. Because the underlying problem of ataxia is systemic, the coordination of all the motor systems for speech is a difficult task. Additionally, the demand for coordination can change based on the speaking task, context, even the emotional state of the speaker. As such, articulatory disruptions are irregular and perhaps unpredictable; for example, a word that may be produced perfectly in one sentence may be distorted in another.

The effects of ataxia also may disrupt movements of the respiratory system, more specifically, the coordination between respiration and phonation. Phonation occurs on the exhalation cycle of breathing, and when the systems are in sync, speech is an efficient, almost effortless product. When the two systems are not well coordinated, the result may be speech that is not so easy. As an illustration, try the following: Breathe in, and as you breathe out, begin counting at a comfortable rate. How far did you get? Counting to 10 should be relatively easy for an intact system. Now count to 10 again but breathe in and before you begin to count let about half of the air escape before you begin to count. How did that go? Counting to 10 on less air is more difficult, isn't it? You probably had to push harder at the end of the utterance to keep speech going. That concept of "pushing harder" means that you were engaging additional muscle systems (probably the abdominals) just to complete the utterance. This simple comparison of using air efficiently and not so efficiently shows how "out of sync" systems can impact speech. During that task you may also have noticed that stress patterns were atypical. Did you notice stressing each number equally? Abnormal stress patterns that overlie speech are another of the features that differentiate ataxic dysarthria from the other dysarthria types. Careful orchestration of all the systems working together is what makes speech so easy for most individuals. For individuals with cerebellar damage, however, imagine systems that are out of sync and working less efficiently all the time (Murdoch, Chenery, Stokes, & Hardcastle, 1991). Ataxia is a condition that makes that scenario a reality. Speech for individuals with ataxic dysarthria, then, is hard work!

The conditions that contribute to cerebellar damage resulting in ataxic dysarthria are similar to what you might find with the other dysarthrias with a few exceptions. First, the primary contributors are degenerative conditions. Examples include unspecified cerebellar degeneration, olivopontocerebellar atrophy, multiple systems atrophy, and Shy-Drager syndrome to mention a few. Demyelinating diseases, such as multiple sclerosis, can also cause cerebellar damage. Stroke or CVA is another cause that is actually common across almost all dysarthria types. Of interest to note, however, is that if a stroke occurs in one cerebellar hemisphere, the prognosis for rapid recovery is favorable. Strokes that occur in the vermis (midline) or that affect both hemispheres will have more lasting effects and disability. One cause of ataxic dysarthria that is unique relates to toxic or metabolic disturbances. Alcohol toxicity, alluded to earlier, is one example, but there are other substances/medications that can reach toxic levels and result in ataxia. For the most part, the ataxia that comes from toxic or metabolic influences can be reversed. However, if the toxicity continues or is severe, there may be permanent damage with irreversible effects.

Hypokinetic Dysarthria

The diagnosis "hypokinetic dysarthria" is similar to some of the other dysarthrias in that the name itself describes what to expect in speech features. As a reminder, "hypo-" means *a lack of*, or *less than expected*, and "kinetic" means *movement*. Right away, understanding the meaning of the diagnosis reveals that individuals who suffer from hypokinetic dysarthria will demonstrate generally less movement, as seen throughout the components of the motor speech mechanism. The general lack of movement stems from disruptions with the basal ganglia control circuit as described in Chapter 1. The basal ganglia and its connections really function to regulate muscle tone, support motor behaviors, make postural adjustments during movement, respond to environmental changes, and assist with the initiation of motor movements and new motor learning. A listing of these functions illustrate that

damage to the basal ganglia circuit definitely will impact motor control and movement. In hypokinetic dysarthria, damage to the basal ganglia is secondary to a depletion of the neurotransmitter dopamine, which is provided by the substantia nigra. The prototype example for this diagnosis is Parkinson disease. Cardinal features of Parkinson disease include resting tremor, rigidity, bradykinesia (also known as hypokinesia or akinesia), and reduced or lack of postural reflexes. Considering these features, bradykinesia/hypokinesia is perhaps the condition that contributes the most to the clinical signs of hypokinetic dysarthria.

Muscle rigidity in the speech musculature will restrict movements. You might see parallels between the muscle rigidity as a feature of hypokinetic dysarthria and the hypertone seen in spastic dysarthria. Indeed, the impact on speech systems can be similar, but there is an underlying difference in muscle rigidity and spasticity. Increased muscle tone or spasticity is a condition that results in muscle tightness. However, spasticity can be alleviated through deep massage or range of motion (ROM) activities. When a structure with spasticity is moved, the initial resistance of spasticity will ease as the structure continues through the movement. Although muscle rigidity also results in muscle tightness, it does not respond to massage or ROM exercises. The tightness demonstrated by muscle rigidity will resist all the way through a movement.

The speech characteristics that best represent hypokinetic dysarthria reflect the underlying primary features of Parkinson disease. The most common speech impairments include reduced pitch, loudness and stress variation, short rushes of speech, dysphonia, and the perception of rapid speech. (It is worth noting that hypokinetic dysarthria is the *only* motor speech impairment in which speech rate is perceived as fast rather than slow.) Muscle rigidity is another muscle condition that is systemic in nature. Thus, components of speech production may have decreased functionality because of the "tightness" of the musculature. With regard to respiration, the symptoms are similar to what may be present in spastic dysarthria. The restricted movements of the respiratory muscles result in a reduced lung capacity. Reduced capacity, and thus air support for speech, will result in an overall reduced intensity (volume) as well as less variation of intensity (used for stress patterns). The phonatory system also demonstrates the effects of muscle rigidity in a general lack of pitch variation. The muscles that manipulate laryngeal structures to change vocal fold tension (thus pitch) are tight, not making the fine adjustments to the system for normal pitch contours, like the rising pitch you typically hear at the end of an utterance when an individual asks a question. Muscle rigidity leading to the lack of pitch variation is somewhat expected in these individuals. However, another aspect of laryngeal function in hypokinetic dysarthria has been a bit perplexing. Dysphonia commonly has been listed as a feature of the diagnosis. Dysphonia is a voice quality also known as hoarseness, which includes some degree of breathiness. Any presence of breathiness in a system with rigidity in the musculature is counterintuitive. If the muscles of phonation are rigid, then you might expect an excessive or hyperadduction of the vocal folds, which would lead to more of a "strained" vocal quality. Instead, the vocal folds actually are hypoadducted, which results in that hoarse, breathy voice quality. The underlying mechanism for this unexpected clinical sign is unclear and keeping some researchers busy trying to find an explanation. Articulatory function also is affected by the nature of the muscles in hypokinetic dysarthria. The effects of Parkinson disease lead to articulators that are restricted in their range of motion; thus, they tend to undershoot targets. The imprecision in meeting articulatory contacts results in speech that is difficult to understand. The strength of the articulators may be in the normal range (at least until the advanced stages of the disease) but muscle rigidity limits movements. The restricted movement also is noted in the muscles of facial expression. The lips are an active articulator of the face, but the rest of the face also adds content to what we express through speech. Individuals with hypokinetic dysarthria have what is known as "masked facies" or a general lack of facial expression during speech or to express emotion. The face may have features that are still, like the immovable features on a mask.

Degenerative conditions are by far the primary cause of hypokinetic dysarthria. Parkinson disease is the major contributor, but there are other conditions that share some of the characteristics of Parkinson disease that have additional symptoms as well. Those diseases are often called Parkinson-plus syndromes and contain such diagnoses as multiple systems atrophy, progressive supranuclear palsy (PSP), and corticobasal degeneration. Involvement of the substantia nigra and dopamine depletion are all common elements, although most of these other diagnoses demonstrate more of a mixed dysarthria (hypokinetic plus another dysarthria type).

Hyperkinetic Dysarthria

As you have just learned, the diagnosis hypokinetic dysarthria means too little or reduced movement of the speech musculature resulting in impairment. At the other end of the spectrum is *"hyperkinetic dysarthria,"* which is defined as excessive movement of the speech musculature also resulting in disrupted speech. A large number of movement disorders result in excessive, involuntary movements of the body. When those movements affect the components of speech, hyperkinetic dysarthria is the result. Depending on the movement disorder, a single speech component (as in the jaw opening dystonia in Figure 8–4) may interfere with speech, or it is possible that the entire system will be

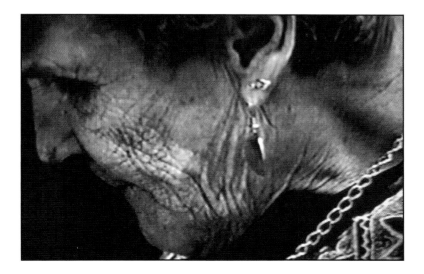

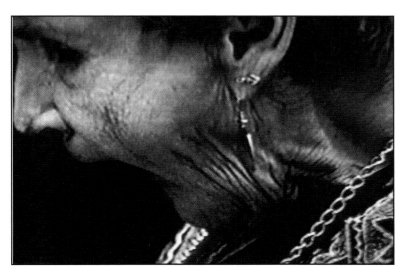

FIGURE 8–4. An example of jaw opening dystonia, one type of hyperkinetic dysarthria.

affected by the involuntary movements making speech difficult to produce.

The movement disorders that result in hyperkinetic dysarthria range from slow to fast movements, small tics of a single body part to whole body movements. Each diagnosis demonstrates a unique pattern of movements. The wide range of disturbance makes it difficult to predict speech characteristics based on simply "hyperkinetic dysarthria" as you can with other dysarthria types (flaccid, spastic). However, there is one unifying symptom that spans the diagnoses: involuntary movement.

The movement disorders that result in hyperkinetic dysarthria are often associated with damage to the basal ganglia. Remember that *hypokinetic* dysarthria also is linked to the basal ganglia; however, the mechanism for hypokinetic dysarthria (i.e., depletion of the neurotransmitter dopamine) is fairly well understood and is isolated to basal ganglia connections, specifically the substantia nigra. The mechanisms for the wide range of movement disorders linked to hyperkinetic dysarthria are not as well understood. The importance of the basal ganglia in regulating the movements planned by the motor cortex is not disputed, but the mechanism of injury/disease that results in such a wide variety of impairments remains a question and a source of ongoing inquiry.

Exactly how the speech mechanism is affected by movement disorders really depends on the type and extent of the condition. As previously mentioned and illustrated in Figure 8–4, an individual may have a fairly focal (isolated) dystonia that only interferes with one structure. In the case of the jaw opening dystonia, an individual might be talking and suddenly (often where there is an open mouth posture for a vowel) the jaw begins to open and perhaps stays

open on its own accord. Imagine how even a relatively isolated impairment such as this might disrupt speech. Just try saying the days of the week, and when you get to Wednesday, open your jaw slowly to an extreme open posture. Were you able to keep talking? If the jaw opening was not extreme, speech might be possible. However, remember that these are *involuntary* movements so it is unlikely that you will have a choice in how wide the jaw opens. Now let's consider a more extreme movement disorder that affects the entire body. Huntington's chorea is a genetic disorder characterized by random movements of the head, neck, trunk, and even the limbs. It is difficult to even simulate such a condition for the purposes of illustration as you did just now with a jaw opening dystonia. Imagine, though, what a sudden hard rotation of your entire trunk would do to the careful balance of breathing, phonation, . . . speech production in general. If you have never seen this condition, the impact can be quite dramatic. Some individuals have so little control that their flailing limbs can even strike them in the face, sending glasses flying. In spite of the wide range of impairments, there are speech features that seem to predominate in hyperkinetic dysarthria. Those features include imprecise consonants, variable speaking rate, prolonged speech segments and pauses, harsh vocal quality, distorted vowels, variable loudness, and voice interruptions. To further review how speech systems might be affected by hyperkinesias, view Table 8–2.

Mixed Dysarthria

The dysarthrias are a group of disorders, each single diagnosis with a unique set of features that include muscle charac-

Table 8–2. Characteristics of the More Common Movement Disorders

Movement Disorder	Movement Characteristics	Systems
Chorea	Rapid, unpredictable, jerky involuntary movements	This is a progressive disease that will likely impact the entire speech mechanism
Dystonia	Slower, more gradual movements	May impact all systems; however, resonance is not typically implicated
Myoclonus	Rhythmic, periodic muscle contraction	Can affect multiple systems; however, the resonance and articulatory systems are often implicated
Tics	Brief involuntary movements (can also be sounds) during normal activity	May be isolated or inclusive of all speech components
Essential tremor	Periodic movements occurring at around 4 to 7 Hz (cycles per second)	Phonation and articulatory systems are often implicated
Spasmodic dysphonia	Involuntary muscle spasms/contractions	The phonatory system

teristics, nervous system lesions, and motor behaviors. Although the list is well described, there are some individuals who may not fit neatly into the characteristics of just one diagnosis. In fact, because damage to the brain is not always specific to one system, many individuals show signs of more than one dysarthria type. Typically, they suffer from widespread or diffuse nervous system damage. For these individuals there is a "mixed dysarthria" category. For example, the disease amyotrophic lateral sclerosis (ALS or Lou Gehrig's disease) is a demyelinating condition that affects the CNS as well as the PNS. People who have been diagnosed with ALS frequently show signs of both spastic dysarthria (often in phonation) and flaccid dysarthria (resonance and articulation). To conclude our overview of

the dysarthrias, the mixed dysarthria category completes the group of dysarthrias. When an individual suffers from nervous system injury that is diffuse or widespread, then many features of the diagnoses discussed above may be seen in combinations, rather than fitting neatly into an isolated category.

Apraxia of Speech

We are going to move away from the focus on dysarthria onto another motor speech disorder, apraxia of speech. The common thread of impairment that spanned the dysarthrias was muscle or motor impairment, which resulted in speech disturbance. The manifestation of speech disruption in apraxia of speech is from neurologic disruption between the formulation of the motor plan that is needed to convey a message and its execution. In apraxia of speech, there often is no muscle impairment, but rather an inability to get the muscles to "cooperate" and carry out the planned message. As an illustration of the concept, picture the following. You are a director at the local community theater. At rehearsal, you have a variety of actors on stage, each perfectly capable of carrying out your every direction. Being the hotshot director, you stay in your seat in the auditorium and ask your ever present assistant to pass along your instructions to the actors on stage. After receiving the instructions, the actors proceed to play out the scene, incorporating none of the directions you thought had been provided. In fact, there was no cooperation at all! The nerve! What happened? The instructions were explicitly conveyed, and the actors were certainly able to carry out the plan. Something must have occurred to the plan as it was conveyed by the director.

Such is the situation in apraxia of speech. The director (brain) formulates a plan for executing speech sounds→words→conversation and the actors (muscles) may be perfectly capable of carrying out that plan. Unfortunately, there is a disruption in the message or plan somewhere between the brain and the muscles that results in impaired an impaired "production," sounds may be in the wrong order, and at times it may be difficult to get the muscles to perform at all. Apraxia of speech occurs with damage to the motor speech area in the left hemisphere. There is wide variation in the area of damage that can occur yet still demonstrate the signs and symptoms of apraxia (there are some who would like to blame it on a very

small area buried in the left hemisphere called the insula). The fact that such variation exists is a testament to the wide degree of individual differences that often occur with damage to the brain. The motor speech area also is heavily implicated with language function, thus, apraxia frequently co-occurs with aphasia (most often Broca's aphasia). As apraxia of speech is frequently concurrent with Broca's aphasia, some of the speech characteristics may relate in part to that language impairment. The most notable speech features include consonant and vowel distortions, slow halting speech rate, error patterns that are unpredictable, and errors that increase with an increase in utterance length and complexity.

The impact of apraxia on the speech mechanism is as you might expect—unpredictable. The unpredictable nature of speech production is an interesting feature of apraxia of speech. In some instances, speech may be executed perfectly, to the delight of the speaker. Then, as often happens, the individual will attempt the utterance again, only to have the production come out all wrong. As you can imagine, this feature of apraxia is a frustrating one for individuals. Although not easy to predict, context does show some influence on speech production for those with apraxia. If the context of speech is automatic (e.g., a greeting as someone enters the room), then successful production is more likely. As the degree of speech automaticity decreases the chances for accurate, fluent speech decline as well.

A review of the speech characteristics associated with apraxia indicates that, when the speech mechanism is considered, the most affected component is the articulatory system (all those actors running around without a plan).

The coordinated smooth movement of the many articulators is not the typical pattern for those with apraxia. Instead, often every word is a struggle and small victories are followed by defeat after crushing defeat. Apraxia may impact additional components of the speech mechanism (there have been reports of voice or phonatory apraxia), but those situations are not the typical presentation for apraxia.

Assessment of Motor Speech Disorders

To assess the speech mechanism, the primary focus for the speech-language pathologist is on the individuals' control of the oral motor system. It is important to assess the structures (when applicable) both at rest and during functional tasks to fully understand the potential for underlying problems. To examine motor control, exploration of muscle strength, speed of movement, range of movement, direction of movement, and the accuracy of movement (precision) is necessary (Netsell, 1996; Tomblin et al., 2000). Careful observation will differentiate between CNS and PNS damage (Appendix 8-B). Additional differential diagnosis across the dysarthria types can be achieved by noting motor steadiness (involuntary/unexpected movements) and muscle tone. Although standardized assessments are available, motor speech disorders include one aspect of communication impairment in which your eyes, ears, and your clinical knowledge are really your best tools. What you learn about the individual, what you know about the mechanism, and what you are able to observe across a variety of diag-

nostic tasks will allow you to differentially diagnose motor speech disorders. For a more comprehensive review of assessment of motor speech disorders, you are directed to Chapter 11.

Treatment of Motor Speech Disorders

The sociologic as well as psychologic impact of disordered speech is dramatic. Individuals with motor speech disorders may feel embarrassment about their speech, and the constant need to revise and repeat their utterances to facilitate understanding can be exhausting. Consequently, individuals may isolate themselves from the activities and people that they enjoy. Such actions impact not only the individual but their significant others or family members as well. The downward spiral of those behaviors can lead to depression, apathy, and a drastic change in the quality of life. The purpose of treatment is to improve speech—more generally communication—working to address the communication goals of the individual. It is possible that oral speech/communication is not a feasible option, either due to declining function or because of the severe nature of the impairment. In those situations, treatment might entail exploring alternative and augmented communication (AAC) options. However, the study of AAC is too large a topic to tackle here. As the focus of this chapter has been specific to speech, let's address the issues of remediating oral communication.

When the focus of rehabilitation is on achieving intelligible speech, the primary treatment purpose for individuals with motor speech disorders is to address the physiologic issues that underlie their communication impairments. In the case of the dysarthrias, there are a number of treatment approaches that address neuromuscular issues (Clark, 2003). Thermal treatments can alleviate spasticity and pain, improving mobility for better function. There are also prosthetic devices that can be used to support structures that no longer function well. Figure 8–5 is an example of a prosthetic device used to support a weak velum. In addition, although its use has been controversial, there is growing evidence to support exercise for strengthening weakened speech musculature.

The growing evidence has to do with applying long-standing principles of exercise into treatment of the oral motor system. For example, to gain strength, exercise must occur at a high intensity level, with increased resistance as strength improves. Think of it this way: if you went to the gym every day for a month and lifted 2-lb dumbbells for 10 repetitions, what do you think the result would be? Well, it probably wouldn't hurt, but you certainly wouldn't get much stronger. So keeping intensity and resistance principles in mind, treatments that incorporate strengthening to remediate speech are changing, and the trend is supported by evidence that it is working. Another principle worth mentioning (with regard to exercise) is task specificity. The more specific the exercise is to the target activity, the better. So imagine an individual with flaccid dysarthria who has lip weakness, which interferes with the ability to produce bilabial sounds (m, b, p). A very "task-specific" exercise would be to request that he or she compress the lips (as you must do to make the sound) as hard as possible, with increasing numbers of repetitions. With such a good degree of task specificity (the exercise incorporates exactly the movements you need for production of the sounds) and applying good exercise principles, the outcome should be rapid and positive.

In addition to working on underlying impairment (muscle tone, weakness), there are treatment techniques that can be incorporated to increase intelligibility. Techniques to improve breathing for speech for those with movement disorders, to relax muscles that demonstrate increased tension, and to bring speech under conscious control to improve articulation, are readily available and easy to incorporate (Robin, Yorkston, & Beukelman, 1996). Many of these can be adopted in certain situations to improve communication (talking on the phone). Little victories go a long way in providing a boost of confidence and motivation.

Therapeutic applications in the treatment of apraxia of speech also are

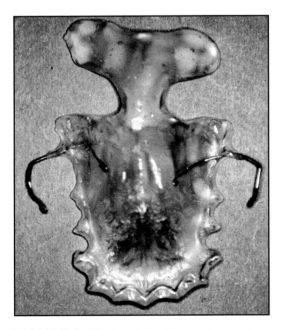

FIGURE 8–5. A palatal lift prosthesis that clips onto the teeth with an extension at the back of the device to support velar closure for speech.

changing. Once again, the field of speech-language pathology has been influenced by our friends and researchers in motor learning and kinesiology. Because the underlying problem in apraxia of speech has to do with the speech program or plan, we have begun to incorporate principles of *motor learning* into our remediation program. In studying how motor sequences are learned and retained in a normal system, we can apply the same principles to help individuals who are having difficulty with motor movements. There is no feeling in the world like knowing you played a role in facilitating communication for an individual who has struggled to produce even the simplest utterance. These therapy techniques are just a few examples of what might be employed in remediation. A review of Chapter 12 will provide more detail on treatment.

References

Clark, H. M. (2003). Neuromuscular treatments for speech and swallowing: A tutorial. *American Journal of Speech Language Pathology, 12,* 400–415.

Duffy, J. R. (2005). *Motor speech disorders: Substrates, differential diagnosis, and management.* St. Louis, MO: Elsevier Mosby.

Freed, D. B. (2000). *Motor speech disorders: Diagnosis and treatment.* San Diego, CA: Singular, Thomson Learning.

Murdoch, B. E., Chenery, H., Stokes, P., & Hardcastle, W. (1991). Respiratory kinematics in speakers with cerebellar disease. *Journal of Speech and Hearing Research, 34,* 768–780.

Netsell, R. (1986). *A neurobiologic view of speech production and the dysarthrias.* San Diego, CA: College-Hill Press.

Robin, D. A., Yorkston, K. M., & Beukelman, D. R. (Eds.). (1996). *Disorders of motor speech:*

Assessment, treatment, and clinical characterization. Baltimore, MD: Paul H. Brookes.

Tomblin, J. B., Morris, H. L., & Spriestersback, D. C. (2000). *Diagnosis in speech-language pathology* (2nd ed.). San Diego, CA: Singular Publishing Group.

Recommended Reading

Adams, S. G. (1997). Hypokinetic dysarthria in Parkinson's disease. In M. R. McNeil (Ed.), *Clinical management of sensorimotor speech disorders* (pp. 261–286). New York, NY: Thieme.

Brookshire, R. H. (1992). *Introduction to neurogenic communication disorders* (4th ed.). St. Louis, MO: Mosby.

Cannito, M. P., & Marquardt, T. P. (1997). Ataxic dysarthria. In M. R. McNeil (Ed.), *Clinical management of sensorimotor speech disorders* (pp. 217–248). New York, NY: Thieme.

Darley, F. L., Aronson, A. E., & Brown, J. R. (1969a). Differential diagnostic patterns of dysarthria. *Journal of Speech and Hearing Research, 12,* 246–269.

Darley, F. L., Aronson, A. E., & Brown, J. R. (1969b). Clusters of deviant dimensions in the dysarthrias. *Journal of Speech and Hearing Research, 12,* 462–496.

Darley, F. L., Aronson, A. E., & Brown, J. R. (1975). *Motor speech disorders.* Philadelphia, PA: W.B. Saunders.

Dworkin, J. P. (1991). *Motor speech disorders: A treatment guide.* St. Louis, MO: Mosby.

LaPointe, L. L., & Wertz, R. T. (1974). Oral-movement abilities and articulatory characteristics of brain-injured adults. *Perceptual Motor Skills, 39,* 39–46.

Ludlow, C. L., Hoit, J., Kent, R., Ramig, L. O., Shrivastav, R., Strand, E., . . . Sapienza, C. M. (2008). Translating principles of neural plasticity into research on speech motor control recovery and rehabilitation. *Journal of Speech, Language, and Hearing Research, 51,* S240–S258.

Moore, C. A., Yorkston, K. M., & Beukelman, D. R. (Eds.). (1991). *Dysarthria and apraxia of speech: Perspectives on management.* Baltimore, MD: Paul H. Brookes.

Murdoch, B. E., Gardiner, F., & Theodoros, D. G. (2000). Electropalatographic assessment of articulatory dysfunction in multiple sclerosis: A case study. *Journal of Medical Speech-Language Pathology, 8,* 359–367.

Rosenbek, J. C., Kent, R. D., & LaPointe, L. L. (1984). Apraxia of speech: An overview and some perspectives. In J. Rosenbek, M. McNeil, & A. Aronson (Eds.), *Apraxia of speech: Physiology, acoustics, linguistics, management.* San Diego, CA: College-Hill Press.

Rosenbek, J. C., & LaPointe, L. L. (1985). The dysarthrias: Description, diagnosis, and treatment. In D. F. Johns (Ed.), *Clinical management of neurogenic communicative disorders* (pp. 251–310). Boston, MA: Little, Brown.

Swigert, N. B. (1997). *The source for dysarthria.* East Moline, IL: LinguiSystems, Inc.

Webster, D. B. (1995). *Neuroscience of communication.* San Diego, CA: Singular Publishing Group.

Zraick, R. I., & LaPointe, L. L. (1997). Hyperkinetic dysarthria. In M. R. McNeil (Ed.), *Clinical management of sensorimotor speech disorders* (pp. 249– 260). New York, NY: Thieme.

Appendix 8-A
Cranial Nerve Information Sheet:
Oral Peripheral Mechanism Examination

Cranial Nerve	Type	Function
I—Olfactory	Sensory	Smell
II—Optic	Sensory	Vision
III—Oculomotor	Motor	Eye movement
IV—Trochlear	Motor	Eye movement (superior oblique)
V—Trigeminal	Sensory	Facial sensation—3 branches • Ophthalamic • Maxillary • Mandibular Anterior tongue sensation
	Motor	Muscles of mastication
VI — Abducens	Motor	Eye Movement—lateral rectus
VII—Facial	Sensory	Taste—anterior 2/3 tongue
	Motor	Facial expression
VIII—Vestibulocochlear	Sensory	Hearing Balance
IX—Glossopharyngeal	Sensory	Pharyngeal sensation
	Motor	Pharyngeal muscles
X—Vagus	Sensory	Pharynx, larynx, esophagus
	Motor	Muscles of palate, pharynx, and larynx
XI—Spinal Accessory	Motor	Shoulder, head movement
XII—Hypoglossal	Motor	Tongue movement

For the purpose of screening, the functions listed above are the primary functions of the cranial nerves. This is not meant to serve as an exhaustive list of cranial nerve function.

Source: From "Cranial Nerve Information Sheet," by J. A. G. Stierwalt, 2003. Copyright 2003 by Stierwalt, J. A. G. Reprinted with permission.

Cranial Nerve Screening

Cranial Nerve	Function	Screening Task
I—Olfactory	Sensory—Smell	Odors
II—Optic	Sensory—Vision	Vision chart/acuity
III—Oculomotor	Motor—Eye movement	"Follow the moving finger"
IV—Trochlear	Motor—Eye movement (superior oblique)	Look at the nose
V—Trigeminal	Sensory—facial sensation/anterior tongue	Have the individual close their eyes: touch the face
	Motor—muscles of mastication	Palpate muscles that clench the teeth
VI—Abducens	Motor—lateral rectus	Look to the side
VII—Facial	Sensory—taste	Sweet, sour, bitter, salt
	Motor—facial expression	Smile, raise the eyebrows
VIII—Vestibulocochlear	Sensory—hearing	A tuning fork
	balance	Look for vertigo
IX—Glossopharyngeal	Sensory—pharynx sensation	Gag reflex
	Motor—pharyngeal muscles	Gag reflex
X—Vagus	Sensory—pharynx, larynx, esophagus	Check phonation
	Motor—muscles of palate, pharynx, and larynx	Assess vocal quality
XI—Spinal Accessory	Motor—Shoulder, head movement	Shoulder shrug and/or turning the head to resistance
XII—Hypoglossal	Motor—Tongue movement	Assess tongue movement

Source: From "Cranial Nerve Screening," by J. A. G. Stierwalt, 2003. Copyright 2003 by Stierwalt, J. A. G., Florida State University. Reprinted with permission.

9

Motor Speech Disorders in Childhood

Case 1—Dysarthria

Richard was a 14-year-old, right-handed male who sustained a severe closed head injury when hit by a motor vehicle. A computed tomographic (CT) scan performed on the day of admission to hospital revealed a large soft tissue hematoma (blood clot) over the temporal regions of his left and right cerebral hemispheres. A small lesion was also identified in the region of the left basal ganglia. Richard was mute for 5 months postinjury. Although from that time speech did begin to return, Richard remained moderately dysarthric until referred to the Centre for Neurogenic Communication Disorders Research at 8 months postinjury. Perceptual analyses of Richard's speech conducted at that time revealed the presence of deficits in all five aspects of the speech production process (prosody, respiration, articulation, resonance, and phonation). A comprehensive instrumental assessment using a range of physiological instruments capable of assessing the functioning of the various components of the speech production apparatus confirmed the presence of impairments at all five levels. In particular, the major features contributing to Richard's dysarthria included severely reduced tongue function and moderately reduced lip, velopharyngeal, and laryngeal function and a mild to moderately reduced respiratory function. His speech was moderately unintelligible with decreased rate of speech, reduced variability of pitch, and imprecision of consonants. The single greatest contributor to Richard's unintelligibility appeared to be the dysfunction in the articulatory system, especially the impaired tongue function. Following an intensive 3-month period of traditional therapy supplemented with biofeedback therapy aimed at improving Richard's tongue and lip function, his speech had improved to a level where intelligibility was rated as being only mildly impaired. Subsequently, Richard was able to return to school with renewed confidence in his spoken output and to pursue a more active and natural social life.

Case 2—Apraxia

Lisa, at 7 years, 2 months of age suffered a cerebrovascular accident involving the left middle cerebral artery shortly after an operation to repair a faulty heart valve. Unfortunately for Lisa, the operation had triggered a blood clot that traveled up the left internal carotid artery to lodge in her left middle cerebral artery (note: a blood clot that has traveled from one part of the body to another is called an embolus). Before the neurologic episode, Lisa had been developing normally and was enjoying second grade at school. Initially, Lisa presented with a severe right hemiparesis (weakness down the right side of the body), which affected both her upper and lower limbs. Her arm was more severely affected than her leg, her right hand having no functional grasp and release. Lisa was unable to walk without assistance and her visual-perceptual abilities were affected. She also had a severe oral and verbal apraxia with a suspected expressive aphasic component. Her right upper motor neuron weakness was associated with drooling from the right side of her mouth. Lisa's range of tongue movement appeared adequate for eating and speech. When she was required to imitate oral movements, gross attempts and groping movements were noted. She was unable to repeat single sounds and her spontaneous speech output consisted of a single vowel and an attempt to say "no." Tests indicated that Lisa's auditory comprehension skills were intact and she responded appropriately to conversation and was able to follow four-stage commands. Lisa used facial expression, gross gestures, and vowel sounds for expressive communication. She was provided with a communication board to aid her communication. Eight months after her stroke, Lisa's speech was intelligible in all situations and her oral and verbal apraxia had resolved to being mild. Her right lower facial muscle weakness had also resolved. She was unable to volitionally elevate her tongue tip but when eating a cookie she cleaned her top lip without effort. Imitations of single sounds revealed only an inability to make voiced and voiceless /the/ and mild distortions of /l/ and /r/. Repetition of phoneme sequences and syllable sequences were still marked by delayed responses and slow rate of repetition with some visible searching behaviors but these problems did not appear to hamper her functional communication. A mild prosodic impairment, mainly a reduced rate of speech, was present when her syntactic construction was complex or when a polysyllabic word she used was new to her vocabulary. There was little detectable muscle weakness. Mild word-retrieval problems remained. Lisa was able to return to school 8 weeks poststroke. Her teacher reported that she was coping with the work in grade 2 and was just below the average in a class of 25.

Introduction

As outlined in Chapter 1, dysarthria and apraxia of speech both are motor speech disorders involving disruption of the processes that occur within the nervous system responsible for the motor control of speech. This chapter focuses on discussion of motor speech disorders occurring in children as a result of injury to the brain or peripheral nerves following head trauma, cerebrovascular accidents (strokes), neoplasms (tumors), anoxic episodes, and so forth. The latter speech disorders are referred to as "acquired" motor speech disorders. Discussion of motor speech disorders associated with congenital condition (i.e., developmental motor speech disorders) such as cerebral palsy are not included.

Although both dysarthria and apraxia of speech are classified as motor speech disorders, the two conditions differ in several ways. Whereas in dysarthria the speech disorder results from either paralysis, weakness, or incoordination of the muscles of the speech mechanism, apraxia of speech is thought to be a disorder of motor speech programming in which individuals have difficulty speaking because of a cerebral lesion that prevents them from executing voluntarily, or on command, the complex sequence of muscle contractions involved in speaking. In the speaker with apraxia of speech, the muscles of the speech production mechanism are neither weak nor paralyzed, as can be demonstrated by the child's ability to carry out movements of the face, tongue, and so forth during reflex activities such as licking the lips to retrieve a crumb when eating a cookie.

Acquired Childhood Dysarthria

Classification of Acquired Childhood Dysarthria

Traditionally, acquired childhood dysarthria has been described and classified according to criteria pertaining to the adult dysarthric population. It is important, however, to remember that children, depending on age, are either beginning to develop or are still developing speech concurrent with damage to the central nervous system. Consequently, interactions between the acquired and developmental mechanisms of motor speech disorders in children may complicate the use and application of adult dysarthria classifications in the pediatric population (Murdoch & Hudson-Tennent, 1994).

The difference in potential for the central nervous system to recover from, or compensate for, brain injury exhibited by children and adults is also a significant factor that limits the application of adult criteria to childhood dysarthria. Specifically, the potential of the central nervous system to recover from brain trauma sustained at a young age has often been reported as favorable relative to the recovery expected following brain damage in adults. It also is possible that the relationship between site of lesion and type of dysarthria determined in adults may not be readily applicable to the developing central nervous system. The most commonly used system for classification of the dysarthrias, at least with respect to adult disorders, was devised by Darley, Aronson, and Brown. (1975). Their system, also known as the Mayo Clinic classification system, identifies six different types of dysarthria (flaccid, spastic, hypokinetic, hyperkinetic, ataxic, mixed dysarthria), which presumably reflect underlying pathophysiology (i.e., spasticity, weakness, etc.) and correlate with the site of lesion in the nervous system. Whether or not the same system can be used for the developing central nervous system, however, is still in debate. Comparisons between the deviant speech characteristics identified for adults and children with acquired dysarthrias have revealed some overlap, but differences that require further investigation also have been evident (Murdoch & Hudson-Tennent, 1994). Unfortunately, currently there is a paucity of literature available that provides a clear description of the nature and course of specific forms of childhood dysarthria. Consequently, until empirical speech data are available to enable derivation of a classification system specific to childhood dysarthria, it would seem appropriate that a system of classification, such as the Mayo Clinic system, be used to define dysarthria in children in the same way it is used to define the equivalent speech disorders in adults. Furthermore, because the same components of the neuromuscular system, namely, the lower motor neurons, upper motor neurons, extrapyramidal system, cerebellum, and the neuromuscular junction as well as the muscles of the speech mechanism, can be affected by neurologic disorders in children as in adults, it would seem appropriate to use the Mayo Clinic system for describing acquired dysarthrias manifest in children.

Flaccid Dysarthria in Children

Damage to the motor cranial nerves and spinal nerves represent lower motor neuron lesions. These lesions interrupt the conduction of nerve impulses from the central nervous system to the skeletal muscles. When either the cranial nerves arising from the bulbar region of the brainstem (i.e., pons and medulla oblongata) (V, VII, IX, X, XI, and XII) and/or the spinal nerves that supply the muscles of respiration are involved, changes in speech collectively referred to as flaccid dysarthria may result. In the case of the bulbar cranial nerves, the damage may involve the nerves either in their peripheral course or in their nuclei in the brainstem.

Trigeminal Nerve Disorders (V). The trigeminal nerves (cranial nerve V) supply the muscles of mastication (temporalis, masseter, pterygoids), which in turn regulate the movement of the mandible. In children with unilateral trigeminal lesions, the mandible deviates toward the paralyzed side when they are asked to open their mouth widely. This deviation is brought about by the unopposed contraction of the muscle responsible for opening the jaw (pterygoid muscles) on the active side (i.e., the side opposite to the lesion). In addition, children will show a loss or reduction of muscle tone and atrophy in the muscles of mastication on the side of the lesion. Only minor alterations in speech occur, however, as a result of unilateral trigeminal lesions, in that movements of the mandible are impaired to only a small extent. Unilateral trigeminal lesions in children may result from traumatic brain injury (TBI) and brainstem tumors involving the pons. A much more devastating effect on speech occurs following bilateral trigeminal lesions (as may occur in bulbar poliomyelitis), the muscles responsible for the elevation of the mandible being too weak in many cases to approximate the mandible and maxilla. This inability, in turn, may prevent the tongue and lips from making the necessary contacts with oral structures for the production of labial and lingual consonants and vowels.

Facial Nerve Disorders (VII). The muscles of facial expression (e.g., orbicularis oris, buccinators, etc.) are supplied by the facial nerves (cranial nerves VII). Unilateral facial nerve lesions cause flaccid paralysis of the muscles of facial expression on the same side of the lesion. Consequently, children with such lesions present with drooping of the mouth on the affected side and saliva may constantly dribble from the corner. In addition, as a result of loss of muscle tone in the orbicularis oculi muscle, the lower eyelid also may droop. During smiling, the mouth is retracted on the active side but not on the child's affected side. Likewise, during frowning, the frontalis muscle on the side contralateral to the lesion will corrugate the forehead; however, on the side ipsilateral to the lesion, no corrugation will occur. In cases of bilateral facial nerve paralysis, saliva may drool from both corners of the mouth and the lips may be slightly parted at rest.

Both unilateral and bilateral facial nerve lesions affect speech production. Children with facial nerve lesions are unable to seal their lips tightly and during speech air escapes between their lips during the buildup of intraoral pressure. Consequently, unilateral facial nerve lesions cause distortion of bilabial and labiodental consonants. Speech impairments associated with bilateral facial nerve lesions range from distortion to complete obliteration of bilabial and labiodental consonants.

A number of different acquired disorders can cause malfunctioning of the facial nerves in children. In some cases the facial palsy may have idiopathic origin, such as in Bell's palsy, which usually causes unilateral facial paralysis. Prognostically, in the region of 80% of Bell's palsy cases recover in a few days or weeks. Unilateral facial paralysis also can result from closed head injuries, damage to one or other facial nerve during the course of forceps delivery, compression of the facial nerve by tumor (e.g., acoustic neuroma), and damage to the facial nucleus by brainstem tumors (e.g., glioma). Bilateral facial paralysis may occur in idiopathic polyneuritis (Guillain-Barré syndrome).

Vagus Nerve Disorders (X). The vagus nerves supply the muscles of the larynx and the levator muscles of the soft palate. Lesions of the vagus nerves, therefore, can affect either the phonatory or resonatory aspects of speech production or both, depending on the location of the lesion along the nerve pathway. Lesions that involve the nucleus ambiguus in the medulla (as occurs in lateral medullary syndrome) or the vagus nerve near the brainstem cause paralysis of all the skeletal muscles supplied via the vagus. Children with this type of lesion present with a voice disorder characterized by moderate breathiness, harshness, and reduced volume due to paralysis of the vocal fold on the same side as the lesion. In addition to the voice problem, these children also present with hypernasality due to paralysis of the soft palate on the affected side.

Lesions of the vagus that involve the nerve at a point distal to the exit of the pharyngeal nerve (which supplies the levator of the soft palate) but proximal to the exit of the superior laryngeal nerve have the same effect on phonation as brainstem lesions. These lesions, however, do not cause hypernasality as the functioning of the soft palate is not compromised.

Hypoglossal Nerve Disorders (XII). The hypoglossal nerves (cranial nerve XII) control the muscles of the tongue. Unilateral hypoglossal nerve damage is associated with flaccid paralysis, atrophy (shrinkage), and fasciculations (small muscle twitches) in the ipsilateral (same side as the nerve damage) of the tongue. On protrusion, the tongue deviates to the affected side.

In bilateral hypoglossal involvement, both sides of the tongue may be atrophied and show fasciculation. Although protrusion occurs in the midline in this case, the degree of protrusion may be severely limited. In addition, elevation of the tip and body to contact the alveolar ridge or hard palate may be difficult or impossible.

Although both phonation and resonation remain normal, lesions of the hypoglossal nerves therefore cause disturbances in articulation by interfering with normal tongue movement. The articulatory imprecision occurs especially during production of linguadental and linguapalatal consonants. In the case of unilateral lesions, the articulatory imprecision may be temporary in that most patients learn to compensate for unilateral tongue weakness within a few days. More serious articulatory impairments, however, are associated with bilateral hypoglossal nerve lesions. As indicated above, tongue movement in such cases may be severely restricted and speech sounds such as high front vowels and consonants that require elevation of the tongue tip to contact the upper alveolar ridge or hard palate (e.g., /t/, /d/, /l/, etc.) may be grossly distorted. Hypoglossal nerve lesions are rare in children.

Spastic Dysarthria in Children

Persistent spastic dysarthria is caused by bilateral disruption of the upper motor neuron supply to the bulbar cranial nerve nuclei. Lesions of upper motor neurons that can cause dysarthria may be located in the cerebral cortex, the internal capsule, the cerebral peduncles, or the brainstem. Clinical signs of upper motor neuron lesions include: spastic paralysis or paresis of the involved muscles, little or no muscle atrophy, hyperactive muscle stretch reflexes (e.g., hyperactive jaw-jerk), and the presence of pathologic reflexes (e.g., positive Babinski sign, positive rooting reflex, etc.).

The general name given to spastic paralysis of the bulbar musculature as a result of bilateral upper motor neuron lesions is pseudobulbar palsy (supranuclear palsy). Pseudobulbar palsy, which takes its name from its clinical resemblance to bulbar palsy, may be associated with a variety of neurologic disorders that bilaterally affect the upper motor neurons anywhere from their cell bodies, located in the motor cortex, through to their synapses with the appropriate lower motor neurons. Bilateral cerebrovascular accidents, multiple sclerosis, motor neuron disease, extensive neoplasms, congenital disorders, encephalitis, and severe brain trauma are all possible causes of this syndrome. All aspects of speech production, including phonation, resonation, articulation, and respiration, are affected in pseudobulbar palsy, but to varying degrees. Overall, pseudobulbar palsy is characterized by features such as bilateral facial paralysis, dysphagia, hypophonia, bilateral hemiparesis, incontinence, and bradykinesia. The most common cause of spastic dysarthria in childhood is hypoxic ischemic encephalopathy (reduced oxygen supply to the brain) usually associated with asphyxia during birth. Spastic dysarthria in children also can be the result of severe head injuries.

Dysarthria Associated With Extrapyramidal Syndromes in Children

Extrapyramidal syndromes are associated with pathologic changes in the basal ganglia and manifest as movement disorders that may also involve the muscles of the speech production mechanism. Classical examples of extrapyramidal syndromes are Parkinson's disease and Huntington's disease. Parkinson's disease is associated with hypokinetic dysarthria. Patients with hypokinetic dysarthria exhibit difficulty initiating speech, reduced loudness, variable speech rate between individuals (some patients speaking at a slower than normal rate and others speaking at a slightly faster than normal rate, and disturbed prosody [e.g., monopitch, reduced stress, and monoloudness]). Although Parkinson's disease is a condition most commonly associated with adult and elderly people, some Parkinsonian-like syndromes also occur in childhood. The most common of these is hypokinetic dyskinesia. In addition, subacute meningitis (infection of the meninges), as may occur in measles, also may present with a Parkinsonian-like profile. In past years, Parkinson's disease occurring secondary to epidemic encephalitis (infection of the brain) was common in children.

Hyperkinetic dysarthria is characterized by the presence of abnormal involuntary movements that disturb the rhythm and rate of the normal motor activities involved in speech production. The major extrapyramidal syndromes that cause hyperkinetic dysarthria include myoclonic jerks, tics, chorea, athetosis, dyskinesia, and dystonia. Myoclonic jerks are sudden, abrupt, unsustained muscle contractions that occur irregularly. The muscles of the speech production mechanism may be involved. The condition is seen in children in association with diffuse metabolic, infectious and toxic disorders of the central nervous system. Tics are recurrent, but brief unsustained involuntary movements usually affecting only a small part of the body. One condition that involves tics and affects speech production is Gilles de la Tourette's syndrome. In this syndrome, which usually manifests between the age of 2 and 15 years, uncontrolled vocalizations (e.g., grunting, coughing, barking, hissing, snorting, etc.) occur as a result of involuntary contractions of the muscles of the speech mechanism.

Slower than myoclonic jerks, choreic contractions involve a single, unsustained, isolated muscle action that produces a short, rapid, uncoordinated jerk of part of the body, such as the trunk, limb, face, tongue, and so forth. These contractions are random in their distribution and their timing is irregular and unpredictable. When superimposed on the normal movements of the speech mechanism during speech production, choreiform movements can cause momentary disturbances to the course of contextual speech. In fact, all aspects of speech can be disrupted in patients with chorea and the hyperkinetic dysarthria of chorea is characterized by a highly variable pattern of interference with articulation, phonation, resonation, and respiration. There are two major diseases in which choreic movements are present: Syndenham's chorea and Huntington's disease. The onset of Sydenham's chorea usually occurs between 5 and 10 years of age, females being affected more than males. In many instances, Sydenham's chorea appears to be associated with either streptococcal infections (strep throat) or rheumatic heart disease. Huntington's disease is an inherited disorder that, although it can manifest in childhood, usually has its onset in adult life.

Athetoid movements are characterized by a continuous, arrhythmic, slow, writhing type of muscle movement. These movements are always the same in the same patient and cease only during sleep. Although athetoid movements primarily involve the limbs, the muscles of the speech mechanism, including the muscles of the face, tongue, and so forth, may also be affected, causing facial grimacing, protrusion and writhing of the tongue, and difficulty in speaking and swallowing. Athetoid movements disrupt these functions by interfering with the normal contraction of the muscles involved. In most cases, athetosis forms part of a complex of neurologic signs, including those of cerebral palsy, that result from disordered development of the brain, birth injury, or other etiologic factors.

The major forms of dyskinesia represent side effects of various drug treatments applied to adults including antipsychotic drugs (tardive dyskinesia) and levodopa therapy for Parkinson's disease (levodopa-induced dyskinesia) and consequently rarely affect children. In dystonia, the involuntary movements are slow and sustained for long periods of time and may produce grotesque posturing and bizarre writhing movements. Conditions that lead to dystonia include encephalitis, head trauma, vascular diseases, and drug toxicity (e.g., tranquilizers).

Ataxic Dysarthria

Damage to the cerebellum or its connections leads to a condition called ataxia in which movements performed by skeletal muscles become uncoordinated. If the muscles of the speech mechanism are involved, speech production may become abnormal leading to a cluster of deviant speech dimensions collectively called ataxia dysarthria. A breakdown in the articulatory and prosodic aspects of speech are the predominant features of ataxic dysarthria. The imprecise articulation results in improper formation and separation of individual syllables leading to a reduction in intelligibility, whereas the disturbance in prosody is associated with loss of texture, tone, stress, and rhythm of individual syllables. The dysprosody results in slow, monotonous, and improperly measured speech, often termed "scanning speech."

There are a number of different causes of acquired ataxia in childhood, including: posterior fossa tumors (e.g., medulloblastomas, cerebellar astrocytomas, etc.), traumatic head injury, infections (cerebellar abscess), degenerative disorders (e.g., metachromatic leukodystrophy), and toxic, metabolic, and endocrine disorders (e.g., heavy metal poisoning, etc.).

Mixed Dysarthria

Some disorders of the nervous system affect more than one level of the neuromuscular system. Consequently, in addition to the more "pure" forms of dysarthria outlined above, clinicians also may be confronted by patients who exhibit "mixed dysarthrias." These may be caused by a variety of conditions including cerebrovascular accidents, head trauma, brain tumors, inflammatory diseases, and degenerative conditions. A mixed ataxic-hypokinetic-spastic dysarthria may be seen in children with Wilson's disease.

Etiology of Acquired Childhood Dysarthria

The major etiologies of acquired childhood dysarthria include traumatic brain injury, intracerebral tumors, cerebrovascular accidents (strokes), and infectious disorders.

Traumatic Brain Injury

Traumatic brain injury (TBI) is the leading cause of death and permanent disability in children and adolescents. Epidemiologic studies indicate that the incidence of TBI in childhood is approximately 200 per 100,000 per year, with male children having a higher incidence of TBI than female children in a ratio around 1.8 to 1. Disabilities demonstrated by children who survive TBI range from persistent vegetative state through mental and physical disabilities, language disorders, academic difficulties, and dysarthria.

The prognosis for recovery shown by children who have suffered mild head injuries has been reported to be excellent. Although the prognosis for recovery from severe head injuries is less certain, it is reported to be better than for adults. This difference may be the outcome of two factors. First, it may be due to the different nature of the impacts causing TBI in children versus adults; second, it may be related to differences in the basic mechanisms of brain damage following TBI in two groups, which in turn are related to differences in the physical characteristics of children's heads and adult heads. The majority of instances of childhood TBI result from falls (this is particularly the case for infants and toddlers) or low-speed (20 to 40 mph or 30 to 60 km/h) pedestrian or bicycle accidents that involve a motor vehicle. Consequently, many pediatric head injuries are associated with a lesser degree of injury resulting from rotational acceleration. Adults, on the other hand, are more likely to sustain TBI as a result of high-speed motor vehicle accidents, which by their nature are more likely to yield greater diffuse brain injury. Road traffic accidents are considered to be the most common cause of long-term morbidity following TBI in childhood. Evidence is available indicating that the type of brain injury resulting from severe head trauma depends on the physical properties of the individual's brain and skull. These physical properties are known to differ in a number of ways between children and adults, thereby contributing to different patterns of brain injury following head trauma in each group. First, an infant's brain weight is 15% of body weight progressing through to only 3% of body weight in adults. Second, the existence of unfused sutures and open fontanelles makes the skull of an infant and young child pliable, allowing a greater degree of deformation and possibly a greater ability to absorb the energy of physical impact.

Although persistent dysarthria is a commonly reported sequelae of severe TBI in children, few studies have investigated the incidence and nature of dysarthria following TBI acquired in childhood. The small number of the studies that have attempted to define the nature of dysarthria subsequent to TBI in children have been case studies (Cahill, Murdoch, & Theodoros, 2000; Murdoch & Horton, 1998; Murdoch, Pitt, Theodoros, & Ward, 1999). Each of these studies identified a range of impairments across the speech production mechanism of each child. In the most comprehensive series of studies completed to date, Cahill and colleagues (2002, 2003, 2005) examined 24 children who had acquired a TBI, using both perceptual and instrumental measures. Consistent with the case studies identified above, they found that each child presented with a differing profile of speech subsystem deficits, ranging from no dysarthria through to moderate-severe dysarthria.

These findings are not unexpected given that the diffuse, nonspecific nature of TBI can lead to damage in many areas of the central nervous system, resulting in impairment in one or more of the motor speech subsystems. More specifically, the perceptual and instrumental analysis of speech function in the group of children with TBI examined by Cahill, Murdoch, and colleagues identified substantial impairments in prosody, velopharyngeal and articulatory function, as well as reduced lung capacity and impaired respiratory-phonatory control for speech but little impairment in laryngeal function.

Brain Tumors

Brain tumors are a recognized cause of acquired dysarthria in childhood (Murdoch & Hudson-Tennent, 1994). The nature and distribution of brain tumors differs, however, in children compared to adults. Tumors located in the posterior cranial fossa (i.e., tumors involving the cerebellum, fourth ventricle, and/or brainstem) account for up to 70% of all pediatric intracranial neoplasms. Consequently, the majority of reported literature relating to pediatric intracranial neoplasms has focused on tumors involving the cerebellum, fourth ventricle, and/or brainstem.

Neurologic symptoms produced by brain tumors include both general and local symptoms. General symptoms result from increased intracranial pressure, which results directly from progressive enlargement of the tumor within the limited space of the cranial cavity. Local symptoms result from the effects of the tumor on contiguous areas of the brain. In that a tumor located in the posterior cranial fossa will inevitably involve the cerebellum, ataxic features may be anticipated in any associated speech disorder. Indeed, the occurrence of "cerebellar dysarthria" has been reported subsequent to surgical excision of posterior fossa tumors in children (Murdoch & Hudson-Tennent, 1994).

Treatment for posterior fossa tumors is by way of surgical excision of the tumor. Children with malignant tumors also may undergo a course of radiotherapy and, in the case of highly malignant tumors, a course of chemotherapy as well. Those children with low-grade tumors (e.g., low-grade astrocytomas) may be spared both radiotherapy and chemotherapy, a factor that has been suggested as a reason for their lower incidence of neuropsychological sequelae.

The most common posterior fossa tumors are medulloblastomas, astrocytomas, and ependymomas. Medulloblastomas are highly malignant brain tumors derived from primitive neurons, the neuroblasts. In particular, the majority of these tumors are thought to arise from embryonal cells in the posterior medullary velum of the cerebellum. Although these tumors originate from the cerebellum, they subsequently invade the subarachnoid space, fourth ventricle, and spinal canal. The primary concern for children with medulloblastoma is the risk of tumor recurrence in the posterior cranial fossa and/or development of supratentorial, spinal cord, or systemic metastases. The prognosis for children with recurrent medulloblastoma is poor.

Astrocytomas are derived from the astrocytic neuroglial cells. When located in the posterior cranial fossa, they can arise from either the vermis or lateral lobes of the cerebellum. Cerebellar astrocytomas are usually low grade with regard to malignancy, and therefore, associated with a favorable prognosis after surgical removal, with tumor recurrence being rare. Ependymomas are derived from the ependymal cells lining the ventricles of the brain with the roof and floor of the fourth ventricle being the most common origins for these tumors. From there, the tumor grows to occlude the cavity of the fourth ventricle, protrudes through the cisterna magna or may extend through the foramen magnum to overlap the cervical segments of the spinal cord. Ependymomas are slow growing and predominantly benign tumors. Because of their origins in the roof or floor of the fourth ventricle, however, complete surgical resection is not possible, so recurrence rates for these tumors is high. Development of metastases (i.e., other tumors resulting from tumor cells that have traveled from the primary tumor site) in other sites, however, is unusual. Overall, the prognosis for a child with an ependymoma is poor in terms of ultimate cure.

Dysarthria has been reported to occur subsequent to the diagnosis and treatment of posterior fossa tumors, with the presentation of the speech impairment ranging from transient mutism, to mild dysarthria, through to a persistent developmental speech disorder. The literature, to date, predominantly documents the presence of transient cerebellar mutism subsequent to surgery for a posterior fossa tumor, and that resolution to normal speech involves a period of dysarthria. There is some evidence, however, that in some individuals treated for posterior fossa tumors, speech does not return to premorbid levels, implying the presence of a persistent dysarthria. However, the majority of reports not only are based on small numbers of children, but also restricted to descriptions of the speech impairment based on perceptual speech analyses. A number of studies have labeled the speech disorder evident as cerebellar or ataxic dysarthria utilizing the Mayo Clinic classification. Unfortunately, in many of these studies, the actual clinical features of the speech disorder were not elaborated, using the overall term of ataxic dysarthria only as a descriptor.

In a recent published series of studies based on perceptual, acoustic, and physiologic assessment, Cornwell, Murdoch, and Ward (2003, 2005) and Cornwell, Murdoch, Ward, and Kellie (2004) determined that, although not all children treated for posterior fossa tumors exhibit a persistent dysarthria, in cases where it does occur, the nature of the deviant perceptual features usually reflects those associated with dysarthria in adults with cerebellar or lower motor neuron damage, dependent on tumor location within the posterior cranial fossa. In particular, where the tumor is primarily cerebellar in location, the child usually exhibits a predominance of phonatory, articulatory, and prosodic disturbances. Examination of the individual components of the speech musculature revealed that there was impairment to lip, tongue, and laryngeal function both at rest and during performance of non-speech and speech tasks, along with more minor deficits in palatal and respiratory function.

Cerebrovascular Accidents

Cerebrovascular disorders constitute a much smaller proportion of neurologic diseases of childhood than of adulthood. However, they occur more frequently than generally thought and are a significant cause of morbidity and mortality in the childhood population. Although dysarthria associated with cerebrovascular accidents (CVA) is, therefore, less common than in adults, cerebrovascular disorders are an acknowledged cause of dysarthria in children being observed in both occlusive and hemorrhagic conditions (Horton, Murdoch, Theodoros, & Thompson, 1997).

The majority of the diseases of blood vessels that affect adults may also at some time affect children. The causes of vascular diseases of the brain in children, however, differ from those in adults. Although some vascular diseases of the brain, such as embolism arising from subacute or acute bacterial endocardial vascular disease, occur at all ages, others such as cerebrovascular disorders associated with congenital heart disease, are peculiar to childhood. At the other extreme, degenerative disorders of the vascular system such as atherosclerosis affect primarily middle-aged and elderly people and are rare in childhood.

Vascular anomalies are the most common cause of primary central nervous system hemorrhage in infants and children. The most important of these are angiomas. Rather than being vascular neoplasms, angiomas represent developmental malformations and can be classified as arteriovenous, venous, cavernous, or capillary. In addition to vascular abnormalities, cerebral hemorrhage in children can occur secondary to hematologic diseases such as leukemia, sickle cell anemia, hemophilia, and thrombocytopenic purpura as well as traumatic head injury.

Arterial occlusion in childhood is most frequently the consequence of congenital dysplasia of the vessels, cerebral arteritis, trauma or thromboembolic disease, the latter condition usually occurring in infants or children with congenital heart disease. Occlusive vascular disease in children has been observed in cases of sickle cell disease and Moyamoya disease and as an outcome of complications of certain hereditary metabolic diseases such as homocystinuria and Fabry's disease.

Despite being a recognized sequelae of cerebrovascular disorders, very few detailed descriptions of dysarthria resulting from cerebrovascular disorders in children have been reported. Horton et al. (1997) provided the only detailed description of a child with dysarthria associated with basilar artery stroke based on comprehensive assessment using both perceptual and physiologic techniques. The physiologic assessments indicated the most severe motor speech deficits to be in the respiratory and velopharyngeal subsystems with significant deficits also being apparent in the articulatory subsystem, collectively resulting in severely reduced intelligibility. Bak, van Dongen, and Arts (1983) also described the perceptual features of the speech disorder exhibited by a child with a brainstem infarct following occlusion of the basilar artery. Specifically, the dysarthria in their case was characterized by imprecise consonants, distorted vowels, hypernasality, and a breathy voice.

Infectious Disorders

Infectious disorders of the central nervous system are a recognized cause of dysarthria in both children and adults.

These infectious disorders include those caused by bacterial, spirochetal, viral, and other less common microorganisms. In particular, major infectious disorders that have been documented in the literature as causing dysarthria in children include: meningitis, encephalitis, bulbar polioencephalitis (bulbar form of poliomyelitis), Reye's syndrome, Sydenham's chorea, and cerebellar abscesses.

Acquired Apraxia of Speech

Acquired apraxia of speech is a motor speech programming disorder characterized primarily by errors in articulation and secondarily by alterations in prosody. Although most of what we know about this disorder comes from studies on adult subjects, it has been speculated that acquired verbal dyspraxia also can occur in children with brain injuries. Unfortunately, only scant information regarding the nature and occurrence of this disorder in childhood is available in the literature, with the presence of apraxia of speech occasionally being noted by authors as one of the speech-language disorders to occur among others following brain injury, but with few details being provided. As in adults, it appears that acquired apraxia of speech usually occurs in combination with an acquired aphasia and/or dysarthria. One possible reason for the lack of attention paid to acquired apraxia of speech in the literature is that the condition appears to resolve quickly.

This is true whether the apraxia is oral or verbal in nature. The only two articles which make reference to acquired apraxia of speech in children either document its recovery or note its presence in the early stages postonset. Aram, Rose, Rekate, and Whitaker (1983) described the oral apraxia seen in a 7-year-old right-handed girl with acquired capsular/striatal aphasia. On day four after onset, the child was totally mute and unable to produce nonspeech oral movements on command but could produce them on imitation. Two days later, these nonspeech movements were initiated on command, as was phonation. Within another two days a full range of tongue movements was possible and vowel sounds could be imitated. At this time, two-word phrases were spontaneously produced. Some weakness of the right facial muscles was present but no dysarthria was noticeable. No further mention of speech disturbances was made, although aphasic symptoms were still present.

Three of the 15 cases of children with acquired aphasia described by Cooper and Flowers (1987) presented with apraxia of speech one month after onset. One case was head-injured whereas the other two had suffered hematomas. All three cases were communicating orally at the time the apraxia was noted. Therefore, an apraxia of speech can be assumed. No information on the apraxia symptoms or their recovery was given. In the absence of detailed descriptions of apraxia of speech symptoms in children, one must again turn to the adult literature.

Features of apraxia of speech seen in adults include:

1. Visible and audible groping to achieve correct individual articulatory postures and sequence of postures to produce sounds and words.
2. Highly variable articulatory errors (e.g., /v/ may at different times be produced /v/, /z/, /p/, /f/, /r/, /b/, /h/, and /w/).

3. Based on perceptual analysis with the naked ear, articulatory errors appear to involve substitutions rather than distortions of individual phonemes as occurs in dysarthria.
4. A greater number of articulatory errors occur during repetition than during conversational speech.
5. The number of articulatory errors increases as the complexity of the articulatory exercise increases—few errors are made on single consonants whereas more errors occur on consonant clusters.
6. In addition to articulatory disturbances, as these patients speak, they slow down their rate of speech, space their words and syllables more evenly, and stress them more equally.
7. Speech output is nonfluent because of pausing and hesitating while the individual gropes for articulatory placement and makes repeated efforts to produce words correctly.

The case description of a child with acquired apraxia of speech provided at the beginning of this chapter illustrated the presence of a number of these features.

References

Aram, D. M., Rose, D. F., Rekate, H. L., & Whitaker, H. A. (1983). Acquired capsular/striatal aphasia in childhood. *Archives of Neurology, 40,* 614–617.

Bak, E., van Dongen, H. R., & Arts, W. F. M. (1983). The analysis of acquired dysarthria in childhood. *Developmental Medicine and Child Neurology, 25,* 81–94.

Cahill, L. M., Murdoch, B. E., & Theodoros, D. G. (2000). Variability in speech outcome following severe childhood traumatic brain injury: A report of three cases. *Journal of Medical Speech-Language Pathology, 8,* 347–352.

Cahill, L. M., Murdoch, B. E., & Theodoros, D. G. (2002). Perceptual analysis of speech following traumatic brain injury in childhood. *Brain Injury, 16,* 415–446.

Cahill, L. M., Murdoch, B. E., & Theodoros, D. G. (2003). Perceptual and instrumental analysis of laryngeal function following traumatic brain injury in childhood. *Journal of Head Trauma Rehabilitation, 18,* 268–283.

Cahill, L. M., Murdoch, B. E., & Theodoros, D. G. (2005). Articulatory function following traumatic brain injury in childhood: A perceptual and instrumental approach. *Brain Injury, 19,* 41–58.

Cooper, J. A., & Flowers, C. R. (1987). Children with a history of acquired aphasia: residual language and academic impairments. *Journal of Speech and Hearing Disorders, 52,* 251–262.

Cornwell, P. L., Murdoch, B. E., & Ward, E. C. (2003). Perceptual evaluation of motor speech following treatment for childhood cerebellar tumour. *Clinical Linguistics and Phonetics, 17,* 597–615.

Cornwell, P. L., Murdoch, B. E., & Ward, E. C. (2005). Differential motor speech outcomes in children treated for midline cerebellar tumour. *Brain Injury, 19,* 119–134.

Cornwell, P. L., Murdoch, B. E., Ward, E. C., & Kellie, S. (2004). Acoustic investigation of vocal fold quality following treatment of childhood cerebellar tumour. *Folia Phoniatrica et Logopaedica, 56,* 93–107.

Darley, F. L., Aronson, A. E., & Brown, J. R. (1975). *Motor speech disorders.* Philadelphia, PA: W. B. Saunders.

Horton, S. K., Murdoch, B. E., Theodoros, D. G., & Thompson, E. C. (1997). Motor speech impairment in a case of childhood basilar artery stroke: treatment directions derived from physiological and perceptual assessment. *Pediatric Rehabilitation, 1,* 163–177.

Murdoch, B. E., & Horton, S. K. (1998). Acquired and developmental dysarthria in childhood. In B. E. Murdoch (Ed.), *Dysarthria: A physiological approach to assessment and treatment* (pp. 373–427). Cheltenham, UK: Stanley Thornes.

Murdoch, B. E., & Hudson-Tennent, L. J. (1994). Speech disorders in children treated for posterior fossa tumours: Ataxic and developmental features. *Euro-pean Journal of Disorders of Communication, 29,* 379–397.

Murdoch, B. E., Pitt, G., Theodoros, D. G., & Ward, E. C. (1999). Real-time visual biofeedback in the treatment of speech breathing disorders following childhood traumatic brain injury: A report on one case. *Pediatric Rehabilitation, 3,* 5–20.

▌▐ ▌ 10 ▌ ▐▌

Acquired Neurologic Swallowing Disorders in Children and Adults

"Jerry, there is nothing more that can be done. You should be prepared to have that tube for the rest of your life."

"I can't believe that, just can't accept it. I am only 59 years old, are you saying I'll never eat again?" Following a brainstem stroke, Jerry had a gastrostomy tube surgically placed in his stomach to receive nutrition and hydration. The tube was inserted because since his stroke, when he attempted to swallow either food or liquid it "went down the wrong pipe," into the lungs. As a result, Jerry had suffered several bouts of aspiration pneumonia, a lung infection directly caused by an inability to swallow safely.

At the time of his stroke, Jerry was an active 59-year-old entrepreneur. He owned several businesses even had a pilot's license so that he could fly himself (using his own plane) when he needed to travel. Sure, he had high blood pressure, but at his age didn't everyone? He had that three vessel coronary artery bypass graft (triple bypass) surgery on his heart a couple of years ago. Didn't that make him as good as new? These are thoughts that ran through Jerry's mind once it cleared several weeks after that fateful day in October when he suffered a devastating ischemic stroke to the brainstem.

It was now April, roughly 6 months after the stroke. There are some remaining motor speech issues, including flaccid dysarthria, and a unilateral vocal fold paralysis, and although it takes extra effort, he can produce intelligible speech. The swallowing impairment that he thought was a temporary condition, however, has not resolved. And, from what he just heard from the physician, it is not going to. What will life be like now? I can't take my wife out to dinner. I can't toss back a few beers with the guys watching football on Sunday afternoon. I can't even enjoy a simple Diet Coke.

The situation is difficult to imagine. Swallowing is a biologic function that develops before birth and we swallow food, liquid, and saliva hundreds of times a day (and night). Yet, the automatic task that is so essential to life, can go very wrong after damage to the nervous system. The medical term for swallowing impairment is *dysphagia*, a condition that can be medically, socially, and psychologically devastating.

Introduction

Eating and drinking are essential components of our daily lives. Not only are these activities necessary for survival, we have also learned to enjoy them. Incorporating eating and drinking into social activity is a standard practice. Think about the last time you were at a gathering with friends. No doubt, a central feature of that gathering was food and drink. Throughout each day, we eat several meals, munch on snacks in between, drink coffee or tea in the morning, and drink sodas or water throughout the day. Okay, so you get the point, right? We eat and drink a *lot*! (Figure 10–1). So much so that it has become highly automated task, a function that we invest very little thought into. We just open our mouths, pop in a morsel, and assume everything will get to the stomach without incident.

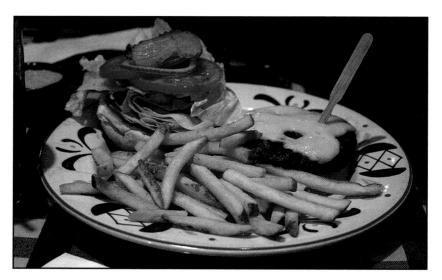

FIGURE 10–1. Typical meal.

You have learned from reading through the chapters of this textbook, that damage to the nervous system can make even the simplest tasks difficult or even impossible to do. When the act of swallowing is affected, the medical term is *dysphagia*. Dysphagia occurs as a symptom of a multitude of medical conditions but is particularly prevalent in those who have sustained damage to the CNS, the PNS, or both. What exactly is a *swallowing problem*? Well, that is a good question, one that will be explored in this chapter. Simply put, dysphagia is any disruption in the process of moving food or liquid from the mouth to the stomach. Examine Figure 10–2, and note that we use a shared pathway for both breathing and eating. For breathing, we use the nasal passages and the mouth, the pharynx. In the lower pharynx, notice there is a bifurcation (or split) into two passageways with one path leading forward into the respiratory tract and the other traveling behind into the digestive tract. The fact that there is a common path is a bit problematic. We have to breathe most of the time, so the respiratory passage must remain wide open for good air exchange. During eating, however, that passage must close off to protect the airway. The process of *swallowing* offers a primary protection for the respiratory system. During the swallow, the entrance to the larynx and airway is sealed off temporarily. As you are reading this, notice your breathing and then initiate a swallow. During the instant of the swallow, you stopped breathing. It is during that precise instant when the airway is sealed. This careful coordination is necessary to maintain balance between the two systems.

You probably have experienced when the balance goes awry. Have you ever been eating or drinking and some-

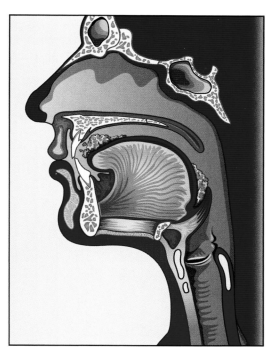

FIGURE 10–2. An illustration of eating in which part of the bolus continues to be chewed while another part moves into the pharynx. Reprinted with permission from *Preclinical Speech Science* (p. 589), by T. J. Hixon, G. Weismer, and J. D. Hoit, 2008, Plural Publishing. Copyright © 2008 by Plural Publishing, Inc.

thing or someone makes you laugh? What happens in that situation? Well, you cough and sputter and your friends start pounding you on the back. Your respiratory system is an important one and when there is intrusion, there is a pretty dramatic attempt to clear it (the coughing). Coughing while eating or drinking is an indication that substance you are swallowing (let's call it a bolus) is going in the wrong direction. A misdirected bolus that enters the airway is called *aspiration* and can pose a serious health risk. Individuals who have dysphagia may suffer from aspiration or other conditions that make it difficult to swallow safely.

Scope of the Problem

Dysphagia is a problem that crosses the lifespan. Premature infants, babies born with a syndrome or other fragile medical conditions, often have difficulty swallowing safely. At the other end of the age continuum (the elderly), there is a greater incidence of neurologic conditions (e.g., stroke or disease), even the natural process of aging can contribute to the presence of dysphagia. Regardless of the setting of your employment, if you become an SLP, you will work with people who experience dysphagia. The incidence of dysphagia is difficult to pin down because there are a number of variables to consider. For example, the population (stroke patients versus head and neck cancer), the method of identifying dysphagia (instrumental assessment or survey), and even how dysphagia is defined. In a number of large studies that have reviewed entire hospitals, it has been reported that roughly one third of the hospitalized population at any one time, regardless of etiology, has swallowing impairment. That is a big group of people (Groher, 1997).

The incidence of dysphagia increases when we consider only individuals who suffer from brain damage. The oral motor system that we use for speech is the same one that we rely on for eating/swallowing (with the exception of the esophagus, which typically is not used for speech). Therefore, the many neurologic etiologies you have been reading about that result in speech impairment also impact swallowing function. Take, for example, the population of individuals who have experienced a stroke. Reports on the percent of individuals who experience dysphagia following a stroke range from 25% to over 80%

(Daniels & Huckabee, 2008). The reason for the wide range in reports relate to the same reasons listed above (population, measurement techniques, definitions). Similarly, in children who experience neurologic conditions such as cerebral palsy, if the speech mechanism is impaired. it is likely that dysphagia will also be a concern.

The Normal Swallow

The act of swallowing is a series of actions and events that take place to manipulate a bolus, move it through the mouth, the pharynx, and safely into the esophagus where it will travel to the stomach. Historically, swallowing has been described as a four-phase process with each phase distinct from the others. More recently, however, researchers have noted that there is overlap to some of the phases, with events from phases occurring simultaneously rather than sequentially (Hixon, Weismer, & Hoit, 2008; Stierwalt & Youmans, 2007). Although we know that overlap exists, it remains easiest to explain and understand the process as occurring in phases. Once you have a comfortable understanding of the process, it will be easier to see and comprehend the areas of overlap.

Oral Preparatory Phase

The first phase of swallowing calls for preparation of the bolus. When food or liquid is taken into your mouth, care is taken to contain it in the oral cavity while it is prepared for the remaining phases. Containment at the front of the mouth occurs primarily by the lips, although the teeth might assist if no chewing is involved. On the sides of the mouth, the buccal (cheek) muscles will increase tension against the teeth to keep the bolus from falling into the cheek cavity (yes, that is why you occasionally bite your cheek). At the back of the mouth, the tongue will elevate and come into contact with the velum, providing posterior containment. The tongue/velum contact also allows breathing to continue while oral preparation is underway (Figure 10–3). Bolus containment is important so the bolus does not fall into the pharynx and the airway that, as mentioned, is open for breathing. With the bolus securely contained in the mouth, preparation can occur. How much preparation is required depends

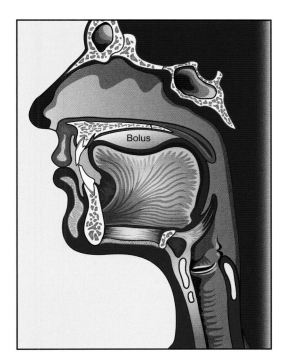

FIGURE 10–3. Oral preparatory phase of swallowing. Reprinted with permission from *Preclinical Speech Science* (p. 585), by T. J. Hixon, G. Weismer, and J. D. Hoit, 2008, Plural Publishing. Copyright © 2008 by Plural Publishing, Inc.

largely on the bolus. Certainly, a chunk of meat, ripped off a turkey leg will take more preparation than a sip of water. The function of oral preparation is to make sure the bolus is masticated (chewed) and broken down. In addition, the bolus is mixed with saliva to help keep it cohesive and easy to control. When the bolus is broken down to a manageable size and consistency, it is gathered by the tongue and brought to the middle of the oral cavity.

There is a good deal of variation in the oral preparatory phase according to the consistency of the bolus. As mentioned, a chunk of meat is prepared differently than a sip of water. Let's follow that process from start to finish. When you have torn that bit of meat off that turkey leg (no doubt purchased from a vendor at a Renaissance fair), you will seal off the lips to contain it in the mouth (lateral and posterior containment is also in place). Now your tongue will go to work, moving the meat over to the teeth that will grind and mix it with saliva. The sensory input from the tongue constantly sends information about the consistency of the bolus, is it manageable for swallowing, or is more chewing necessary? When the bolus is "just right," the tongue will gather it in the middle of the tongue in one cohesive unit. The amount of muscle activity and time it takes to prepare a bolus that requires mastication clearly is greater than what is necessary for a liquid bolus. It is important to point out, however, that a liquid bolus is not without its challenges. Although mastication or chewing is not required, the fluid nature of the bolus requires an incredible amount of motor ability just to keep it under control. Once it enters the mouth, the greatest challenge is to contain it and gather it together. To illustrate that point, consider the following. You have a cup of water, and a cup of mashed potatoes and you drop each onto the floor. Which one is the easiest to pick up or clean up? The water, when not contained, will flow all over the floor, whereas a more solid substance will just plop onto the surface in one blob. So, although fluid is considered an "easy" consistency, that fact is only true if motor/muscle control is intact. Because of these consistency effects, the oral preparatory phase is under voluntary control, meaning you can choose to chew as long as is necessary or not chew at all if the bolus doesn't require breakdown. The voluntary nature of this phase makes it highly variable in terms of timing and muscle activity.

Oral Transit Phase

Once the bolus has been prepared and gathered at the center of the tongue, the oral transit phase begins. The purpose of the oral transit phase is to deliver the bolus from the oral cavity to the pharynx so it can begin its descent to the esophagus. To initiate bolus transit, the tongue is anchored at the front of the oral cavity behind the teeth. The tongue then begins a contraction against the hard palate that begins right behind the teeth and moves back along the hard palate to the back of the mouth. This front-to-back contact between the tongue and hard palate serves to push or strip the bolus through the mouth and back to the pharynx (Figure 10–4). As reviewed in the previous section, bolus containment continues to be important here. The lips will remain closed and the cheek muscles against the teeth, but as the bolus moves to the back of the mouth, the soft palate will begin to lift in preparation for the swallow.

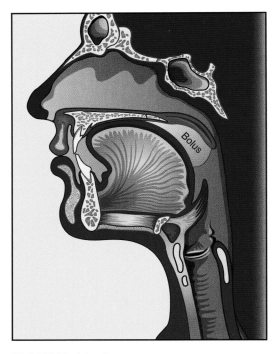

FIGURE 10–4. Oral transport phase of swallowing. Reprinted with permission from *Preclinical Speech* Science (p. 586), by T. J. Hixon, G. Weismer, and J. D. Hoit, 2008, Plural Publishing. Copyright © 2008 by Plural Publishing, Inc.

As with the oral preparation phase, there is some change in the transit because of bolus consistency. Although, the variation that occurs in the oral transit phase is due to consistency, the change is not as great as that seen in oral preparation. The variation that does occur has to do with pressures exerted by the tongue to force the bolus back to the pharynx. For a bolus that is more solid, the tongue must exert greater pressure (Kahrilas, & Logemann, 1993; Youmans & Stierwalt, 2006; Youmans, Youmans, & Stierwalt, 2009). When you think about it, that makes a lot of sense. For fluids, little pressure would be generated because it already moves so easily, requiring little pressure from the tongue.

When you consider the *timing* aspect of oral transit, however, there is little variation across consistencies. The time it takes to move a solid bolus is essentially the same as a liquid bolus.

The Pharyngeal Phase

In the pharyngeal phase of swallowing (Figure 10–5), there is an orchestrated series of events, the purpose of which are to protect the airway from aspiration as the bolus moves through the pharynx and enters the esophagus. The events are triggered as the bolus enters the pharynx at the end of bolus transit through the mouth. The velum, which

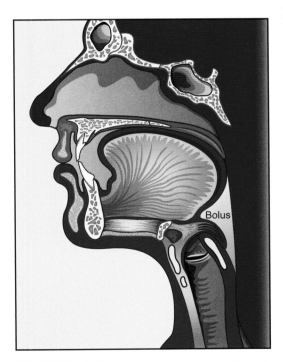

FIGURE 10–5. Pharyngeal phase of swallowing. Reprinted with permission from *Preclinical Speech* Science (p. 587), by T. J. Hixon, G. Weismer, and J. D. Hoit, 2008, Plural Publishing. Copyright © 2008 by Plural Publishing, Inc.

started to elevate at the end of the oral transit phase, makes contact with the posterior pharyngeal wall. The tongue continues to push the bolus back into the pharynx. The base of the tongue then also serves as a foundation for the pharyngeal muscles, which contract to squeeze the bolus through the pharynx. There are actually three primary pharyngeal muscles that contract sequentially from the top to the bottom to accomplish bolus movement through the pharynx.

Bolus movement through the pharynx is only one aspect of the pharyngeal phase. The important role of protecting the airway is another vital function that occurs during this phase. When the tongue pushes the bolus back into the pharynx, the muscles in the floor of the mouth begin to contract. Tightening those muscles pulls the framework of the larynx up and forward, also pulling the opening to the airway forward. The up and forward excursion of the larynx causes a downward movement of the epiglottis, closing the opening to the larynx. This seal at the entrance to the larynx, which sits on top of the trachea, completes the first of three levels of protection for the airway. The additional levels of protection occur when the false (ventricular) folds and the true vocal folds simultaneously adduct, sealing the airway at two more levels. Redundancy in the system (three layers of protection) really points out the importance of closing off the airway to potential intrusion of food or liquid.

At the bottom of the pharynx lies the esophagus. The boundary between these two structures is the cricopharyngeus muscle. The cricopharyngeus muscle is a circular muscle at the top of the esophagus that is in tonic contraction, which simply means that it acts as a sphincter (also known as the upper esophageal sphincter or UES) and opens only to allow a bolus to enter the esophagus. The opening of the UES occurs as a consequence of two actions. The primary action is the nerve impulse that travels to the cricopharyngeus that says, "Relax man, food's coming." The muscle does indeed "relax" or open, allowing the bolus to pass through the UES to the esophagus. The secondary action that opens the UES is a result of the movement of the laryngeal framework. The UES (remember this is also the cricopharyngeus muscle) is attached to the cricoid cartilage (the lower border of the laryngeal framework), so as the framework moves up and forward, it stretches the cricopharyngeus muscle pulling it open. Once the bolus has passed through the UES, the muscle returns to tonic contraction. With the return of the UES to its resting state, the structures above are all returning to their original positions opening the airway so breathing can resume.

When consistency effects are considered, variations in the pharyngeal phase are similar to those experienced in the oral transit phase. Greater muscle pressure is necessary to move a thicker bolus, but fluid follows gravity and flows easily through the pharynx. With respect to the time it takes to move a bolus through the pharynx, it is similar across consistencies, but understandably a little longer for a more solid bolus. There is one other "consistency" effect worth mentioning. Liquids, because of their fluid properties, can sneak into

Boyle's Law Revisited

In Chapter 2, we discussed several physics principles as they relate to respiration? One of them, specifically Boyle's law, applies to swallowing as well.

As a reminder, Boyle's law states that, in a container, the variables of volume and pressure are inversely proportional and have a constant product, simply meaning that as one increases the other decreases. As we discussed, its application to respiration is the following. When the volume of the lungs increases, the air pressure within them will experience a corresponding decrease. At that time, the air pressure *within* the lungs is negative relative to atmospheric air pressure outside the body. The negative pressure in the lungs will function like a suction force, pulling air into the lungs through the upper respiratory passageways.

So what exactly is the application to swallowing? Well, in swallowing, our "container" is the pharynx. As the bolus moves into and through the pharynx and the UES opens, the volume of the container will increase with the addition of the open esophagus. Again, the increased size of the container will cause a drop in pressure. The negative pressure, which is in front of the bolus as it travels into the esophagus, will create a suction force that functions to assist bolus movement into the esophagus.

Just another illustration of the importance of the pharyngeal phase of swallowing!

every nook and crevice in the pharynx. Remember that the entrance to the airway, which is located in the pharynx, is sealed off during this phase. When that process is intact, a bolus will not penetrate that seal. However, if the closure is incomplete or if it occurs slowly, then fluid can flow into the larynx, thus, airway. A more solid consistency is less likely to do so because it tends to hold together better (remember the mashed potatoes).

The Esophageal Phase

The esophageal phase begins with closure of the UES. Once in the esophagus, the bolus travels down the tube through a combination of gravity and muscle contraction. Muscle contraction that occurs in the esophagus is peristaltic in nature. Peristalsis is a wavelike contraction with relaxation ahead of the bolus and contraction behind, efficiently moving the bolus to the lower esophagus. At the end of the esophagus is a sphincter muscle similar the UES (in fact, they call this one the lower esophageal sphincter or the LES). The LES is also in tonic contraction (this keeps stomach contents, which contain acid from entering the esophagus). Once the bolus has entered the esophagus, however, the LES will open, allowing the bolus to pass into the stomach where it can be broken down and digested further.

Consistency effects in the esophageal follow the pattern of the pharyngeal phase. A bolus that is more substantial will move a little slower and require more work from esophageal muscles. Have you ever swallowed a bite of peanut butter sandwich and felt like it got stuck about halfway down to the stomach? It takes a substantial force to move some consistencies through the esophagus, especially if it is a large bite of a more solid consistency. Usually, a swallow of liquid behind the bite that "got stuck" will help to push it through the esophagus, alleviating the problem.

Age-Related Differences

With a better understanding of the normal swallowing process, it is important to note that differences occur across the age spectrum. Although the process of swallowing is essentially the same from around school age until old age, there are some differences in the very young and the elderly.

Let's first address the anatomical differences. Infant structures are very small and in some instances underdeveloped, which changes the orientation of oral motor structures for swallowing. The mandible, for example is much smaller and has yet to develop into the adult model. The ramus, which is the portion of the mandible that travels down from the temporomandibular joint until it turns at the angle of the jaw, is very small. In addition to its small size, the ramus slopes forward; there is no clear vertical portion of the bone as there is in the adult mandible. Because the mandible supports the tongue, the small size and sloping orientation of the ramus results in a tongue that literally fills the oral cavity and is carried in a more forward position. Other differences relate to the location of structures in the neck. The larynx is carried very high in babies, located almost directly behind the point of the chin. The "compact" nature of structures in the pharynx provides protection for the infant who generally feeds in a reclined position. Finally, the infant has additional muscle filaments in the lips to help achieve a good seal around a bottle or breast nipple, and the cheeks contain "sucking pads" that support the tension that is needed for nipple feeding. Each of these variations in muscle disappears as the child grows and transitions away from nipple feeding (Arvedson & Brodsky, 2002).

In addition to the developmental differences in anatomy just described, the process of swallowing in the infant varies from that of an older child or an adult. The normal process of swallowing goes through an evolution that begins well before birth. Suckling, which is a developmental precursor to sucking, begins to emerge in the fetus around 18 weeks gestation and matures around 32 weeks. During the suckling pattern, the mandible is stabilized for tongue movement, which consists primarily of a back-and-forth motion. Remember, the tongue literally fills the oral cavity so the back-and-forth motion against a nipple helps to express milk. Suckling is a pattern that continues until around 6 months of age when a more developed sucking pattern emerges. In the sucking pattern, more structures are active. The mandible moves up and down, and the tongue blade moves down and forward, then up and back to more actively draw milk from a nipple. This movement is closer to the movements that will be required for bolus manipulation and transit as the baby grows and begins to attempt more solid foods. The last skills to develop are chewing patterns, which may not be fully matured until the child reaches 3 to 6 years of age.

So, from approximately school age to old age, the swallow process and mechanism is fairly stable, keeping in mind there is a lot of growth yet to occur. The age-related changes that occur in the elderly have to do with the aging body and the increased likelihood that disease or other neurologic events may be experienced. With aging comes sarcopenia, which is the term for an age-induced loss of muscle mass, which can lead to a decline in muscle strength as well. The elderly person also swallows less frequently, has less sensory awareness of the bolus in the oral cavity, the "trigger" of the swallow is slower to initiate, and the respiratory system declines. All of these factors that affect the anatomy or physiology of the swallowing mechanism contribute to the potential for swallowing impairment to occur in elderly populations (Logemann, 1998).

The incidence of neurologic conditions also increases as we age. The chances for stroke, progressive neurologic diseases, and cancer, all elevate due to advancing age. Of course, there are preventative measures that can be taken, as discussed in Chapter 3, to decrease the risk. Sadly, many do not make lifestyle changes that decrease their risk for these conditions, and just as unfortunately, they may occur in spite of a healthy lifestyle.

Dysphagia

Dysphagia is any disruption in the process of moving food or liquid from the mouth to the stomach. Now that you know more detail about swallowing, let's expand our definition to say that dysphagia occurs when there are impairments in any one or combination of the phases of the swallow. A serious implication of dysphagia is when the bolus is misdirected into the airway. When a bolus enters the larynx, it has started down the wrong path (the term for this is penetration). Typically, we would cough at that point and clear the bolus. If the cough is ineffective or absent, then the bolus may travel further, below the vocal folds and into the trachea (this is considered aspiration). In those cases, it is likely that the bolus will travel all the way down to the lungs where it has the potential to cause an infection (aspiration pneumonia), which in an ill or weakened person may be life threatening.

The presence of dysphagia can result in poor nutritional and hydration status (conditions that can cause general health problems), lead to a reduced capacity to heal from injury or illness, or even pose serious health risk in the case of aspiration pneumonia. Take, for example, an infant who feeds from a bottle or breast. If you have ever been around an infant at feeding time, you know that they can typically "down" a bottle in very little time. The feeding experience is an enjoyable time between infant and feeder as they experience positive social closeness, with eye contact, sometimes some cooing and sound play, and when the baby is finished, they experience a satisfied satiated feeling. On the other hand, a baby who is weak may struggle just to express milk from a nipple. Mom reports that it takes 45 minutes to an hour just to get 4 ounces down. Because the process is hard work for the baby, there is neither time nor inclination to "bond" or engage in social interaction with the feeder; in fact, the whole process is a frustrating experience, one that leaves the baby fatigued and still hungry. The result is an infant who does not want to eat, possibly earning the diagnosis "failure to thrive." Dysphagia in the infant or child typically is related to impairment that is either structural or neurologic from underlying congenital conditions or from accident or disease processes that may occur in childhood (Table 10–1).

On the adult side, the effects of dysphagia can look like the following.

Table 10–1. Common Etiologies That Often Result in Pediatric Dysphagia

Diagnosis	Nature of the Diagnosis
Cerebral palsy	Congenital, neuromuscular
Cleft lip/palate	Congenital, structural
Other craniofacial anomalies/ syndromes	Congenital, structural, neuromuscular
Premature birth (low birth weight)	Congenital, neuromuscular
Developmental delays	Congenital, neuromuscular
Exposure to toxic substances (drugs, alcohol)	Congenital, neuromuscular
Traumatic brain injury	Acquired, neuromuscular
Traumatic injury	Acquired, structural
Brain tumor (neoplasm)	Acquired, neuromuscular

A 66-year-old woman with Parkinson disease visits your clinic with a recent history of a 30 lb weight loss. When asked about the weight loss, she reported that she just didn't understand it, she felt like she was ". . . eating all the time, but that she just couldn't seem to get anything down." Upon examination, it was clear why she felt she was eating all the time, with just one bite she struggled just to move it through the oral cavity and then through the pharynx. The muscles of the swallowing mechanism were very weak. Part of the difficulty also came from ineffective tongue movements (festination) that are a symptom of Parkinson disease. This woman was suffering from malnutrition and dehydration from a general lack of food and liquid intake and needed a feeding tube to return to a healthy nutritional status.

These examples illustrate how serious a swallowing impairment can be in children and adults. There is, of course, a range in the severity of dysphagia symptoms (Table 10–2). There are indi-

Table 10–2. Examples of Warning Signs for Dysphagia in Children and Adults

Age	Signs and Symptoms
Infant to School Age	Disinterest in food
	Avoidance posturing (turning head away from food/bottle) during feeding
	Arching the trunk, pushing away from the feeder
	Food aversions (avoidance of certain foods or textures
	Lengthy meal times
	Increased fussiness during feeding
	Lethargy (excessive) during feeding
	Coughing during eating/feeding
	Difficulty coordinating respiration and swallowing
	Delays in development (cognitive and motor)
Older Children and Adults	Unexplained weight loss
	Decreases cognitive status
	Wet/gurgly sounding vocal quality during eating
	Chronic respiratory conditions (i.e., COPD, asthma, bronchitis)
	Polypharmacology (taking multiple medications)
	Lengthy mealtimes
	Presence of neurologic disease/trauma
	Diet modification (avoiding certain foods)
	Food preparation (changing how food is prepared to make it easier to manage)
	Coughing, throat clearing during mealtime
	Respiratory changes while eating

viduals with mild impairment who may just have to avoid certain foods or liquids but are otherwise unaffected by the fact that they have dysphagia. For many of these individuals, dysphagia is a temporary condition, one that will resolve as their illness subsides, or as they grow, or even recover from an event such as a stroke. Some individuals, however, may have medical conditions that result in dysphagia that will remain until their death.

Neurologic Bases of Swallowing

The act of swallowing is a vital function for day-to-day life. Therefore, the underlying neurologic basis of swallowing is distributed and encompasses aspects from both the CNS and the PNS. Many of the CNS components were introduced in Chapter 1 of this text. Clearly, based on the description of the normal swallowing process, both motor and sensory aspects are integral to successful completion of eating. Therefore, cortical and subcortical structures that function to initiate, regulate, and refine motor signals to the head and neck regions, as well as to the digestive tract are important. Sensory signals also are important; they are responsible for awareness of the bolus in the oral cavity, the pharynx, and if it intrudes into the larynx. The sensory system also initiates or "triggers" the swallow. Therefore, the sensory pathways through the CNS contribute to successful eating. In addition to the higher cortical and subcortical pathways, the brainstem portion of the CNS regulates many of our body's vital functions, including such activities as, respiration, cardiac output,

and swallowing. The swallowing center of the brainstem is located in the medulla (right above the spinal cord). The brainstem control of swallowing is primarily involved in the swallow initiation (trigger), and the careful balance of timing and coordination of the structures for protecting the airway.

Contributions of the PNS are included as well in the swallowing process. Because the structures involved are utilized in both speech and swallowing functions, you might notice a good deal of overlap in the cranial nerves that contribute to successful eating. Although it is important to see and smell food (CN I, II, III, IV, VI) as a part of the eating process, the cranial nerves that actually contribute to the swallowing *process* include cranial nerves V-trigeminal, VII-facial, IX-glossopharyngeal, X-vagus, XI-spinal accessory, and XII-hypoglossal. See Table 10–3 to review these nerves and their contributions to swallowing.

Assessment

A number of assessment techniques can be used to evaluate swallowing across the age span. These techniques include observation during systematic administration of a variety of foods and liquid. The observations may take place in any environment, at the bedside, in a hospital setting, a radiology suite, in the person's home, or even in your clinic. The assessment techniques include those that require only your keen observation skills coupled with your knowledge of the swallowing process (clinical swallowing examination), or those that incorporate instrumentation that allows you to visualize swallowing events (videofluoroscopy or other imaging techniques).

Table 10–3. Cranial Nerves That Contribute to Swallowing Function

Cranial Nerve	Name	Motor/ Sensory Mixed	Primary Function for Swallowing
5	Trigeminal	Mixed	(S) Facial sensation, sensation of a bolus on the anterior 2/3 of the tongue (M) Jaw movement, chewing or mastication
7	Facial	Mixed	(S) Oral cavity sensation, taste function on the anterior 2/3 of the tongue (M) Facial expression, lip seal and containment
9	Glossopharyngeal	Mixed	(S) Pharyngeal sensation (M) Pharyngeal movement
10	Vagus	Mixed	(S) Laryngeal sensation, sensation of penetration, aspiration (M) Phonation, cough, velar elevation
11	Spinal-Accessory	Motor	Head and shoulder movement, assists with pharyngeal function of CN IX, and X
12	Hypoglossal	Motor	Tongue movement, bolus manipulation, formation, and transit

Clinical Swallowing Examination

The clinical swallowing examination (CSE) is the only assessment technique available to all SLPs because it doesn't require additional instrumentation. In a CSE, the SLP with training in the process of swallowing observes an individual while he or she takes in and swallows a variety of consistencies of food and liquid. Although this technique may seem limited (after all, everything is going on inside the body!), a number of observations and measurements take place that might indicate problems (see Table 10–4 for specific examples). The purposes of the CSE include the following:

1. to rule out those who are not good candidates, even for further evaluation,
2. to recommend a more comprehensive instrumental evaluation,
3. to determine appropriate recommendations regarding the consistency of food/liquid that is safe for consumption,
4. to determine treatment directions.

Benefits of the CSE, are that it can take place anywhere and does not require anything other than the individual being assessed and the SLP. In addition, there is no exposure to x-ray and no invasive procedures that are difficult to tolerate.

Table 10–4. Clinical Observations That Indicate Dysphagia During a CSE

Swallowing Phase	Structures Involved	Functional Impairments
Oral Preparatory Phase	Lips	Lack of lip seal around utensils/cups/glasses
	Teeth	
	Hard palate	Food/liquid leaking from the lips during bolus manipulation
	Soft palate	Increased time to prepare a bolus
	Tongue	Coughing during bolus manipulation
	Jaw/Mandible	Disorganized chewing
	Cheeks	Lengthy chewing time
		Food in the cheek after the swallow
		Multiple swallows (more than two) for each bite
Oral Transit Phase	Lips	Leakage of food liquid during transit
	Hard palate	Food remaining on the hard palate after the swallow
	Tongue	
	Cheeks	Food in the cheek after the swallow
		Multiple swallows (more than two) for each bite
		Coughing during bolus manipulation
Pharyngeal Phase	Velum	Nasal regurgitation (food or liquid coming from the nose)
	Tongue	
	Pharyngeal muscles	Effortful swallow
	Laryngeal framework	Coughing during the swallow
	Epiglottis	Wet/gurgly voice quality
	True vocal folds	Extended breath hold during the swallow
	False vocal folds	
	Cricopharyngeus muscle (UES)	Multiple swallows for every bite
		Changes in respiration
Esophagus	Esophagus	Feeling that food is "stuck in the chest"
	Lower esophageal sphincter (LES)	

The primary drawback to the CSE is that you must rely on your clinical knowledge, intuition, and observation skills without the benefit of the additional information that instrumental procedures might provide.

Videofluoroscopic Examination of the Swallow

An instrumental technique to assess swallowing function that is considered the "gold standard" is videofluoroscopy, also known as a modified barium swallow (MBS) evaluation. Fluoroscopy is a dynamic x-ray, so internal structures can be viewed in action. This technique is utilized for many applications in medicine (joint movements, lower digestive function). The addition of "video" to the term reveals that the assessment procedure has been captured, either on videotape, or more recently, as digital media, which usually means you can view it immediately following the procedure and as many times as is desirable. To apply this instrumental technique in swallowing function, we utilize the videofluoroscopy equipment in a radiology suite of a hospital or clinic to view an individual while he or she is swallowing a variety of consistencies of barium (a substance that is easily seen on x-ray). If you view an individual in the lateral plane (from the side), you can view the manipulation of barium in the oral cavity and the pharynx, and it can even be followed to the stomach (Figure 10–6). Therefore, you can view all the internal aspects of the swallow that are not visible in a CSE. The individual also can be viewed in the anteroposterior view (facing the camera). This view offers information regarding symmetry of bolus travel through the pharynx. If there is a unilateral (one-sided) weakness, the bolus will travel on that side (because the strong side will contract and push the bolus over to the weak side). Figures 10–7A through 10–7F illustrate a unilateral weakness and, thus, asymmetrical travel of a bolus through the pharynx during the swallow.

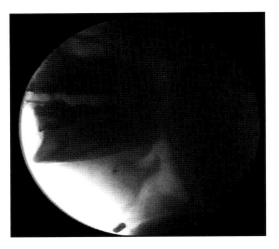

FIGURE 10–6. The lateral image which is typically viewed during a videofluoroscopic evaluation of the swallow.

Benefits of the videofluoroscopy are that each of the phases of the swallow can be viewed, penetration and aspiration can be clearly identified if they occur, and other swallowing impairments that might add to the risk of aspiration (pooling of material in the pharynx, delayed trigger of the swallow) can be determined. The drawbacks include the exposure to radiation, the taste of barium is not altogether pleasant so it may not provide a realistic sample of swallowing, and that it provides only brief sample of behavior with just a few bites of each consistency.

Other Instrumental Techniques

There are a number of additional instrumental techniques that offer imaging capabilities so that one or more swallowing structures can be viewed. Although it is not utilized nearly as frequently as videofluoroscopy, another technique that is growing in popularity is the fiberoptic endoscopic evaluation of the swallow

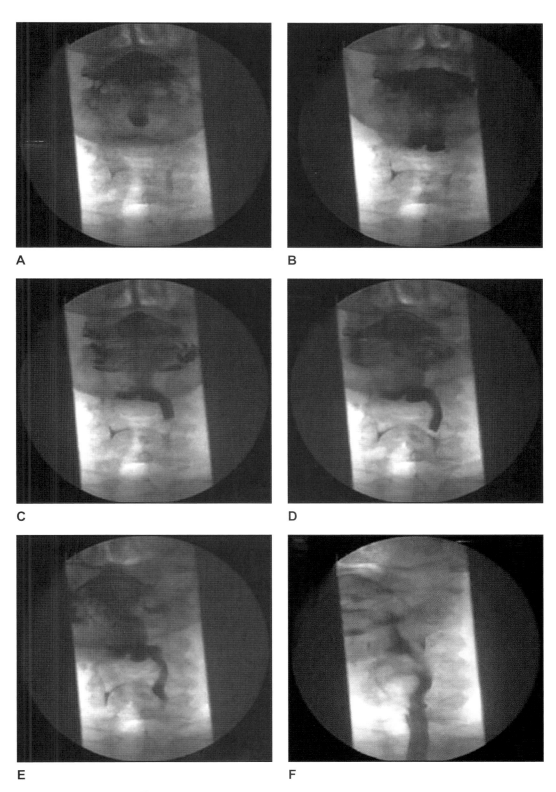

FIGURE 10–7. A–F. Anteroposterior (AP) view during a videofluoroscopic evaluation illustrating unilateral weakness of the pharynx.

(FEES). For this technique a flexible fiber-scope (a tube containing a light source and camera) is passed through the nasal passages, over the velum, and down to the pharynx. With the camera, the structures in the pharynx and the larynx can be clearly viewed before and after the swallow. During the swallow, because of the degree of muscle contraction, the camera view is obscured. This visualization technique offers a good deal of information about penetration, aspiration and overall function in the pharynx. However, the oral cavity cannot be viewed, and tolerance for placement of the scope through the nose and into the pharynx can be problematic.

Another imaging technique that may be utilized is ultrasound. You may have seen the application of ultrasound in viewing an embryo or fetus. The same technique can be used to examine swallowing. However, because this technique uses sound waves, it can be used only over soft tissue (sound waves will not travel well through cartilage or bone). The only view of swallowing that is possible with ultrasound, then, is what can be obtained from the soft tissue under the tongue (because of the teeth and mandible). The pharyngeal phase is not well viewed because of the cartilages of the larynx and the cervical spine. Thus, the information obtained through ultrasound is limited to tongue function. The limited application of this technique has led to application primarily in the research laboratory.

Treatment

Treatment of dysphagia involves a wide range of activities that vary according to the age of the individual with swallow-ing impairment. In the infant or very young child, the primary focus of treatment is on managing the environment to make the eating experience as successful as possible. With the older person, environmental factors also may need to be addressed, but you can focus more directly on specific impairments with an individual who can understand the issues and follow therapeutic instructions. Regardless of the person's age, treatment of swallowing impairment typically involves direct treatment, indirect treatment, or perhaps a combination of the two. A thorough discussion of these techniques is beyond the introductory scope of this chapter. However, a definition with examples should provide a good overview.

Direct Treatment

Direct treatment includes techniques that are incorporated during the act of swallowing that will make the process safer. For example, we discussed earlier in this chapter the fluid, fast moving nature of liquids. Because they are so difficult to control and they move so fast, liquids in their natural state can be difficult to manage, and are thus, easily aspirated (*especially* for the person who has neurologic impairment). A direct treatment application for this problem is to thicken the liquids so they are easier to manage. Using manufactured products designed specifically for this purpose, a thin liquidlike water or juice can be thickened to syrup or a honey consistency, which makes it much easier to control. Another example of a direct treatment technique is the effortful swallow. For the individual who has had damage to the nervous system, muscle weakness often is an issue, making bolus transit through the oral cavity and pharynx problematic. When a person is directed to consciously focus on the swallow and "swallow hard, with effort," the muscles will work harder and transit will be more effective. This technique has to be selected carefully, however, because it would not be a useful technique for individuals who fatigue easily. The purpose of direct treatment is to carefully examine the impairments that are demonstrated by each individual and apply strategies for improving those problems while eating or drinking.

Indirect Treatment

Not every individual with dysphagia is a candidate for direct treatment techniques. For example, there are some patients who are not eating or drinking by mouth, either due to aspiration or the high risk of aspiration. For these individuals, there are indirect treatment techniques. Indirect techniques address underlying problems that result in swallowing impairment, for example, weakness (Clark, 2003). To remediate weakness, exercise is often used (the reader is referred back to the general discussion of sound exercise principles reviewed in Chapter 8). In the case of swallowing, the exercise often is isometric in nature (pushing against a stationary object). Let's take, for example, an individual with tongue weakness. Tongue weakness will result in problems in the oral phases as well as the pharyngeal phase of swallowing. Utilizing exercise to strengthening the tongue, then, would offer a good deal of benefit. Exercises might include pushing the tongue against the roof of the mouth, against a tongue blade, or against a device that could offer feedback (i.e., Iowa Oral Performance Instrument

[IOPI]). If the optimal principles of exercises are incorporated, benefits should be demonstrated quickly (in a matter of days/weeks). As with application of direct treatments, the adoption of indirect treatment strategies should be selected carefully to fit the needs of the person with dysphagia. In some cases, a combination of the two approaches works well in addressing the individual needs of swallowing impairment.

References

Arvedson, J., & Brodsky, L. (2002). *Pediatric swallowing and feeding: Assessment and management* (2nd ed.). Clifton Park, NY: Thompson Learning

Clark, H. M. (2003). Neuromuscular treatments for speech and swallowing: A tutorial. *American Journal of Speech Language Pathology, 12,* 400–415.

Daniels, S. K., & Huckabee, M. (2008). *Dysphagia following stroke.* San Diego, CA: Plural Publishing.

Groher, M. E. (1997). *Dysphagia: Diagnosis and management* (3rd ed.). Boston, MA: Butterworth-Heinemann.

Hixon, T. J., Weismer, G., & Hoit, J. D. (2008). *Preclinical speech science: Anatomy, physiology, acoustics, perception.* San Diego, CA: Plural Publishing.

Kahrilas, P., & Logemann, J. (1993). Volume accommodation during swallowing. *Dysphagia, 8,* 259–265.

Logemann, J. (1998). *Evaluation and treatment of swallowing disorders.* San Diego, CA, College-Hill Press.

Stierwalt, J. A. G., & Youmans, S. R. (2007). Tongue measures in individuals with normal and impaired swallowing. *American Journal of Speech Language Pathology, 16*(2), 148–156.

Youmans, S. R., & Stierwalt, J. A. G. (2006). Measures of tongue function related to normal swallowing. *Dysphagia, 21,* 102–111.

Youmans, S. R., Youmans, G. L., & Stierwalt, J. A. G. (2009). Differences in tongue strength across age and gender: Is there a diminished strength reserve? *Dysphagia, 24,* 57–65.

Suggested Readings

Bosma, J. (1986). Development of feeding. *Clinical Nutrition, 5,* 210–218.

Corbin-Lewis, K., Liss, J., & Sciortino, K. (2005). *Clinical anatomy and physiology of the swallow mechanism.* Clifton Park, NY: Thomson Delmar Learning

Crary, M. A. (1995). A direct intervention program for chronic neurogenic dysphagia secondary to brainstem stroke. *Dysphagia, 10,* 6–18.

Daggett, A., Logemann, J., Drademaker, A., & Pauloski, B. (2006). Laryngeal penetration during deglutition in normal subjects of various ages. *Dysphagia, 21,* 270–274.

Ding, R., Logemann, J., Larson, E., & Redemaker, A. (2003). The effects of taste and consistency on swallow physiology in younger and older healthy individuals: A surface electromyographic study. *Journal of Speech, Language and Hearing Research, 46,* 977–989.

Hirst, L., Ford, G., Gibson, G., & Wilson, J. (2002). Swallow-induced alterations in breathing in normal older people. *Dysphagia, 17,* 152–161.

Horner, J., & Massey, E. (1988). Silent aspiration following stroke. *Neurology, 38,* 317–319.

Johnson, A., & Jacobson, B. (1998). *Medical speech-language pathology: A practitioner's guide.* New York, NY: Thieme Medical Publishers.

Justice, L. M. (2010). *Communication sciences and disorders: A contemporary perspective* (2nd ed.). Boston, CA: Allyn & Bacon

Koenig, J., Davies, A., & Thach, B. (1990). Coordination of breathing, sucking, and swallowing during bottle feedings in human infants. *Journal of Applied Physiology, 69,* 1623–1629.

Langmore, S., Schatz, K., & Olson, N. (1988). Fiberoptic endoscopic evaluation of swallowing safety: A new procedure. *Dysphagia, 2,* 216–219.

Langmore, S., Schatz, K., & Olson, N. (1991). Endoscopic and videofluoroscopic evaluations of swallowing and aspiration. *Annals of Otology, Rhinology and Laryngology, 100,* 678–681.

Langmore, S. E. (1991). Managing the complications of aspiration in dysphagic adults. In *Seminars in Speech and Language.* New York, NY: Thieme Medical Publishers.

Linden, P., & Siebens, A. (1983). Dysphagia: Predicting laryngeal penetration. *Archives of Physical Medicine and Rehabilitation, 64,* 281–284.

Logemann, J. (1986). *Manual for the videofluorographic study of swallowing.* Waltham, MA: College-Hill Press, Little Brown.

Ludlow, C. L., Hoit, J., Kent, R., Ramig, L. O., Shrivastav, R., Strand, E., et al. (2008). Translating principles of neural plasticity into research on speech motor control recovery and rehabilitation. *Journal of Speech, Language, and Hearing Research, 51,* S240–S258.

McConnel, F. (1986). Analysis of pressure generation and bolus transit during pharyngeal swallowing. *Laryngoscope, 98,* 71–78.

McConnel, F., & Cerenko, D. (1988). Timing of major events of pharyngeal swallowing. *Archives of Otolaryngology, Head and Neck Surgery, 114,* 1413–1418.

Miller, A. (1986). Neurophysiological basis of swallowing. *Dysphagia, 1,* 91–100.

Murry, T., & Carrau, R. L. (2006). *Clinical management of swallowing disorders* (2nd ed.). San Diego, CA: Plural Publishing.

Perlman, A., & Schulze-Delrieu, K. (1997). *Deglutition and its disorders.* San Diego, CA: Singular Publishing Group.

Sonies, B. C., & Baum, B. J. (1988). Evaluation of swallowing pathophysiology. *Otolaryngology Clinics of North America, 21,* 4.

Sonies, B. C., Parent, L. J., Morrish, K., & Baum, B. J. (1988). Durational aspects of the oral-pharyngeal phase of swallowing in normal adults. *Dysphagia, 3,* 1.

Splaingard, M. L., Hutchins, B. & Sulton, L. D. (1988). Aspiration in rehabilitation patients: Videofluoroscopy vs. bedside clinical assessment. *Archives of Physical Medicine and Rehabilitation*, *69*, 637–640.

Stierwalt, J. A. G. (2009). Dysphagia in the tracheostomized, ventilator dependent. In H. N. Jones & J. C. Rosenbek (Eds.), *Dysphagia in rare conditions*. San Diego, CA: Plural Publishing.

11

Principles of Assessment of Child and Adult Neurologic Speech-Language Disorders

Careful and detailed assessment of acquired neurologic speech disorders is essential to aid clinicians in their formulation of a diagnosis and for determination of specific treatment priorities. A range of assessment techniques are available to the clinician to assist in these processes. A comprehensive assessment of persons affected by neurologic speech impairments usually includes the following components: a detailed case history, an oromotor examination, determination of the key features of the speech disorder, and identification of their neurologic substrates.

Case History

Prior to undertaking any formal tests it is informative and necessary for the clinician to first collect a case history from the client. A detailed case history can inform the clinician of the salient features of the disorder from the perspective of the client. It is not unusual that a skilled clinician can arrive at a tentative diagnosis based on information gained from the case history alone. Essential background information to be collected as part of the case history should include the following client details: age, education level, occupation; marital and family status; prior history of speech-language impairments (including developmental conditions experienced in childhood); onset and course of the disorder (how long has the client had the condition? Is it progressive or stable? etc.); associated deficits (e.g., drooling, swallowing impairments, hemiplegia, etc.); emotional disturbances; prior treatment and management regimens; client's awareness and understanding of the disorder; consequences of the disorder for the client (e.g., disruption to work, school, or social activities, etc.).

Oromotor Examination

An oromotor examination primarily involves visual and tactual observation of the speech production mechanism during performance of a range of non-speech activities and provides important information about the size, strength, symmetry, range, tone, steadiness, speech, and accuracy of movements of the face, jaw, tongue, and velum (soft palate). Each of these four components of the speech production system is observed in the following conditions: at rest; during sustained postures (e.g., retraction of the lips, protrusion of the tongue, etc.); and during movement (e.g., alternate pursing and retraction of the lips). While each structure is at rest the clinician should observe whether or not the structure is symmetrical or deviated to one side (e.g., at rest does the face, tongue, jaw, and velum appear symmetric). Furthermore, while at rest the presence of any involuntary movements (e.g., twitching of the tongue muscle) and muscle wastage (atrophy) need to be noted as both of these features may be indicative of the presence of a neurologic impairment such as a lower motor neuron lesion. The strength of the tongue and jaw can be tested by having the client move these structures against a force applied by the clinician (e.g., the client can be asked to press his or her tongue against the cheek to oppose a force imposed externally on the cheek by the hand of the clinician). The presence and absence of both normal and pathologic reflexes also can be good indicators of the presence of disease in either the peripheral or central nervous systems. For example, the absence of a normal reflex such as the gag reflex or jaw jerk can indicate the presence of pathology. Likewise, the presence of primitive or pathologic reflexes (i.e., reflexes absent in non-neurologically-impaired individuals) such as the sucking reflex also is indicative of neurologic impairment.

Determination of the Principal Features of the Speech Disorder

Techniques available for determining the principal features of the neurologic speech disorder exhibited by a client and their neuropathologic substrates can be broadly divided into three major categories: perceptual techniques (these assessments are based on the clinicians impression of the auditory-perceptual attributes of the client's speech); acoustic techniques (assessments in this category are based on the study of the generation, transmission, and modification of sound waves emitted from the vocal tract); and physiologic techniques (these methods are based on instrumental assessment of the functioning of the various subsystems of the speech production mechanism in terms of their movements, muscular contractions, and so forth).

Perceptual Assessment

Perceptual analysis of neurologic speech disorders has been the "gold standard" and preferred method by which clinicians have made differential diagnoses and defined treatment programs for their clients for many years. In fact, many clinicians still rely almost exclusively on auditory-perceptual judgments of speech intelligibility, articulatory accuracy, or subjective ratings of various speech dimensions on which to base their diagnosis of dysarthria and apraxia of speech and plan their intervention. The use of auditory perceptual assessments to characterize the different types of dysarthria and to identify the spectrum of deviant speech characteristics associated with each was pioneered by Darley, Aronson, and Brown (1969a, 1969b; 1975). It was from the findings of their auditory-perceptual studies of dysarthria that the system of classification of dysarthria most frequently used in clinical settings was developed. Darley et al. (1969a, 1969b) assessed speech samples taken from 212 dysarthric speakers with a variety of neurologic conditions on 38 speech dimensions that fell into 7 categories: pitch, loudness, voice quality (including both laryngeal and resonatory dysfunction), respiration, prosody, articulation, and two summary dimensions relating to intelligibility and bizarreness. A key component of their research was the application of the "equal-appearing intervals scale of severity," which utilized a seven-part scale of severity.

Rating scales also have been used by a number of other researchers to determine the deviant speech characteristics of various neurologic speech disorders. For example, a modification of Darley's original seven-point rating scale developed by FitzGerald, Murdoch, and Chenery (1987) has been used to investigate speech disorders in patients with multiple sclerosis, Parkinson disease, pseudobulbar palsy, stroke, and ataxic dysarthria, among others. Another example of how symptoms of dysarthria are assessed and measured on a rating scale is the Frenchay Dysarthria Assessment (FDA) (Enderby, 1983). The FDA is the only published diagnostic test of dysarthria and utilizes a nine-point rating scale presented vertically as a bar graph (Figure 11–1). As in the Darley et al. (1975) seven-point rating scale, a rating of 1 corresponds to more severe disruption with 9 representing normal function.

The 28 dimensions rated in the FDA are grouped under the headings of reflex, respiration, lips, jaw, palate, laryngeal, tongue, and intelligibility.

In addition to rating scales, other perceptual assessments used to investigate neurologic speech disorders include the application of intelligibility measures, phonetic transcription studies, and articulation inventories. According to Duffy (2005), "intelligibility is the degree to which a listener understands the acoustic signal produced by a speaker," (p. 96). Quantifiable intelligibility measures are clinically important because they can monitor change during treatment and document functional level or adequacy of communication. Although most comprehensive perceptual assessments, such as those developed by Darley et al. (1975) and FitzGerald et al. (1987) mentioned above, provide a single measure of overall intelligibility, this measure represents a global rating of the overall impact of the speech on the listener and considers how much effort is involved by the listener in understanding the speech sample. Thus, these global measures are based on the entire sample of speech, usually a spoken paragraph such as the "Grandfather Passage" (Darley et al., 1975). A more valid method of estimating dysarthric speech intelligibility is to obtain a number of more detailed and comprehensive measures of intelligibility. The Assessment of Intelligibility of Dysarthric Speech (ASSIDS) (Yorkston & Beukelman, 1981) provides an index of severity of dysarthric speech by quantifying both single-word and sentence intelligibility as well as the speaking rate of individuals. It requires the client to read or imitate 50 randomly selected words and 22 randomly selected sentences that range in length from 5 to 15 words.

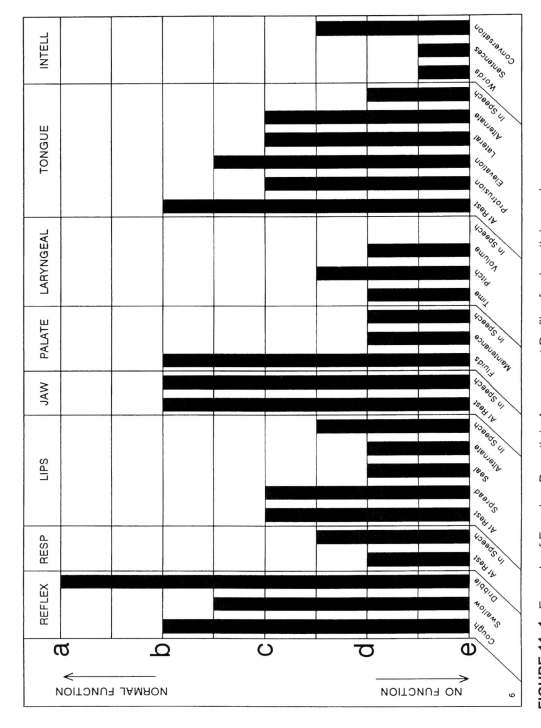

FIGURE 11–1. Example of Frenchay Dysarthria Assessment Profile of a dysarthric speaker.

228

A number of dimensions are calculated in the ASSIDS, including: a percentage intelligibility for single words, a percentage intelligibility for sentences, a total speaking rate, a rate of intelligible speech expressed as intelligible words per minute, and a communication efficiency ratio.

Where necessary, such as for research purposes, more detailed perceptual analyses of neurologic speech disorders can involve the use of phonetic transcription of selected speech stimuli (e.g., production of a series of single-syllable real and nonsense words) to provide detailed information about the pattern of articulatory deficits. In addition, articulatory inventories can be used to characterize the articulation abilities of individuals with dysarthria and apraxia of speech. For example, an articulation test such as the Fisher-Logemann Test of Articulation Competence (Fisher & Logemann, 1971) can be used to provide an articulation profile and may be analyzed further to establish the presence of developmental features such as phonological processes.

The major advantages of perceptual assessment are those that have led to its preferred use as the tool for characterizing and diagnosing dysarthric speech. Perceptual assessments are readily available and require only limited financial outlay. In addition, all students of speech-language pathology are taught how to test for and identify perceptual symptoms. Finally, perceptual assessments are useful for monitoring the effects of treatment on speech intelligibility and the adequacy of communication.

Clinicians need to be aware, however, that a number of inherent inadequacies in perceptual assessment may limit its use in determining treatment priorities. First, accurate, reliable perceptual judgments often are difficult to achieve as they can be influenced by a number of factors including the skill and experience of the clinician and the sensitivity of the assessment. In particular, raters must have extensive structured experience in listening prior to performing perceptual ratings.

Second, perceptual assessments are difficult to standardize both in relation to the patient being rated and the environment in which the speech samples are recorded. Patient variability over time and across different settings prevents maintenance of adequate intra- and interrater reliability. Furthermore, the symptoms may be present in certain conditions and not others. This variability is also found in the patients themselves such that characteristics of the person being rated (e.g., their age, premorbid medical history, and social history) may influence speech as well as the neurologic problem itself.

A third factor that limits reliance on perceptual assessments is that certain speech symptoms may influence the perception of others. This confound has been well reported in relation to the perception of resonatory disorders, articulatory deficits, and prosodic disturbances.

Probably the major concern of perceptual assessments, particularly as they relate to treatment planning, is that they have restricted power for determining which subsystems of the speech motor system are affected. In other words, perceptual assessments are unable to accurately identify the pathophysiologic basis of the speech disorder manifest in various types of dysarthria. It is possible that a number of different physiologic deficits can form the basis of perceptually identified features, and that different patterns of interaction within a patient's overall symptom complex can result in a similar perceptual deviation (e.g., distorted consonants can result from reduced respiratory support for speech, from inadequate velopharyngeal functioning or from weak tongue musculature). When crucial decisions are required in relation to optimum therapeutic planning, an overreliance on only perceptual assessment may lead to a number of questionable therapy directions.

Acoustic Assessment

Acoustic analyses can be used in conjunction with perceptual assessments to provide a more complete understanding of the nature of the disturbance in dysarthric speech. In particular, acoustic assessment can highlight aspects of the speech signal that may be contributing to the perception of deviant speech production and can provide confirmatory support for perceptual judgments. For example, they may confirm the perception that speech is slow and demonstrate that the reduced rate of speech may be the result of increased interword durations and prolonged vowel and consonant production. As a further example, an acoustic analysis might be used to confirm the perception of imprecise consonant production and to show that such imprecision is the result of spirantization of consonants and reduction of consonant clusters. In addition to altered speech rate and consonant imprecision, other perceived deviant speech dimensions that can be confirmed by way of acoustic analysis include, among others, breathy voice, voice tremor, and reduced variability of pitch and loudness. Acoustic analysis also is useful for providing objective documentation of the effects of treatment and disease progression on speech production.

Acoustic measurements can be taken primarily from two different types of acoustic displays: oscillographic displays and spectrographic displays. An oscillographic display is a two-dimensional waveform display of amplitude (on the y-axis) as a function of time (x-axis). Oscillographic displays are easy to generate and can provide information on a variety of acoustic parameters such as segment duration (e.g., vowel duration, word duration, etc.), amplitude, fundamental frequency, and the presence of some acoustic cues of articulatory adequacy such as voice onset time, spirantization, and voiced-voiceless distinctions. Measurements from oscillographic displays can be made either manually or alternatively, by using computer-controlled acoustic analysis software. Some of the commonly used computerized systems and dedicated devices for acoustic speech analysis include: C Speech, CSL (Computerized Speech Lab), CSRE (Canadian Speech Research Environment); ILS-PC (Interactive Laboratory System), and MSL (Micro Speech Lab).

In contrast to the two-dimensional oscillographic display, a spectrographic display is actually a three-dimensional display of both frequency and amplitude as a function of time, where time is on the x-axis and frequency is displayed on the y-axis. There are two different types of spectrographic displays: wideband displays (also called broadband displays) and narrowband displays. Wideband spectrographic displays are used to determine accurate temporal measurements whereas narrowband spectrograms are useful for making measurements of fundamental frequency and the prosodic aspects of speech.

Although there is no "standard" set of parameters included in all acoustic analyses, there are a number of different acoustic measures that can provide important information about the acoustic features of dysarthric speech. These parameters can be loosely arranged into groups of measures including: fundamental frequency measures, amplitude measures, perturbation measures, noise related measures, formant measures, temporal measures, measures of articulatory capability, and evaluations of manner of voicing.

Physiologic Assessment

Although perceptual evaluations contribute valuable information to the process of diagnosing and interpreting neurologic speech disorders, instrumental observation and measurement of speech and its physiological correlates offers significant advantages over unaided perceptual judgments. By including the use of instrumental procedures in the process of diagnosing speech disorders, clinicians are able to extend their senses and objectify their perceptual observations. In particular, instrumentation has given the clinician the ability to determine the contributions of malfunctions in the various components of the speech production mechanism to the production of disordered speech. Indeed, modern instrumentation enables the clinician to assess and obtain information about the integrity and functional status of the muscle groups at each stage of the speech production process from respiration through to articulation. It is not surprising, therefore, that clinicians are beginning to appreciate the considerable advantages of instrumental analysis which provides quantitative, objective data on a wide range of different speech parameters far beyond the scope of an auditory-based impressionistic judgment. Instrumental assessment can enhance the abilities of the clinician in all stages of clinical management, including:

- increasing the precision of diagnosis through more valid specification of abnormal functions that require modification
- providing positive identification and documentation of therapeutic efficacy
- expanding options of therapy modalities, including the use of instrumentation in a biofeedback modality.

To be of value in determining treatment priorities, instrumental assessment should be comprehensive, covering as many components of the speech production mechanism as possible. A wide variety of different types of physiologic instrumentation has been described in the literature for use in the assessment of the functioning of the various components of the speech production apparatus. Each of these instruments has been designed to provide information on a specific aspect of speech production including muscular activity, structural movements, airflows, and air pressures generated in various parts of the speech mechanism. The features of the most commonly used physiological instruments used to assess the functioning of the respiratory system, larynx, velopharynx (soft palate), and articulators (e.g., lips, tongue, etc.) are briefly outlined below.

Instrumental Assessment of Speech Breathing. The respiratory system provides the basic energy source for all speech and voice production, regulating such important parameters as speech and voice intensity (loudness), pitch, linguistic stress, and the division of speech into units (e.g., phrases). Physiologic instruments used in the assessment of speech breathing can be divided into two major types: those that directly measure various lung volumes, capacities, and airflows (e.g., spirometers) and those that indirectly measure respiratory function by monitoring movements of the chest wall, the so-called kinematic assessments (e.g., mercury strain gauges, magnetometers, respiratory inductance plethysmographs, strain-gauge belt pneumographs).

Spirometers are specifically designed for the evaluation of respiratory volumes. The basic principle of a spirometer is to measure and record the volumes of air blown into either a tube or a fitted face mask, which is attached to the machine (Figure 11–2). By using this type of assessment, the investigator can obtain a number of valuable respiratory/airflow measures, including vital capacity, forced expiratory volume, functional residual capacity, inspiratory capacity, expiratory and inspiratory reserve volumes, as well as volume/flow relationships and tidal volume and respiration rate.

Kinematic devices allow the clinician to infer the airflow volume changes during respiration from rib cage and abdominal displacements. In that they do not require the need for restrictive mouth pieces and nose clips that can interrupt natural speech production and respiratory patterns, the kinematic method allows for more accurate measurements of the breath support during speech production. The rib cage and diaphragm-abdomen displace volume as they move and, as a result, their combined volume displacements equal that of the lungs. In essence, therefore, the kinematic analysis involves the simultaneous but independent recording of changes in the circumference of the rib cage and abdomen.

Investigations of speech breathing using kinematic assessments have predominantly used four main types of kinematic instrumentation. These include magnetometers (e.g., Solomon & Hixon, 1993), strain-gauge belt pneumograph systems (e.g., Manifold & Murdoch, 1993), mercury strain gauges (e.g., Cavallo & Baken, 1985), and respiratory inductance plethysmography (available commercially as the "Respitrace" system) (e.g., Sperry & Klich, 1992). Of these techniques, the Respitrace system is most commonly available in clinical settings. This system senses movements of the chest wall via the changes in electrical inductance of a zigzag of wire attached to elastic bands positioned around the rib cage and abdominal regions (Figure 11–3). Oscillators positioned in the center of the chest wall anteriorly

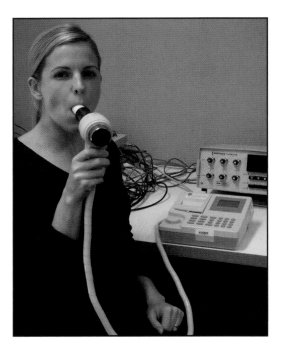

FIGURE 11–2. Respiratory spirometer.

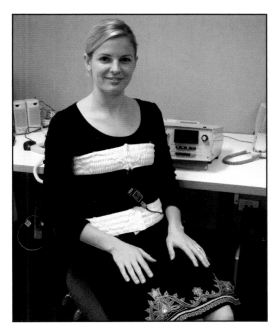

FIGURE 11–3. Respitrace system for kinematic assessment of speech breathing.

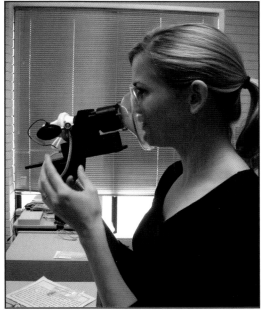

FIGURE 11–4. Aerophone II airflow measurement system.

produce a frequency-modulated signal which passes through the wires of the chest bands, the frequency of which is related to the circumference of the chest wall. Changes in the size of the chest wall circumference alter the shape and, therefore, conductance of the zigzag wires of the straps, and, as a result, change the signal.

One other important indicator of respiratory function for speech production is the ability of the subject to generate subglottal air pressure during speech. Subglottal air pressure is estimated using an Aerophone II (Kay Elemetrics) airflow measurement system (Figure 11–4). The Aerophone II consists of a hand-held transducer module together with a powerful data acquisition and processing software program. The transducer module consists of miniaturized transducers capable of recording airflow, air pressure, and acoustic signals during

speech. A face mask through which a thin flexible tube of silicon rubber is inserted to record intraoral pressure is attached to the hand-held transducer module. To estimate subglottal pressure, the subject is asked to repeat /ipipipi/ into the face mask, with the rubber tube located in the oral cavity, for several seconds. The point of maximum intraoral pressure during the pronunciation of the voiceless stop /p/ is calculated automatically over six repetitions and used as the estimate of subglottal air pressure.

Instrumental Assessment of Laryngeal Function. Physiologic evaluation of laryngeal function is carried out using both direct and indirect techniques. Endoscopy using a rigid endoscope or nasendoscopy using a flexible fiberscope both allow for direct observation of vocal fold movement. Both systems are telescopic-type devices that illuminate the laryngeal area and allow visual inspection of the laryngeal region. The rigid endoscope is inserted through the mouth into the region of the oropharynx, allowing direct observation of the vocal folds during phonation of sustained vowels. In comparison, the flexible fiberscope is inserted through the nasal cavity and then passed down through the pharyngeal area until the tip of the scope is positioned at approximately the level of the epiglottis to allow an unobstructed view of the vocal folds. As the oral cavity is not obstructed using the nasendoscopic technique, visual record of laryngeal function can be obtained during normal speech production. Both the endoscope and nasoendoscope are connected to a video monitoring and recording system, which allows the visual image of the vocal folds to be recorded for later viewing and analysis. Videostroboscopy combines the use of a strobe light source in conjunction with the videoendoscopic procedures outlined above. Using the stroboscopic technique, the movements

of the vocal folds during speech production can be "slowed" or "stopped" through the optical illusion of stroboscopy making identification of vocal fold dysfunction much easier.

The indirect methods of evaluating physiologic functioning of the larynx include electroglottography (electrolaryngography) and aerodynamic examination. Electroglottography is an electrical impedance method of estimating vocal fold contact during phonation that is designed to allow investigation of laryngeal microfunction (cycle-by-cycle periodicity and contact). The electroglottographic assessment is conducted using a Fourcin laryngograph interfaced with a Waveform Display System (Kay Elemetrics Model 6091) (Figure 11–5). The system records the degree of vocal fold contact and the vocal fold vibratory patterns during phonation, these features being displayed in the form of an Lx waveform. The Waveform Display System allows for acquisition and real-time viewing of the Lx waveform on the computer monitor as well as storage and

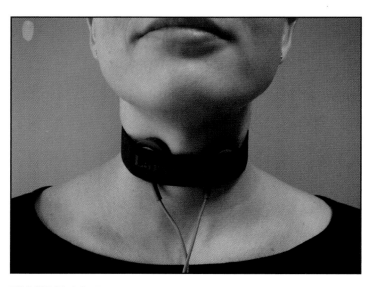

FIGURE 11–5. Client fitted with a Fourcin laryngograph.

analysis of segments of the waveform. Although some caution must be used in interpreting electroglottographic results, a number of authors have acknowledged that this procedure provides a useful estimate of vocal fold contact during the glottal cycle and gives some insight into the regulation, maintenance, and quality of phonation.

Aerodynamic measures allow examination of the macrofunctions of the larynx such as laryngeal airflow, glottal pressures, and glottal resistance. Estimates of these parameters are obtained by way of an Aerophone II Airflow Measurement System (see Instrumental Assessment of Speech Breathing above).

Instrumental Assessment of Velopharyngeal Function (Soft Palate). Two contemporary instruments for assessing velopharyngeal function include an accelerometric procedure and the nasometer. The accelerometric procedure involves the use of two miniature accelerometers to detect nasal and throat vibrations during speech. One miniature accelerometer is attached to the upper side of the nose over the lateral nasal cartilage just in front of the nasal bone, while the other is attached to the side of the neck over the lamina of the thyroid cartilage. The output signals from each accelerometer are amplified by a DC amplifier and the amplified signals are then relayed to a computerized physiologic data acquisition system. The system yields an index of oral/nasal coupling during production of a range of nasal and nonnasal sounds, words, and sentences.

Another instrument available for assessment of nasality is a nasometer (Kay Elemetrics) (Figure 11–6). The nasometer is a computer-assisted instrument that provides a measure of nasality derived from the ratio of acoustic energy output from the nasal and oral cavities during speech. Acoustic energy is detected by

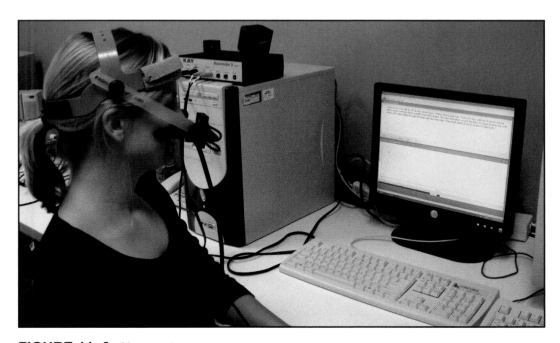

FIGURE 11–6. Nasometer.

two directional microphones (one placed in front of the nares and the other in front of the mouth) separated by a sound separator plate. The instrument yields a "nasalance" score made up of a ratio of nasal to oral plus nasal acoustic energy calculated as a percentage.

Instrumental Assessment of Articulatory Function. The term "articulators" is used to represent collectively the muscle groups of the lips, tongue, and jaw. While these structures are often grouped together due to their common influence over speech production at the articulatory stage, each one functions independently and contributes differently to speech production. Consequently, a variety of instrumental techniques have been developed in order to examine the degree of compression force exerted by each articulator during speech and nonspeech tasks, as well as to investigate force control properties, rate of individual articulatory movements, endurance capabilities of the individual articulators, and the movement patterns during speech production of each separate aspect of the articulatory system

Of the various types of instrumentation used to assess the articulators, strain gauge transducers used to record articulator movement and force generating capacities have been the most frequently used. Because of their high levels of sensitivity, strain gauge transducers are especially suited to detecting the subtle changes in movement that occur in speech production. In addition, they are relatively inexpensive, noninvasive, provide an immediate voltage analogue of movement, and can be adapted to assess lip, tongue, and jaw function during both speech and nonspeech tasks. An example of a strain gauge system for estimating lip strength is shown in Figure 11–7.

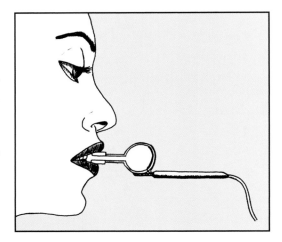

FIGURE 11–7. Example of a strain gauge system for measuring lip strength.

In addition to strain gauge transducers, pressure or force transducers also can provide valuable information regarding the functioning of the articulatory system. For example, a miniaturized pressure transducer frequently is used to assess lip function (Figure 11–8). Because of its small size the transducer can be placed between the lips to generate interlabial pressure measurements during speech production without interfering with normal articulatory movements. The transducer is interfaced with a dedicated software package designed to allow for investigations of combined upper and lower lip pressures, pressure control for maximum and submaximum pressure levels, and endurance and speech pressures during production of bilabial sounds.

An equivalent commercially available instrument for estimating tongue strength and endurance is the Iowa Oral Performance Instrument (IOPI), which consists of an air-filled rubber bulb attached to a pressure transducer (Figure 11–9). For testing, the bulb is placed in the mouth and the subject is instructed

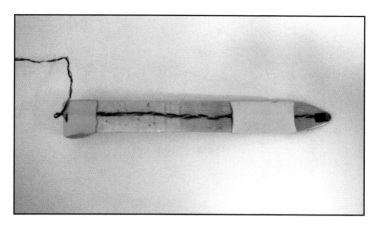

FIGURE 11–8. Miniature pressure transducer for estimating bilabial pressures.

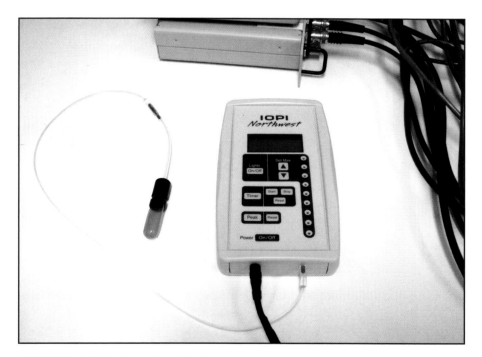

FIGURE 11–9. Iowa Oral Performance Instrument.

to squeeze the bulb against the roof of the mouth with the tongue. When the bulb is squeezed by the tongue, the amount of pressure is displayed on a digital readout.

Electromyography (EMG) is another technique that has commonly been used (primarily by researchers rather than clinicians) to examine articulator function. Using this technique, the momentary changes in electrical activity that occur when a muscle is contracting are recorded by using various types of electrodes (e.g., surface, needle, or hook-wire) placed either overlying (surface electrodes), or within (e.g., hook-wire electrodes and needle electrodes) the muscle. The data obtained from EMG assessment has proven useful for investigating the neurophysiologic bases of various disorders, such as identifying the presence of increased muscle tone (hypertonicity) or abnormal variations in the activation or inhibition of muscle activity. In addition, EMG has been used to record muscle activity simultaneously with the speech movement patterns of the same muscles to examine the motor control of the articulators.

Electropalatography is another technique for examining tongue function, which provides the clinician with information on the location and timing of tongue contacts with the palate during speech. In this technique, the client wears an acrylic palate with an array of contact sensors implanted on the surface (Figures 11–10A and 11–10B). When contact occurs between the tongue and any of the electrodes, a signal is conducted via lead-out wires to an external processing unit, which then displays the patterns of contact on a computer screen (Figure 11–11).

In recent years, the development and introduction of a technique called electromagnetic articulography (EMA) has provided a safe, noninvasive assessment tool with which the dynamic aspects of articulatory dysfunction in various neurologic speech disorders may be investigated. Importantly, the EMA technique does not require the use of ionizing radiation. Rather, the EMA system tracks articulatory movements during speech using weak alternating electromagnetic fields. Transmitter coils, housed in a plastic cube and positioned around the head, generate alternating magnetic fields at different frequencies, which in turn induce alternating signals in small receiver coils temporarily glued to the tongue, upper and lower lip, and jaw (Figure 11–12). The position of the receiver coils in relation to the transmitter coils is sampled over time and plotted on a computer, providing a visual representation of articulator movements in real time. From these data, quantitive kinematic parameters can be derived including the velocity, acceleration, distance, and duration of movements of the lips, tongue, and jaw during speech production. The most recently introduced EMA system, the AG500 is capable of tracking articulatory movements in three dimensions.

Evaluating the movements of the tongue is more difficult than assessing lip or jaw movement primarily because the tongue functions within the confines of the mouth. In addition to the EMA technique described above, imaging techniques such as cineradiography and ultrasound have proved useful for examining the complex patterns of tongue movement during speech. Cineradiography is a high-speed x-ray motion picture technique which records the lateral view of the mouth, nose, and pharynx. Using this technique, it is possible to view the articulatory structures during speech to identify gross deviations of articulatory movement such as reduced mobility of the tongue or soft palate. Unfortunately, due to its reliance on potentially harmful x-rays, cineradiography has fallen out of favor and has little potential for use as a routine clinical tool, especially for child cases. In contrast, ultrasonography involves the transmission of high-frequency sound waves through the body's tissues. Con-

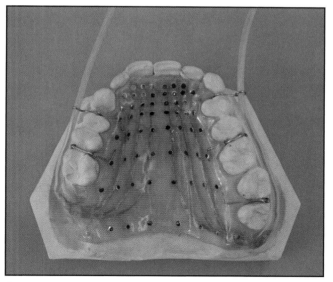

A

FIGURE 11–10. **A.** Acrylic electropalatography palate with embedded touch sensors and **B.** Client fitted with an electropalatography palate.

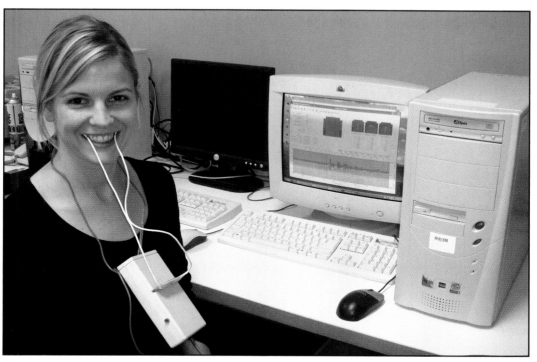

B

sequently, ultrasound is considered harmless and noninvasive, allowing tongue movement to be investigated for longer periods without harm or discomfort to the client. Unlike other imaging techniques, ultrasound reveals not only the

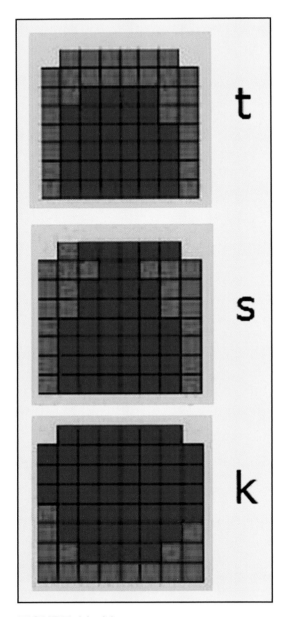

FIGURE 11–11. Electropalatographic contact pattern representing tongue contact with the palate.

surface displacement but also changes in soft tissue organization within the tongue in both the sagittal and coronal planes and can be used to record lingual movements during production of vowels and most consonants.

Limitations with ultrasound include an inability to assess tongue tip movements and to view the movements of other structures (e.g., jaw, lips, etc.) besides the tongue using this technique. In addition, specialist training and some experience in viewing ultrasound scans is required to interpret the information provided by these scans accurately. Furthermore, the need to place the ultrasound source below the lower jaw directly under the floor of the mouth may restrict natural jaw movement during speech. Despite these limitations, however, ultrasound has the potential to be a useful clinical tool for client evaluation.

Summary. In summary, although instrumentation has opened a whole new range of assessment techniques, physiologic data should be integrated with data from other appraisal procedures (i.e., combined information from perceptual, physiologic, and acoustic information) to ensure that an accurate diagnosis is made and that the subsequent remediation techniques are appropriate. In particular, the limitations of each of the instrumental procedures need to be kept in mind when making clinical decisions based on their findings. It also must be remembered that despite the wide variety of objective instrumental measures available for documenting the physiology of speech production, to date, the clinical application of these techniques has been limited. Increasing the use of instrumentation in the clinical setting for the purposes of both assessment and treatment will require the implementation of training programs for the clinicians as well as an increase in clinical research projects designed to

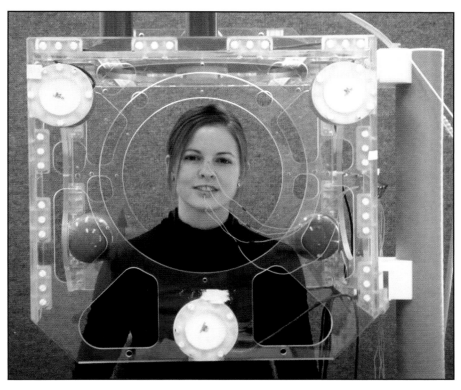

FIGURE 11–12. AG500 electromagnetic articulograph.

demonstrate the clinical utility of instrumental techniques and to validate the role of instrumentation in the management of neurologic speech disorders.

Assessment of Neurologic Language Disorders

As in the case of neurologic speech disorders outlined above, prior to initiation of any treatment for acquired language disorders, the clinician must complete a detailed case history and comprehensive assessment of the communication disorder. In the early stages postonset, a bedside evaluation most often is based largely on observation by the clinician rather than the administration of formal language tests. As part of the bedside assessment the speech-language pathologist should consider factors such as: the patient's ability to comprehend spoken language (e.g., does he or she follow the conversation, can he or she follow one, two, and three-stage commands such as, "point to the floor then to the ceiling"; naming abilities; and the patient's ability to repeat words of increasing complexity and sentences).

Once the client is medically stable, observation can then be supplemented with a range of formal tests. In general, these tests fall into one of two major categories: tests that evaluate basic language skills; and tests of functional and pragmatic language abilities.

Tests of Basic Language Function

These tests identify the presence of language deficits but do not ascertain the impact of these deficits on functional communication abilities. In this way, tests included in this category sample neurologic language disorders such as aphasia at what the World Health Organization (WHO) refers to as the "impairment level." Tests of basic language function can be divided into two groups: tests of general language that assess primary comprehension and production abilities; and high-level language tests that assess more complex language function.

Tests of General Language Abilities

Examples of tests of general language abilities commonly used by speech-language pathologists include: the Neurosensory Center Comprehensive Examination for Aphasia (NCCEA) (Spreen & Benton, 1977), the Boston Naming Test (BNT) (Kaplan, Goodglass, & Weintraub, 1983), the Boston Diagnostic Aphasia Examination (BDAE) (Goodglass, Kaplan, & Barresi, 2001), the Western Aphasia Battery (WAB) (Kertesz, 1982), the Porch Index of Communicative Abilities (PICA) (Porch, 1967), Examining for Aphasia-4 (EFA-4) (LaPointe & Eisenson, 2008), Reading Comprehension for Aphasia (RCBA-2) (LaPointe & Horner, 1988), and the Aphasia Diagnostic Profile (ADP) (Helm-Estabrooks, 1992). The provision of a detailed description of each of these assessments is beyond the scope of the present chapter; however, to demonstrate the range of language tasks covered by this type of assessment, further description of the components of the NCCEA, BNT, EFA-4, and RCBA-2 is provided below.

Neurosensory Center Comprehensive Examination for Aphasia (NCCEA). The NCCEA constitutes a detailed assessment of language functions, incorporating subtests that evaluate primary as well as high-level linguistic abilities. Principally designed for the assessment of aphasic individuals, the NCCEA is comprised of 20 language tasks that specifically evaluate the status of immediate verbal memory, verbal production and fluency, receptive language, reading, writing, and basic articulatory proficiency. Overall, the assessment provides a descriptive versus taxonomic classification of linguistic abilities (Table 11–1 provides description of individual NCCEA subtests).

The Boston Naming Test (BNT). The BNT is a reliable measure of confrontation naming abilities and provides information about the effectiveness of semantic and phonemic cues in facilitating word retrieval. Subjects are instructed to name 60 constituent black and white line drawings of various objects ranging in frequency from *bed* to *abacus* and are permitted up to 20 seconds to respond to each item. A semantic cue is given if the subject provides a response that represents a misinterpretation of the target or a lack of recognition. A phonemic cue is provided subsequent to any failure to respond or incorrect response to a semantic cue, or in the event of recognition of the item but an inability to produce its name.

Examining for Aphasia-4 (EFA-4). Use this test to identify the presence of acquired aphasia, determine the severity of symptoms and their impact on the quality of life, target goals for treatment, and document progress during treatment.

Table 11–1. Description of Individual Neurosensory Center Comprehensive Examination for Aphasia Subtests

1. Visual object naming (VN): requires subjects to verbally label objects presented on a tray.

2. Description of object use (DOU): requires subjects to provide a description of use pertaining to a range of presented objects following the probe, "What do you use this for?"

3. Tactile naming right hand (TNR): a range of objects are individually placed into the subject's right hand under a covering screen, and the subject is instructed to name the objects accordingly.

4. Tactile naming left hand (TNL): as per TNR; however, objects are placed in left hand.

5. Sentence repetition (SR): requires subjects to repeat spoken sentences of increasing length but of minimal grammatical complexity.

6. Repetition of digits (REPD): requires subjects to repeat a series of spoken digit strings ranging from 3 to 7 numbers.

7. Reversal of digits (REVD): subjects are instructed to reverse a series of spoken digit strings ranging from 3 to 7 numbers.

8. Phonemic fluency (WF): requires subjects to generate as many words as possible beginning with the letters F, A, and S, each within 60-second time intervals.

9. Sentence construction (SC): subjects are instructed to produce grammatically correct sentences incorporating 2 or 3 stimulus words provided by the examiner.

10. Object identification by name (IDNAME): subjects are instructed to point to a range of objects on command.

11. Token (TT): subjects are required to point to or move a number of colored tokens relative to a series of spoken instructions of increasing length and grammatical complexity.

12. Oral reading of names (ORNAME): subjects are instructed to read object names from a series of flash cards.

13. Oral reading of sentences (ORSENT): subjects are instructed to read sentences of increasing difficulty extracted from the token test, from a series of flash cards.

14. Reading names for meaning (RNM): typically administered after subtest 12 (ORNAME), subjects are required to point to a range of objects corresponding to written names on a series of flash cards.

15. Reading sentences for meaning (RSM): typically administered after subtest 13 (ORSENT), subjects are required to follow simple commands written on a series of flash cards.

16. Visual graphic naming (VGN: subjects are instructed to write the names of a range of presented objects.

continues

Table 11–1. *continued*

17. Written naming (WN): relates to performance on the VGN task. Items are scored according to accuracy of writing and spelling.

18. Writing to dictation (WD): subjects are required to write their name and 2 dictated sentences.

19. Writing to copy (WC): subjects are instructed to copy 2 sentences presented on flash cards.

20. Articulation (ART): subjects are required to repeat a series of real words and nonwords containing a variety of consonant-vowel blends.

Adapted from Spreen & Benton, 1977.

The subtests include Visual Recognition, Auditory Recognition, Tactile Recognition, Auditory Verbal Comprehension, Silent Reading Comprehension, Nonverbal Tasks, Verbal Tasks, Meaningful Speech, and Meaningful Writing. Components of the test include: examiner's manual, picture book, 25 diagnostic form examiner record booklets, 25 short form examiner record booklets, 25 diagnostic form response forms, 25 short form response forms, 25 diagnostic summary forms, 25 personal history forms, and an object kit.

Reading Comprehension for Aphasia (RCBA-2). RCBA-2 provides a systematic evaluation of the nature and degree of reading impairment in adults with aphasia, including oral-reading comprehension. It measures reading comprehension and guides the direction and focus of the therapy. Materials are in large, bold print.

Individually administered in 30 minutes with 20 subtests covering single-word comprehension for visual confusions, auditory confusions, and semantic confusions; functional reading; synonyms; sentence comprehension; short paragraph comprehension; paragraphs; and morphosyntactic reading with lexical controls. The test kit includes: examiner's manual, stimulus picture book, supplementary picture books, 25 profile/ summary forms, and storage box.

Tests of High-Level Language Function

Tests included in this category assess the aspects of language function most highly dependent on frontal lobe function and in so doing evaluate the processes that permit conscious and effective manipulation of the semantic system via the interaction of primary language, cognitive, and executive processes in the brain. Examples of tests of high-level language function commonly used by speech-language pathologists include: the Test of Language Competence-Expanded Edition (TLC-E) (Wiig & Secord, 1989); the Word Test-Revised (TWT-R) (Huisingh, Barrett, Zachman, Blagden, & Orman, 1990); the Wiig-Semel Test of Linguistic Concepts (WSTLC) (Wiig & Semel, 1974), and semantic fluency tasks. As each of these tests assess a different aspect of high-level language function, the major features of each are briefly summarized below.

The Test of Language Competence-Expanded Edition (TLC-E). The TLC-E is an assessment of language proficiency and metalinguistic ability, consisting of a range of subtests which probe the semantic system, semantic-syntactic interfaces, and pragmatics. Designed and standardized on two levels (i.e., Level 1: children 5 to 9 years and Level 2: preadolescents and adolescents aged 9 to 18+ years), the TLC-E assesses language competence by way of complex tasks that demand divergent language production, cognitive-linguistic flexibility, and planning for production. Subtests included in the TLC-E Level 2 include: Ambiguous Sentences (AS), Listening Comprehension: Making Inferences (MI), Oral Expression: Recreating Sentences (RS), Figurative Language (FL), and Remembering Word Pairs (RWP) subtests.

The AS subtest assesses the ability to identify and interpret the alternative meanings of lexical and structural ambiguities. Lexically, ambiguous sentences contain lexical elements with more than one possible meaning (e.g., *He bought the glasses*, where glasses may refer to *eyeglasses* or *drinking glasses*). Structural ambiguities may be classified as either surface or deep subtypes. Surface structure level ambiguities contain adjacent words that may be grouped in two or more distinct ways (e.g., *Mary likes small dogs and cats*, where *small dogs and cats* may refer to *all small dogs* and *small cats*, or *small dogs* and *cats in general* [regardless of size]). Deep structure level ambiguities contain more than one logical relationship between words and phrases (e.g., *The turkey is ready to eat*, where the *turkey* may *be ready to eat something* or *ready to be eaten*). Subjects are presented with a series of ambiguous sentences in both spoken and written form and

instructed to provide two distinct interpretations for each item. Responses are scored quantitatively according to essential meaning criteria.

The MI subtest assesses a client's ability to utilize causal relationships or chains in short paragraphs to make logical inferences. Clients are provided with a series of paired propositions including a lead-in (e.g., *Jack went to a Mexican restaurant*) and concluding sentence (e.g., *He left without giving a tip*). On the basis of this information they are then instructed to make logical inferences pertaining to the event chain, by selecting two plausible intervening clauses from four possible choices (e.g., (a) *The restaurant closed when he arrived*, (b) *He only had enough money to pay for the meal*, (c) *The food and service were excellent*, or (d) *He was dissatisfied with the service*). All test stimuli are provided in spoken as well as written form. The correct responses for the above example would be (b) and (d).

The RS subtest evaluates the ability to formulate grammatically complete sentences utilizing key semantic elements within defined contexts. Clients are provided with a situational context (e.g., *At the ice-cream store*) and three words (e.g., *some, and, get*) in spoken and written/pictorial form, and instructed to generate a complete sentence that reflects the relevant situational context, utilizing all three words. Responses are scored according to holistic scoring rules pertaining to semantic, syntactic, and pragmatic accuracy, as well as the number of target words successfully used.

The FL subtest evaluates the ability to interpret metaphorical expressions and to correlate structurally related metaphors according to shared meanings. Clients are provided with a series of metaphorical expressions (e.g., *She sure casts a spell over me*) accompanied by defined situational contexts (e.g., *A boy talking about a girl at a school dance*), and instructed to provide a novel verbal interpretation of the metaphor. Once clients have explained the metaphor in their own words, they are then instructed to identify a match for the sample metaphor from four possible choices. Response choices include: a metaphoric match (e.g., *She is totally bewitching to me*), an oppositional foil (e.g., *I am out from under her spell*), a literal foil (e.g., *She spells much better than I*), and a nonrelated foil (e.g., *In her life, every day is Halloween*). All test stimuli are presented in spoken as well as written form. Metaphorical explanations are recorded verbatim and scored according to specified interpretation rules. The final score represents a composite of the verbal interpretation score and the matched selection score.

The RWP supplemental subtest assesses the ability to recall paired word associates. Associations are classified as one of four possible categories, including: paradigmatic (e.g., *coat-sock*), spatial (e.g., *plane-cloud*), temporal (e.g., *moon-bed*), and unrelated (e.g., *antler-egg*). Clients are provided with two presentations (i.e., elicitation lists A and B) of 16 spoken word pairs considered to be representative of common and familiar vocabulary. Subsequent to the oral presentation of each elicitation list, the examiner provides one of the words from each pair. Clients then are instructed to recall its associate. The sum of correctly recalled pairs relative to elicitations list A and B represents the total score.

The Word Test-Revised (TWT-R). The Word Test-Revised (TWT-R) represents an assessment of expressive vocabulary and semantics, originally designed for use with the school-age child. The TWT-R specifically probes the ability to identify and express critical semantic features of the lexicon by way of tasks that involve categorization, definition, verbal reasoning, and lexical selection. Subtests of the TWT-R include: Associations (ASS), Synonyms (SYN), Semantic Absurdities (SEMAB), Antonyms (ANT), Definitions (DEF), and Multiple Definitions (MULDEF).

The ASS subtest requires clients to identify a semantically unrelated word within a group of four spoken words and provide an explanation for the selected word in relation to the category of semantically related words. For example, from the group of words *knee, shoulder, bracelet*, and *ankle*, the word *bracelet* is considered semantically unrelated *because it is not a body part*. Responses are scored according to word choices as well as criteria pertaining to acceptable and unacceptable explanations.

The SYN subtest requires clients to generate synonyms for verbally presented stimuli. Answers are again scored in reference to acceptable and unacceptable response criteria. For example, in response to the stimulus *donate*, acceptable responses include words with similar sets of semantic features such as *give/contribute*, whereas unacceptable responses include *offer/fund*.

The SEMAB subtest evaluates a client's ability to identify and repair semantic incongruities. Clients are presented orally with a series of semantically absurd sentences (e.g., *My grandfather is the youngest person in my family*) and instructed to repair the evident incongruity by generating a semantically appropriate sentence. Scoring is again based on acceptable response criteria. Acceptable responses demand the simultaneous identification of the resident semantic incongruity, the replacement of inappropriate with appropriate vocabulary, and the maintenance of the integrity of essential elements within the generated sentence (e.g., *My grandfather is the oldest person in my family*). Incorrect repairs (e.g., *My grandfather is the biggest person in my family*), explanation of the semantic absurdity despite prompting (e.g., *My grandfather can't possibly be the youngest person in my family*), or semantic negation (e.g., *My grandfather is not the youngest person in my family*), all are classified as unacceptable responses.

The ANT subtest requires clients to generate antonyms for verbally presented stimuli. Answers are scored in reference to acceptable and unacceptable response criteria. In response to stimulus *first, last* would be classified as an acceptable response as it encapsulates reversible critical semantic dimensions of the stimulus word, whereas *second* would be classified as an unacceptable response.

The DEF subtest evaluates a client's ability to identify and describe the critical semantic features of a word. Subjects are provided with a series of stimulus words and instructed to explain their meaning. Answers again are scored according to acceptable and unacceptable response criteria, in relation to specific critical semantic elements. For example, in providing a definition of the word *house*, the attributes *person + lives* are defined as critical semantic elements. *Where my family lives*, therefore, would be classified as a complete/acceptable definition; however, *Where you play* would be classified as an incomplete/unacceptable response.

The MULDEF subtest requires clients to provide two distinct meanings for a series of spoken homophonic words in relation to specific referents, probing flexibility in vocabulary use. Scoring again is based on acceptable and unacceptable response criteria. For example, germane definition references pertaining to the word *rock* include a *stone, music,* or an *action*. Acceptable task responses would include, *It's a hard piece of earth, Music you play,* or *Moving back and forth. A hard thing* or *A thing you throw*, however, would be classified as unacceptable responses, as they fail to incorporate specified semantic referents.

Wiig-Semel Test of Linguistic Concepts (WSTLC). The WSTLC assesses the auditory comprehension of complex linguistic structures. Consisting of 50 yes/no questions, correct responses are contingent on the undertaking of logical semantic operations in the manipulation of a range of complex linguistic relationships, including passive, comparative, temporal, spatial, and familial structures.

Semantic Fluency Tasks. Semantic fluency tasks involve having the client generate as many items as possible within specified semantic categories, in 60-second time intervals. The semantic categories can include items such as exotic animals (e.g., lion, giraffe, etc.), tools (hammer, screwdriver, etc.), vegetables, and so forth. In some cases, a semantic category may be restricted by specifying that named items must start with a particular letter (e.g., Name all the vegetables that start with the letter "c"—cabbage, carrots, cauliflower, etc.).

Tests of Functional and Pragmatic Language Abilities

As indicated above, a key limitation of tests of basic language function is that they focus primarily on the evaluation of language abilities from an impairment perspective (i.e., identify the presence of language deficits but fail to ascertain the impact of these deficits on the functional communication skills). Alternatives or adjuncts to the assessments outlined above include measures of communication activity limitation and participation restriction. Assessments of communication activity limitation encompass measures of functional and pragmatic communication abilities, which enable the evaluation of a client's ability to plan, deliver, and understand communication content within a range of interactive contexts. Pragmatic assessments typically appraise the ability to use language within natural contexts, including knowledge of language structure, knowledge of the environment and social rules, as well as the ability to adapt to changing environmental demands (Penn, 1999). In contrast, functional communication assessments largely aim to evaluate the quality of communication attempts (Manochiopining, Sheard, & Reed, 1992), or the impact of communication disorders on social and vocational roles, otherwise referred to as participation restrictions. Although a more in depth discussion of these assessment tools is beyond the scope of this chapter, the incorporation of such measures is considered critical to any thorough clinical evaluation of language dysfunction, as opposed to an exclusive impairment-driven approach. The reader is referred to Table 11–2 for some suggested functional and pragmatic assessments that may be applied in the management of aphasia and related neurologic lan-

Table 11–2. Suggested Functional and Pragmatic Communication Assessments That May Be Applied to the Management of Subcortical Language Disorders

Functional Assessments	Authors
Functional Communication Profile	(Sarno, 1975)
Everyday Communication Needs Assessment (ECNA)	(Worrall, 1999)
Functional Assessment of Communication Skills for Adults (ASHA FACS)	(Frattali, Thompson, Holland, Wohl, & Ferketic, 1995)
Communicative Effectiveness Index (CETI)	(Lomas et al., 1989)
Communicative Adequacy in Daily Situations	(Clark & White, 1995)
The Communication Profile	(Payne, 1994)
Pragmatic Assessments	Authors
The Profile of Communicative Appropriateness	(Penn, 1985)
The Edinburgh Functional Communication Profile (revised)	(Wirz, Skinner, & Dean, 1990)
Communicative Abilities in Daily Living (CADL)-Revised	(Holland, Frattali, & Fromm, 1999)

guage disorders. In recent years, several scales that aim to evaluate quality of life and burden for aphasic individuals and close relatives (e.g., spouses) have been developed including the Burden of Stroke Scale (Doyle, 2002) and the Quality of Communicative Life Scale (Paul, Frattali, Holland, Thompson, Caperton, & Slater, 2004).

References

Cavallo, S. A., & Baken, R. J. (1985). Prephonatory laryngeal and chest wall dynamics. *Journal of Speech and Hearing Research, 28,* 79–87.

Clark, L. W., & White, K. (1995). Nature and efficiency of communication management in Alzheimer's disease. In R. Lubinski (Ed.), *Dementia and communication* (pp. 238–256). San Diego, CA: Singular.

Darley, F. L., Aronson, A. E., & Brown, J. R. (1969a). Clusters of deviant speech dimensions in the dysarthrias. *Journal of Speech and Hearing Research, 12,* 462–496.

Darley, F. L., Aronson, A. E., & Brown, J. R. (1969b). Differential diagnostic patterns of dysarthria. *Journal of Speech and Hearing Research, 12,* 246–269.

Darley, F. L., Aronson, A. E., & Brown, J. R. (1975). *Motor speech disorders.* Philadelphia, PA: W. B. Saunders.

Doyle, P. J. (2002). Measuring health outcomes in stroke survivors. *Archives of Physical Medicine and Rehabilitation, 83*(12, Suppl. 2), S39–S43.

Duffy, J. (2005). *Motor speech disorders: Substrates, differential diagnosis and management.* St. Louis, MO: Elsevier Mosby.

Enderby, P. (1983). *Frenchay dysarthria assessment.* San Diego, CA: College-Hill Press.

Fisher, H. B., & Logemann, J. A. (1971). *The Fisher-Logemann test of articulation competence.* Boston, MA: Houghton Mifflin.

FitzGerald, F. J., Murdoch, B. E., & Chenery, H. J. (1987). Multiple sclerosis: Associated speech and language disorders. *Australian Journal of Human Communication Disorders, 15,* 15–33.

Frattali, C., Thompson, D., Holland, A., Wohl, C., & Ferketic, M. (1995). *American Speech-Language and Hearing Association functional assessment of communication skills for adults.* Rockville, IN: American Speech-Language Hearing Association.

Goodglass, H., Kaplan, E., & Barresi, B. (2001). *The Boston diagnostic aphasia examination* (3rd ed.). Philadelphia, PA: Lippincott, Williams and Wilkins.

Helm-Estabrooks, N. (1992). *Aphasia diagnostic profile.* Chicago, IL: Riverside Press.

Holland, A., Frattali, C., & Fromm, D. (1999). *Communicative activities of daily living.* Austin, TX: Pro-Ed.

Huisingh, R., Barrett, M., Zachman, L., Blagden, C., & Orman, J. (1990). *The word test-revised: A test of expressive vocabulary and semantics.* East Moline, IL: Linguisystems.

Kaplan, E., Goodglass, H., & Weintraub, S. (1983). *Boston naming test.* Philadelphia, PA: Lippincott, Williams, and Wilkins.

Kertesz, A. (1982). *The western aphasia battery.* New York, NY: Grune & Stratton.

LaPointe, L. L., & Eisenson, J. (2008). *Examining for aphasia-4.* Austin, TX: Pro-Ed.

LaPointe, L. L., & Horner, J. (1998). *Reading comprehension for aphasia-2.* Austin, TX: Pro-Ed.

Lomas, J., Pickard, L., Betser, S., Elbard, H., Finlayson, A., & Zoghaib, C. (1989). The communicative effectiveness index: Development and psychometric evaluation of a functional communication measure for adult aphasia. *Journal of Speech and Hearing Disorders, 54,* 113–224.

Manifold, J., & Murdoch, B. E. (1993). Speech breathing in young adults: Effect of body type. *Journal of Speech and Hearing Research, 36,* 657–671.

Manochiopining, S., Sheard, C., & Reed, V. A. (1992). Pragmatic assessment in adult aphasia: A clinical review. *Aphasiology, 6,* 519–534.

Paul, D., Frattali, C., Holland, A., Thompson, C., Caperton, C., & Slater, S. (2004).

Quality of communication life scale. Rockville, MD: American Speech-Language Hearing Association.

Payne, J. C. (1994). *Communication profile: A functional skills survey.* Tucson, AZ: Communication Skill Builders.

Penn, C. (1985). The profile of communicative appropriateness: A clinical tool for the assessment of pragmatics. *South African Journal of Communication Disorders, 32,* 18–23.

Penn, C. (1999). Pragmatic assessment and therapy for persons with brain damage: What have clinicians gleaned in two decades. *Brain and Language, 68,* 535–552.

Porch, B. E. (1967). *Porch index of communicative ability.* Palo Alto, CA: Consulting Psychologists Press.

Sarno, M. T. (1975). *The functional communication profile.* New York, NY: NYU Medical Center, Institute of Rehabilitation Medicine.

Solomon, N., & Hixon, T. (1993). Speech breathing in Parkinson's disease. *Journal of Speech and Hearing Research, 36,* 294–310.

Sperry, E. E., & Klich, R. J. (1992). Speech breathing in senescent and younger women during oral reading. *Journal of Speech and Hearing Research, 35,* 1246–1255.

Spreen, O., & Benton, A. L. (1977). *Neurosensory center comprehensive examination for aphasia.* Victoria, Canada: University of Victoria.

Wiig, E. H., & Secord, W. (1989). *Test of language competence—expanded edition.* New York, NY: The Psychological Corporation.

Wiig, E. H., & Semel, E. (1974). Development of comprehension of logical grammatical sentences by grade school children. *Perceptual and Motor Skills, 38,* 171–176.

Wirz, S. L., Skinner, C., & Dean, E. (1990). Revised *Edinburgh functional communication profile.* Tucson, AZ: Communication Skill Builders.

Worrall, L. (1999). *The everyday communication needs assessment.* London, UK: Winslow Press.

Yorkston, K. M., & Beukelman, D. R. (1981). *Assessment of intelligibility of dysarthric speech.* Austin, TX: Pro-Ed.

12

Principles of Treatment for Neurologic Communication Disorders

"'Sorry, Jill . . . it's a brain tumor.' Two of the most feared words in the English language. She broke it to me as gently as she could. Brain tumor. Unwanted growth. It wasn't malignant and they said it probably wouldn't grow back. But they had to do surgery to take it out. I hope they got it all. They said it was pretty much confined to the region of my frontal lobes right behind my eyes. What could make that stuff grow in my brain? I need my brain. Dr. Firlik said the surgery was a success, though they had to destroy some healthy brain tissue to get all of the "neoplasm," their term for the unwelcome, infiltrating little bitch that grew in my head and tried to ruin my 33-year-old life. I don't have any trouble walking or with my arms but I'm worried about whether I'll be able to take care of my baby. I can't seem to concentrate. My attention wanders. I don't know why I can't finish the things I start. My speech gets lost a little, too. Sometimes I get lost in the middle of telling them something. Even things I should know like what I did last summer at Lake Ellen during our trip to Upper Michigan. My brother and sisters were there. We made pasties, those little Cornish meat pies. I couldn't even remember the steps. What comes first, the potatoes or the crust? Screwed up pasties. Screwed up following directions. Screwed up life. What's going to happen? They said they could treat it. Maybe further surgery. Maybe some different medications. Maybe some speech therapy. Maybe I'll need some counseling as well. This is not what I had in mind for my life. Maybe I'll get better. Maybe all this treatment stuff will work. It better. I'll need all the help I can get to raise precious little Adrienne with only part of a brain. Oh, well. Such is knife."

Introduction

"Treatment" can have many meanings. In apparel and fashion design, it refers to modifying fabrics or clothing. In film, treatment refers to turning prose into a screenplay. In ecology, sewage treatment refers to processes of removing contaminants from wastewater. In health care, treatment is synonymous with therapy, the process of attempts to remediate medical or behavioral problems to a result that is desirable and beneficial. Treatment of health issues and disorders of communication can range widely from medical, surgical, pharmaceutical, and/or behavioral approaches (Figure 12–1).

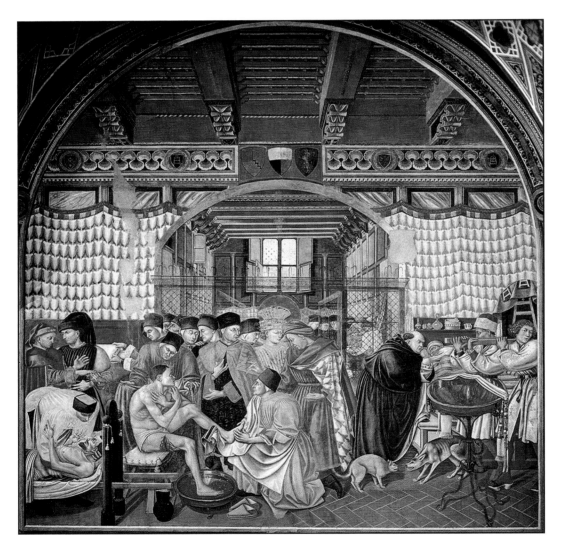

FIGURE 12–1. Care of the sick. From *Care of the Sick*, Domenico di Bartolo, 1441–1442. Public domain on Wikimedia Commons.

In Jill's case, in the scenario listed above, treatment was multimodal and involved several different professions. After complaints to her family physician, her brain tumor was diagnosed by a neurologist, a medical specialist in brain diseases. She then was referred to a neurosurgeon who operated on her to remove the meningioma that had grown slowly in her brain behind her eyes. Her hospital stay necessitated association with several others on the health care team. Nurses, rehabilitation professionals in occupational therapy and physical therapy, specialists in social work who attended to her needs after discharge, the hospital pharmacist, and the speech-language pathologist all entered the picture as part of her treatment team. The focus of Jill's treatment is rehabilitation and the skills she had acquired but were lost or impaired by the tumor.

is maximal function and best possible quality of life. The goal of habilitation and rehabilitation is a noble one: that people with functional impairments should be able to live their lives as independently as possible with the same rights, opportunities, responsibilities, and obligations as the rest of society. Habilitation and rehabilitation usually are used as comprehensive terms to cover all medical, psychological, social, educational, and work-oriented measures undertaken to help children and adults who are suffering from a medical condition or have been injured to develop, or regain, the best possible function and lay the foundations for a good life. In brain-based communication disorders all of the modes and venues of treatment may be necessary. We rely heavily on behavioral treatment, that is, interventions designed to change communication behaviors, but along the way many other professionals get involved.

Rehabilitation

What distinguishes habilitation from rehabilitation is that *habilitation* is intended for people with functional impairments caused by congenital injuries or disease, or to injury or disease acquired early in life. Its objective is to help a person in every way develop the best possible functional ability. *Rehabilitation* involves helping the functionally impaired person in every way regain the best possible functional ability and physical and mental well-being after the reduction or loss of a function due to injury or disease. Habilitation and rehabilitation both aim to prevent and ameliorate the difficulties that functional impairments can cause in daily life. The goal of both

Treatment of Communication Disorders: Fundamentals

Communication is a multidimensional dynamic process that allows people who have learned language to interact with their environment. Through the marvel of communication, we are able to express our thoughts, needs, and emotions. It is so fundamental that it has been characterized as essential ingredients for the "Three Ls," Living, Learning, and Loving (LaPointe, 2005). Without it, we cannot carry out the mundane activities of daily living like ordering a cappuccino with a cranberry bagel, listening to a Stephen Lynch song about beautiful babies, or the hundreds and hundreds of other interactions we engage in every day that require us to write, talk, listen, or speak. We cannot read directions, assignments, medicine labels, or listen to lectures. Most importantly of all, we cannot generate and nurture our interpersonal relationships; without discourse our contact with friends and family would wither and fade away. Communication is an intricate process that involves cerebration, cognition, hearing, speech production, and motor coordination. Evaluation and treatment of a communication disorder includes consideration of all aspects of the normal communication process as brain-based disorders can interrupt, corrupt, and disrupt any or all of these processes.

Language is the transformation of thoughts into meaningful symbols (sounds in the air or squiggles on paper or screen) communicated by speech, writing, or gestures. Thoughts are organized by the brain, specifically the left cerebral hemisphere, and encoded into a sequence according to whatever the learned grammatical and linguistic rules of the culture and language might be. These rules govern the way sounds are organized (phonology), the meaning of words (semantics), how words are formed (morphology), how words are combined into phrases (syntax), and the use of language in context (pragmatics) (Emedicine.medscape, 2010).

Speech involves the coordinated motor activity of muscles involved in respiration, phonation, resonance, and articulation. The entire system is modulated by both central and peripheral connections of brain cell bodies and axons to muscles and organs. Speech is greatly dependent on a specialized network of cranial nerves V, VII, VIII, IX, X, XI, and XII, as well as the phrenic and intercostal nerves. The cranial nerves are traditionally labeled with Roman numerals, but these paired nerves also have names. For speech, the primary cranial nerves are the trigeminal (V), facial (VII), vestibulocochlear (VIII), glossopharyngeal (IX), vagus (X), spinal accessory (XI), and the hypoglossal (XII) (Emedicine.medscape, 2010).

For speech, the respiratory muscles, specifically the muscles associated with expiration, must generate enough air pressure to provide adequate breath support to make speech loud enough to hear (Emedicine.medscape, 2010). The diaphragm is the main muscle of expiration; however, the abdominal and intercostal (between the ribs) muscles help control the force and length of exhalation for speech. A great dance of muscles is necessary to produce the vibrations of phonation and these muscles of the larynx generate vibratory energy during vocal fold approximation so that sound is produced. Say "AHHHH." It happens. Vocal pitch and intensity are modified by air pressure below the level of the vocal folds (subglottic), tension of the vocal folds, and position of the larynx. We can scream and we can whisper. We can sing in falsetto like the Bee Gees of the golden oldies or we can assume our habitual natural pitch level. Articulatory muscles within the pharynx, mouth, and nose modify and valve the tone of the sound and produce all of the little beads on the string of speech that consists of phonemes (speech sounds) and their transitions. The intricate and coordinated action of these muscles produces speech. By altering the shape of the vocal tract, we are capable of producing a tremendous range of sounds. Speech requires the balanced coordination of over 100 muscles at speeds that are a blur. Speech is our most complex, balanced, coordinated human neuromuscular activity. It must be nearly perfectly innervated to create these time-space movement coordinates. No wonder little things, such as strokes, head banging, golf-ball sized tumors, or nasty diseases that strip the nerves of their conductivity, can throw it off.

Sound waves are transformed by the auditory system into neural input for both the speaker and the listener. The outer ear detects sound pressure waves in the air (or even under water, but not nearly as distinctly) and converts them into mechanical vibrations in the middle and inner ear. The cochlea, that magical snail-like shell full of hair cells and fluid, then transforms these mechanical vibrations into vibrations in fluid, which act on the nerve endings of the vestibulocochlear (XIII) cranial nerve. Thus, the process of communication begins and ends in the brain (Figure 12–2). Communication is what makes us human. The brain lends itself to the creation of a never ending list of metaphors. The brain is a computer; the brain is a web; the brain is a river; the brain is an orchestra; the brain is a cookbook; the brain is a snowflake; the brain is a dream factory. No wonder we value it more than, say, our great toe or our appendix.

All of the disorders previously discussed and feared may impair a person's ability to communicate. These disorders may involve voice, speech, language, hearing, cognition, or even the basic task of taking food and swallowing it. Recognizing and addressing communication disorders is important; failure to do so may result in isolation, depression, and loss of independence. Life without communication caused by brain damage has been described as a living death by those who have recovered enough to comment on it. So we do our best to understand the clinical science of brain-based communication disorders interwoven with the clinical science and art of rehabilitation and restoration of this most human and complex function.

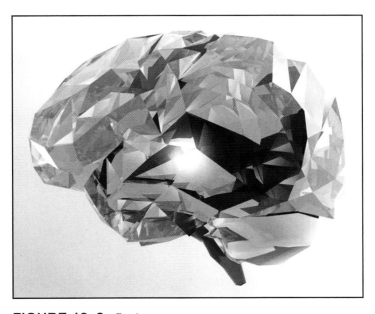

FIGURE 12–2. Brain.

Rehabilitation Assumptions and Principles

In a European Neurology Society Meeting on neurorehabilitation, Butterworth and Howard (1990) articulated some theoretic suppositions that can serve as useful principles for rehabilitation of brain-based disorders. They listed several assumptions, some of which may appear as a firm grasp of the obvious, but nevertheless form an elemental firmament for treatment. Because their suggestions did not include as much emphasis on the acknowledgment of the effects of these impairments on life participation, we have modified them to reflect contemporary approaches to rehabilitation. These basic assumptions oblige reflection and realization.

■ We must identify the exact nature of impairments and determine their impact on acceptable life participation and activities
■ We must match treatment to the identified impairments and life participation needs of each unique individual
■ We must be eclectic in our adoption of treatment approaches. Treatment may encompass any or all of the strategies of:
  □ relearning information or procedures that have been lost
  □ facilitation of access to information or skills that are intact but inaccessible
  □ reconstitution or compensation for lost functions, that is, finding new ways to achieve goals
  □ accommodation, adjustment, and *Aristos* (i.e., making the best of a given situation) (LaPointe, 2005)
■ We must ensure that the person and families with whom we are working

have the opportunity to communicate their treatment objectives and outcomes and that these desires are incorporated overall treatment goals
■ We must incorporate the principles of evidence-based practice and evaluate the effectiveness of treatment (Dollaghan, 2007)
■ We must utilize principles of cross-disciplinary collaboration and cooperation by participating in professional teams.

Other Principles Worthy of Consideration

In their book *Aphasia: A Clinical Approach* (1989), Rosenbek, LaPointe, and Wertz devoted a chapter to "Principles of Clinical Aphasiology." These principles have broader application than just to the disorder of aphasia and may well be germane to most of the brain-based communication disorders. These authors stated:

> We learned our principles from others —other professionals and the [men and women with aphasia] who have agreed over the years to spend time with us.
> We have learned the same things over and over from some, and unique things from a few. Like a code for living, the principles governing our daily activities with [people with aphasia] have evolved, sometimes so subtly that they escape our notice until we sit down, as now, and take stock.

The clinical principles outlined by Rosenbek, LaPointe, and Wertz (1989) included some that have evolved a bit, some that are relatively timeless, and all that seemed to reflect the opinions of deeply committed clinical professionals who had a passion for their work with hundreds of people with communication disorders. For example, they opined:

- Clinical aphasiology requires clinical aphasiologists—Part-time clinicians, if they are full-time clinical aphasiologists, can treat people with aphasia. But simple caring is not enough. Intellect and a subscription to *Brain and Language* also are not enough. Nor is having earned one's 10-year pin or 10 ASHA-approved CEUs in a year. Training in neurolinguistics is not enough, nor is knowing how to run a successful private practice from a garage after working all day in the public schools. [People with aphasia] deserve the care of a clinical aphasiologist. Clinical aphasiologists care about [people with aphasia]; they spend time with them every day; they read, remember, and integrate what they read; they go to workshops to stay abreast; and they specialize in the understanding, diagnosis, and treatment of aphasia and [people with aphasia].

- Treatment has three goals—The goals of treatment are: (1) to assist people to regain as much communication as their brain damage allows and their needs drive them to, (2) to help them learn how to compensate for residual deficits, and (3) to help them learn to live in harmony with the differences between the way they were and the way they are.

- The most important goal usually is to prepare persons with aphasia for a lifetime of aphasia—This is not true in all cases but certainly is true in most of the chronic conditions with which we are confronted. Too many people (and health care professionals) generalize the acute-care medical model concept to the challenge of dealing with chronic conditions. This problem is reflected not only in the misguided or failed expectations of working with people with chronic conditions, but also gravely reflected in the reimbursement and insurance issues that permeate many health care systems. Get 'em in; get 'em out is not an adequate model for dealing with chronic conditions and many brain-based disorders indeed are chronic. Until this philosophy of economic, bottom-line approaches to health care is radically changed, professionals and sufferers must prepare for the frustrations of inadequately allocated reimbursement for chronic conditions. That will indeed "ensure" (no pun intended) that our clients must be prepared for long-term chronicity.

- Treatment should be influenced by an attitude about what a person with aphasia is—Persons with aphasia do not talk at all or nearly as well as before becoming ill, and all their other communicative acts are impaired in varying degrees as well. In addition, they are likely to be more irritable, scared, depressed, and distractible than before they got sick. Despite these changes, they often are unchanged at the core. If they were loving before, they will be again. If they were irascible, they will remain so. If they were making their ways through life, they will continue to do so. If they were dying, regardless of how subtly, the episode causing the disorder will not be an antidote. Above all, if they were doing the best they could before, they will set about doing the best they can to adjust to their disability and to the treatments that are likely to accompany it. All of this is not fatalism or resignation. It is applause for the resiliency of people with brain-based disorders, and it is an appeal for professionals to avoid getting in the way of each person's recovery. It is also the summary of an attitude that profoundly influences what we think. Clinicians should reinforce the client's personal strengths and support their natural processes. They should treat people with aphasia and not aphasia. Knowing what to support, what to change, what to accommodate, and what to ignore are marks of clinical maturity. Many of these thoughts and philosophies about treatment were generated and hatched by the outstanding clinician Jay Rosenbek, and the egg was then warmed if not scrambled by Wertz and LaPointe. These principles guided all three of their clinical lives.

Specific Skills and Knowledge

The skills and knowledge involved in assessing and treating brain-based disorders of communication and swallowing require some general and some very specific competencies. These include:

- assessment, appraisal, and diagnosis skills with emphasis on interviewing proficiency, preparation and test administration, interpretation of the results with subsequent ability to integrate and present what has been learned in both oral and written form
- clear and concise report writing with emphasis on the goal of comprehensible documentation and explanation
- therapy practices that incorporate task analysis, behavioral objectives, and implementation (Figure 12–3),

and integration of information from others on the professional team
- documentation of treatment outcomes, progress, and accountability that conform to the scope of practice and ethical standards of the appropriate discipline
- implementation or referral for appropriate client and family counseling.

Social Models of Treatment

Some of the material in this section has been considered in a chapter on social validation of treatment for aphasia that has appeared in a *Festschrift* for Chris Code in a book edited by Ball and Damico (2006). As LaPointe and Lenius (2006) have reviewed, traditionally, clinicians have used standardized tests such as the Western Aphasia Battery (Kertesz, 1982) to determine areas of impairment, select therapy goals, and possibly document change. This focus on impairment has been consistent with traditional approaches to disease characteristic of the medical model, but may not be the most efficient way to determine socially relevant goals. The seemingly ever changing terminology of the World Health Organization is being integrated into models of aphasia treatment (Rogers, Alarcon, & Olswang, 1999; Threats, 2006), and the concepts involved are important. Changes in social activities and participation are emerging as more relevant goals of treatment and are eroding the stone face of impairment-based approaches to intervention. The Life Participation Approach to Aphasia continues to have an impact on approaches to aphasia intervention and is shaping the very core of the aphasia treatment model (LPAA Group, 2000). Most stan-

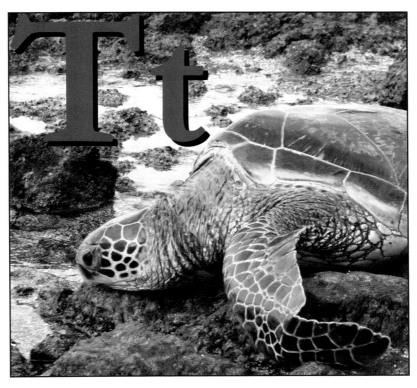

FIGURE 12–3. Example of therapy practice.

dardized tests of aphasia are predominantly impairment based. Recently, some efforts have been made to incorporate the social model of aphasia into assessment procedures. The latest edition of Eisenson's classic *Examining for Aphasia* (LaPointe & Eisenson, 2008) incorporates principles of the social model of aphasia into assessment in an effort to guide clinicians in the quest to develop relevant participation-based treatment goals. This approach does not suggest that we discard the infant with the cleansing aqua, for impairments and cognitive-linguistic processes also may need to be targeted for treatment; but for far too long it has been impairment or nothing, with little emphasis on reintegration of the person into an active, participating milieu. This attitude and

set of values is epitomized by the recent work of Audrey Holland on the importance of counseling in communication disorders from a wellness perspective (Holland, 2008).

The traditional biographic standardized test interview needs to be supplemented or indeed replaced with specific information gathering as to the goals, values, hobbies, likes, dislikes, hopes, fears, anticipations, and motivations of each unique individual for whom we are planning treatment. This will assist the informed clinician with planning, delivering, and evaluating services (Pound, Parr, & Duchan, 2001). The LPAA Project Group (2002), Simmons-Mackie & Damico (2001), LaPointe (2002), and Cruice et al. (2005) all provide social model flesh and humanity to the bones of treatment planning in aphasia. This entire movement of course harkens back to the birth and upbringing of language in context and person-centered concepts of aphasia intervention nurtured and influenced so thoroughly by Audrey Holland (Holland, 1982),

Interview questions appropriate to determining and creating socially relevant and valid treatment goals can be gleaned, inferred, or directly created from all of the above sources and from the assessment protocol of LaPointe and Eisenson (2008). The interview allows the client and any others present to express what life was like before the onset of aphasia, how life is impacted now, and what areas of communication breakdown generate the most stress on relationships.

In an effort to define socially valid aphasia therapy goals, Ross and Wertz (2003) set out to determine the difference in quality of life as rated by people with and without aphasia. Two groups (people with aphasia for at least six months and non-brain-damaged individuals) completed quality of life measures. The greatest difference between the groups was evident in areas of activities of daily living, opportunities to acquire new information and skills, social support, mobility, and sexual activity. Of course, it is imperative to customize treatment planning and weave specific treatment goals around the idiosyncrasies of each person, but this study shows support for language therapy focusing on enhancing communication for specific functional situations and expanding participation in society. Recent work by Ross and her colleagues (Ross, LaPointe, and Katz, 2008) has suggested that loneliness and sense of belonging also are factors that impact people with brain-based communication disorders

and should be a consideration in treatment planning and the attempt at implementing treatment outcomes.

Sometimes we tend to err on the side of overzealous treatment planning and realization. One of the authors of this book (LLL) remembers well an early treatment planning faux pas when a full court press of intervention (twice per day; intensive reading comprehension strategies integrated into the treatment schedule) was probably not in keeping with the personal goals of the person with aphasia. After two weeks of rather intensive treatment, I remember his words well: "Doc, I thank you for all you're trying to do here, but, you know, I never have completely read through a whole book. I don't really care if I ever do. I just want to go up on the St. Johns River and live with my brother in the trailer there, and maybe sit out on the dock and fish a little. I know you're trying real hard Doc, and I appreciate it, but I really don't care if I can't read very good."

If the treatment goals of the person with aphasia are not built into the treatment plan, misguided expenditures of time, effort, and money can be the result. This clinical lesson made it abundantly clear that precise activity and participation therapy must be harmonious with the expectations and needs of the person in therapy. Sometimes the people with whom we work are content to fish, plant kumquats, or join the circus (Figure 12–4).

These principles set the ground for our belief system in interacting with people with brain-based disorders of communication and swallowing. We know not what the future holds, it will surely be trials and tribulations, but just as surely it will contain family holidays, fish curry, happy weddings with henna hands (Figure 12–5), faithful pets, art,

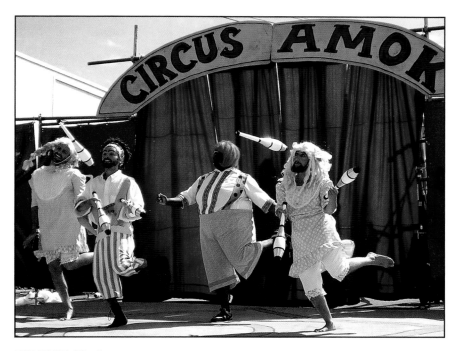

FIGURE 12–4. Circus. From "Circus Amok Jugglers" by David Shankbone, New York City, 2006. Taken from Wikimedia Commons under the Creative Commons Attribution 2.5 License.

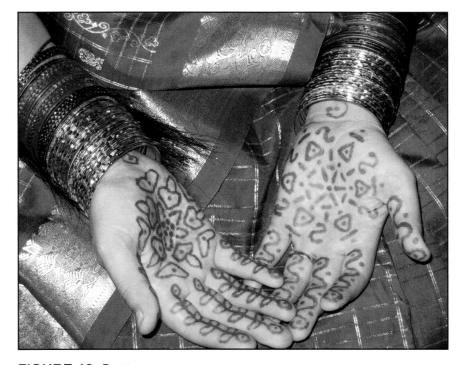

FIGURE 12–5. Henna.

music, and sports peak moments, walks on the beach (Figure 12–6) and new directions and accomplishments. Good treatment in both principle and implementation can help restore or compensate for these joys of living to people with brain-based disorders (Figure 12–7). As Small (2000) has implied, we can expect not only advancement of our understanding of how the brain operates in order and disorder, but also an abundance of new mysteries that will pique our curiosity and motivate our questions. That is one of the many reasons we get up in the morning.

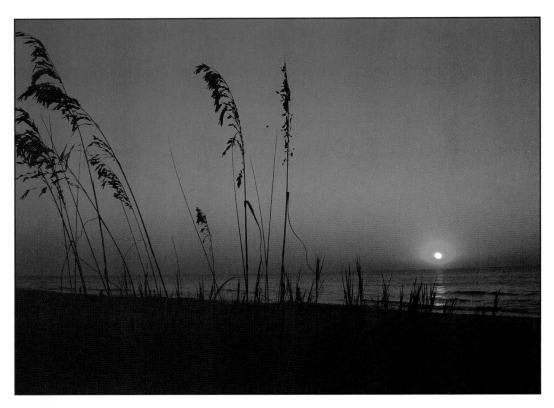

FIGURE 12–6. Sunset on the beach.

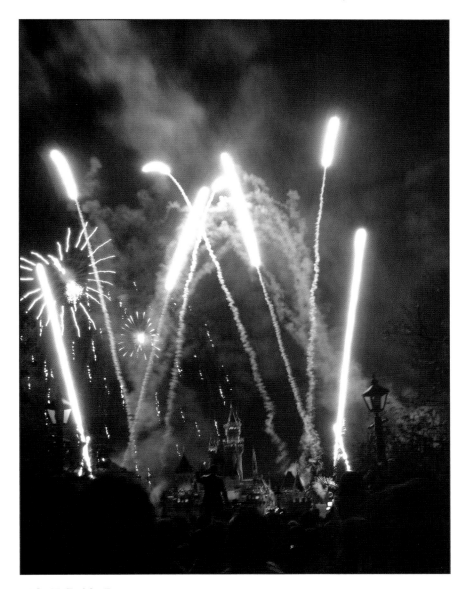

FIGURE 12–7. Fireworks celebrating the joy of life.

References

Ball, M., & Damico, J. (Eds.). (2007). *Clinical aphasiology: Future directions.* New York, NY: Taylor and Francis (Psychology Press).

Chapey, R., Duchan, J. F., Elman, R. J., Garcia, L. J., Kagan, A., Lyon, J. G., & Simmons-Mackie, N. (2001). Life participation approach to aphasia: A statement of values for the future. In R. Chapey (Ed.), *Language intervention strategies in adult aphasia* (4th ed., pp. 235–245). Baltimore, MD: Williams & Wilkins.

Code, C., & Herrmann, M. (2003). The relevance of emotional and psychosocial factors in aphasia to rehabilitation. *Neuropsyhological Rehabilitation, 13,* 109–132.

Cruice, M., Worrall, L., Hickson, L., & Murison, R. (2005). Measuring quality of life: Comparing family members' and friends' ratings with those of their aphasic partners. *Aphasiology, 19*(2), 111–129.

Dollaghan, C. A. (2007). *The handbook for evidence-based practice in communication disorders.* Baltimore, MD: Brookes.

Emedicine.medscape. (2010). Retrieved February 23, 2010, from http://emedicine.medscape.com/article/317758-overview

Holland, A. L. (1982). Observing functional communication of aphasic adults. *Journal of Speech and Hearing Disorders, 47*, 50–56.

Holland, A. L. (2008). *Counseling in communication disorders: A wellness perspective.* San Diego, CA: Plural Publishing.

Kertesz. A. (1982). *The Western Aphasia Battery.* New York, NY: Grune and Stratton.

LaPointe, L. L. (1994). Neurogenic disorders of communication. In Minifie F. (Ed.), *Introduction to communication sciences and disorders* (pp. 351–397). San Diego, CA: Singular Publishing Group.

LaPointe, L. L. (1996). On being a patient. *Journal of Medical Speech-Language Pathology, 4*(1), xi–xiii.

LaPointe, L. L. (1999a). Quality of life with aphasia. In C. Code, (Ed.), Psychosocial issues in aphasia. *Seminars in Speech and Language, 20*(1), 5–15.

LaPointe, L. L. (1999b). An enigma: Outcome measurement in speech and language therapy. *Advances in Speech-Language Pathology, 1*(1), 57–58.

LaPointe, L. L. (2000). Quality of life with brain damage. *Brain and Language, 71*, 135–137.

LaPointe, L. L. (2001). Darley and the psychosocial side. *Aphasiology, 15*(3), 249–260.

LaPointe, L. L. (2002). The sociology of aphasia. *Journal of Medical Speech-Language Pathology, 10*(1), vii–viii.

LaPointe, L. L. (2003). Functional and pragmatic directions in aphasia therapy. In I. Papathanasiou & R. de Bleser (Eds.), *The sciences of aphasia (Vol. 1): From theory to therapy.* Boston, MA: Pergamon.

LaPointe, L. L. (2005). *Aphasia and related neurogenic language disorders* (3rd ed.). New York, NY: Thieme.

LaPointe, L. L., & Eisenson, J. (2008). *Examining for aphasia* (4th ed.). Austin, TX: Pro-Ed.

LaPointe, L. L., & Lenius, K. (2006). Social validation in aphasia recovery. In M. Ball & J. Damico (Eds.), *Clinical aphasiology: future directions.* New York, NY: Taylor and Francis (Psychology Press).

LaPointe, L. L., Maitland, C. G., Stierwalt, J. A. G., Toole, T., & Hancock, A. B. (2006). Distraction, competition, and interference: How do people with brain damage navigate in a sea of distraction? *Neurorehabilitation and Neural Repair, 20*(S2A-2), 58–59.

Lasker, J. P., LaPointe, L. L., & Kodras, J. E. (2005). Helping a professor with aphasia resume teaching through multimodal approaches. *Aphasiology, 19,* 399–410.

LPAA Project Group (Chapey, R., Duchan, J., Elman, R., Garcia, L., Kagan, A., Lyon, J., & Simmons-Mackie, N.). (2000). Life participation approaches to aphasia: A statement of values for the future. *ASHA Leader, 5*, 4–6.

Lyon, J. G. (1998) *Coping with aphasia.* San Diego, CA: Singular Publishing Group.

Morse, J., & Johnson, J. (1991). *The illness experience: Dimensions of suffering.* London, UK: Sage Publications.

Pound, C., Parr, S., & Duchan, J. (2001). Using partners' autobiographical reports to develop, deliver, and evaluate services in aphasia. *Aphasiology*, 15, 477–493.

Rogers, M A, Alarcon, N. B., & Olswang, L. B. (1999). Aphasia management considered in the context of the World Health Organization model of disablements. *Physical Medicine and Rehabilitation Clinics of North America, 10*(4), 907–923, ix.

Rosenbek, J. C., LaPointe, L. L., & Wertz, R. T. (1989). *Aphasia: A clinical approach.* Austin, TX: Pro-Ed.

Ross, K. B., LaPointe, L. L., & Katz, R. C. (2008, May/June). *Loneliness and sense of belonging in aphasia.* Presented at the Clinical Aphasiology Conference, Jackson, WY.

Ross, K. B., & Wertz, R. T. (2003). Quality of life with and without aphasia. *Aphasiology*, 17, 355–364.

Sacks, O. (1984). *A leg to stand on.* New York, NY: Harper and Row.

Sarno, M. (1993). Aphasia rehabilitation: Psychosocial and ethical considerations. *Aphasiology 7*(4), 321–334.

Shadden, B. (2005). Aphasia as identity theft: Theory and practice. *Aphasiology, 19,* 211–223.

Simmons-Mackie, N., & Damico, J. S. (2001). Intervention outcomes: A clinical application of qualitative methods. *Topics in Language Disorders, 21*(4), 21–36.

Small, S. (2000). The future of aphasia treatment. *Brain and Language, 71*, 227–232.

Threats, T. T. (2006). Towards an international framework for communication disorders: Use of the ICF. *Journal of Communication Disorders, 39*(2), 206–215.

Index